Modern Hip Preservation

Reinhold Ganz
Editor

Modern Hip Preservation

New Insights In Pathophysiology And Surgical Treatment

Springer

Editor
Reinhold Ganz
Professor Emeritus, Faculty of Medicine
University of Bern
Gümligen, Bern, Switzerland

ISBN 978-3-030-91966-5 ISBN 978-3-030-91967-2 (eBook)
https://doi.org/10.1007/978-3-030-91967-2

This Springer imprint is published by the registered company Springer Nature Switzerland AG
The registered company address is: Gewerbestrasse 11, 6330 Cham, Switzerland

Foreword

The hip joint has a quite simple anatomy (a spherical head into a hemispheric cup), but it carries the responsibility, shared with the knee and the ankle, of the motion and of all the activities for a normal living including sports. Despite its apparent simplicity, to my mind it deserves the concept of "hip universe" for the following reasons.

The anatomy (neck and femoral head, acetabulum, acetabular lip, capsule) is different for each individual. The diversity does not only concern the dimensions, but mainly the inclination and the version of the acetabulum and the neck, the shape of the head, the covering of the same, the CCD angle and the neck length: hip kinematics and loads are individually variable.

Any anatomical alteration, even of small importance, and the consequent functional dyskinesia that results, causes a non-reversible, unstoppable structural alteration, with negative consequences on the functional complex of the hip, resulting in a crippled and unhappy patient.

Osteoarthritis is the final stage in the evolution of one or more anatomical changes, with derangement of the hip universe, ending in irreversible joint degeneration.

The understanding of the pathogenetic evolution of different pathologies can lead to specific and preventive corrections of the final treatment, which is a valid but irreversible solution (hip prosthetic replacement).

The concept of hip preserving surgery was born in the 1980s, in the mind and in the hands of an open-minded, inspired orthopaedic surgeon, Reinhold Ganz, and it fits well in my concept of "hip universe" that starts from the knowledge of the vascular supply of the femoral head, which has to be mandatorily respected in all procedures of preservation of the natural hip.

Once the vascular supply has been respected, all procedures have been conceived to recreate the natural spherical shape of the femoral head, and when needed, its proper coverage on the acetabular side; it can be defined as a back-to-normal anatomical surgery, implying knowledge, innovation, dedication and surgical skills.

The entire range of hip pre-osteoarthritic pathologies, spanning from pathogenesis to the surgical treatment, is treated in this book, which crowns the masterwork of prof. Ganz, as well as of the GICCA group (Gruppo Italiano di Chirurgia Conservativa dell'Anca), led by Reinhold during many years of cooperation and teaching.

I largely use the concept of "hip universe" during my lessons for the medical students; I have found it well fitting in the spirit of this book, and in the foreword I have had the honour to write, as a member of GICCA.

Orthopaedics and Traumatology
University of Pavia, Pavia, Italy
Francesco Benazzo

Preface

Correction of deformities of the human skeleton is an old desire. It is best depicted by the crooked tree, introduced by the French physician Nicolas Andry (1658–1742) to explain prevention and conservative treatment of spine deformities. Today it serves as logo for numerous societies and journals of orthopaedic surgery. More than a century had to elapse until progress in antisepsis and anaesthesia as well as the invention of radiography allowed surgical corrections of the skeleton to be undertaken. First procedures were simple alignments of the lower limb after fracture or ankylosis; internal fixation was not applied and pseudarthrosis was a desired end result. Internal fixation of the hip was first attempted in the 1920s with the three flanged nail introduced by Smith-Petersen and the first osteotomy for coxarthrosis is attributed to McMurray, who published it in 1939. During the following 30 years orthopaedic centres executed a high number of adult hip osteotomies, mainly as varus correction and nearly exclusively in hips with established osteoarthritis. With the introduction of total hip replacement in the early 1970s offering long-lasting and pain-free function, joint preserving surgery of the adult hip lost its attraction steadily with the result that today young orthopaedic doctors may not even see a hip osteotomy in their training.

The renaissance of attempts to preserve the natural hip started in the 1980s. First unexpected, a growing interest was observed which had much to do with the recognition that more young people suffered from hip problems, and on the other side, the survival of total joint replacement significantly decreases with younger age. Based on studies of the vascular blood supply of hip and pelvis, better understanding of the mechanism of joint degeneration but also new surgical techniques evolved and matured to concepts to successfully treat the young hip joint before major degeneration takes place.

Meanwhile a sustained and worldwide interest can be observed, which shifted from the established osteoarthritis to the symptomatic hip of adolescent and young adult before advanced joint degeneration. Surgical dislocation of the hip was first designed as an approach to treat intraarticular problems and was first executed in 1996 to treat extended chondromatosis of the hip joint. Successively, it came to be a workhorse for a new class of intraarticular surgeries and it allowed to establish the impingement concept, which put the aetiology of coxarthrosis on a new basis. At about the same time the Bernese periacetabular osteotomy received increasing acceptance as a versatile procedure for different dysplasias of the acetabulum. Hip joint preservation burgeons to grow and takes a front seat in the field of hip surgery.

More than 10 years ago, a study group was formed in Northern Italy under the name of Gruppo Italiano di Chirurgia Conservativa dell' Anca (GICCA) in order to apply the principles. Meanwhile several hundred hips have been operated. We report this experience in a book to let the reader deepen the knowledge of the subject in one, single, comprehensive work.

Bern, Switzerland Reinhold Ganz

Acknowledgements

On the initiative of Giorgio Curradini, a study group (GICCA—Gruppo Italiano di Chirurgia Conservativa dell'Anca) was formed in Northern Italy 15 years ago which has applied the principles of modern hip preservation and has treated several hundred hips so far. The creation of this group allowed us to add continuous experience and discover new aspects and evolutions of this rather new type of surgery. Undoubtedly, Curradini's mentorship to the renaissance of conservative hip surgery is of outmost importance. We report this experience in an e-book, a format allowing to add continuously experience, new aspects and further evolution of hip joint preservation.

We are indebted to Stefano Lanfranco for his extraordinary commitment. Without his constant supervision and editing, the book would not have been published.

Last but not least, a special thanks goes to our publisher who has believed in the project and has made its realization possible.

Contents

1 Vascular Anatomy of the Hip: An Update

Morteza Kalhor and Reinhold Ganz

1.1 Introduction

Vascular anatomy of the pelvis and hip joint in general and that of the femoral head, in particular, has been the subject of investigation since many years. General aspects of hip vascular anatomy have been described in anatomy books and literature [1–3]. Tuker in 1949 and Trueta in 1953 following injection studies concluded that MFCA was the main source of blood supply to the femoral head [4–6]. Their findings were confirmed by subsequent studies. Despite the available historical knowledge in hip vascular anatomy, iatrogenic femoral head AVN continued to be a major complication following hip surgery.

The mystery was disclosed when recent arterial injection studies have shown that surgical or traumatic injury of MFCA in its extracapsular course was the usual cause of damage to the femoral head blood supply. Gauthier et al. confirmed the frequent occurrence of this vascular injury in tenotomy of the short hip external rotators during routine hip surgeries [7]. Introduction of surgical hip dislocation provided the orthopedic surgeons an appropriate technique for full access to the hip joint with minimal or no risk of AVN [8].

More recent cadaveric injections have shown precisely the surgical anatomy of the hip vessels and acetabulum [9–15], which finally led to the development of new procedures in hip surgery [16, 17]. The extracapsular approach for intra-articular problems was replaced by direct intracapsular techniques. It is now possible to safely dislocate the hip joint and manage various intra-articular conditions directly, with minimal or no risk of AVN. The prerequisites to obtain favorable results in these complex procedures are protection of the supplying vessels in their extra- and intra-capsular courses.

Our goal in this chapter is to demonstrate the surgical anatomy of the vessels supplying the hip joint and acetabulum. The description is based on our findings in fresh cadaveric dissections following arterial injection studies. The corresponding vessels are followed from the origin to their final distribution.

1.2 Topographic Anatomy

The main vascular supply to the external aspect of the pelvis comes from five vessels: Medial and lateral femoral circumflex arteries (MFCA, LFCA), superior and inferior gluteal arteries (SGA, IGA), and obturator artery (OA).

M. Kalhor (✉)
Department of Orthopedic Surgery, Firoozgar Medical Center, Iran University of Medical Sciences, Tehran, Iran

R. Ganz
Faculty of Medicine, University of Bern, Bern, Switzerland

R. Ganz (ed.), *Modern Hip Preservation*, https://doi.org/10.1007/978-3-030-91967-2_1

1.3 Course and Distribution of the Medial and Lateral Circumflex Femoral Arteries

The circumflex femoral arteries have an extra-pelvic origin branching either from profunda femoris or femoral artery (Fig. 1.1).

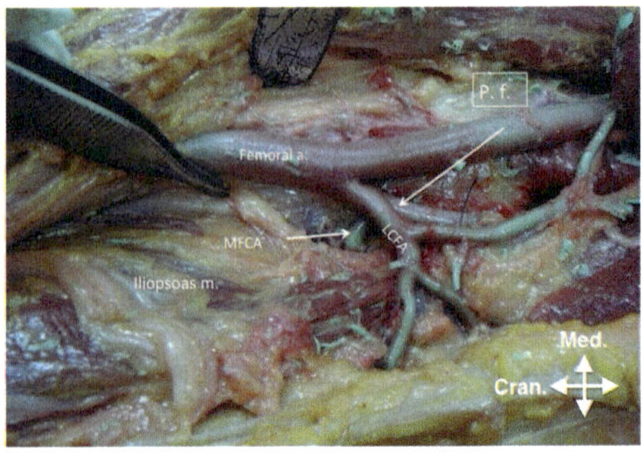

Fig. 1.1 Anterior aspect of right hip distal to the inguinal ligament after distal retraction of sartorius and rectus femoris muscles. *MFCA*: Medial Femoral Circumflex Artery; *LFCA*: Lateral Femoral Circumflex Artery; *P.F.*: Profunda Femoris artery

1.3.1 LFCA: Lateral Femoral Circumflex Artery

Usually originating from the profunda femoris artery, the LFCA courses laterally underneath the rectus femoris muscle. After giving off the descending and transverse branch the LFCA runs laterally toward the tensor fasciae latae muscle as ascending branch (Fig. 1.1). The ascending portion of the artery invariably supplies the anterior capsule by a prominent branch (Fig. 1.2).

Additionally, the ascending part of the artery variably provides one or two small branches to contribute to the femoral head blood supply as anterior retinacular arteries (Fig. 1.3).

After supplying the tensor fascia latae muscle, the ascending branch turns cephalad and cross the hip capsule anterolaterally toward the superior aspect of the acetabulum. In its way the ascending branch supplies the most anterior part of the hip abductor muscles (gluteus medius and gluteus minimus) as well as the anterolateral aspect of the capsule (Fig. 1.4). The ascending branch finally anastomoses with the supra-acetabular branch of the SGA to take part in the periacetabular vascular ring (Fig. 1.5).

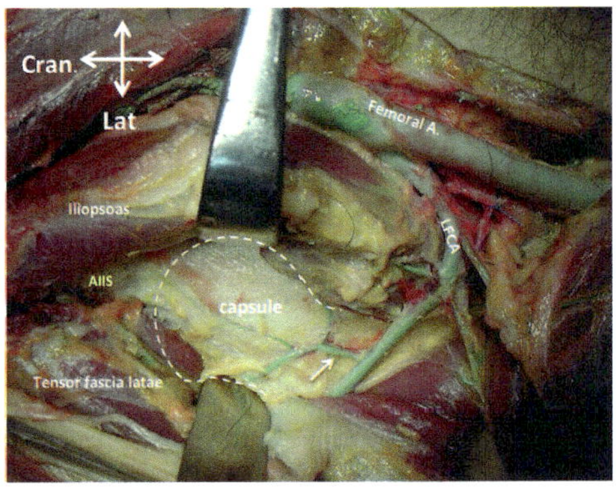

Fig. 1.2 Anterior aspect of right hip after retraction of anterior hip muscles to show the capsular branch of *LFCA* (*arrow*). *AIIS*: Anterior inferior iliac spine. *LFCA*: lateral femoral circumflex artery. *Broken line* indicates to the location of the femoral head. Adapted with permission from [11]

1.3.2 MFCA: Medial Femoral Circumflex Artery

1.3.2.1 Extracapsular Course

It originates from the posteromedial aspect of the profunda femoris and less often from the common femoral artery (Fig. 1.1). It runs medially and then posteriorly lying between iliopsoas and pectineus muscle. In its way posteriorly and before turning laterally, the MFCA supplies the adductor muscles in addition to hip capsule and

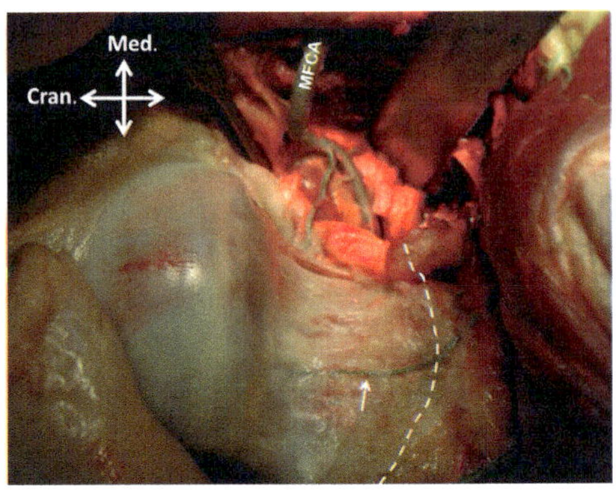

Fig. 1.3 Anterior aspect of right hip after capsulotomy. *Arrow* shows the anterior retinacular artery originating from LFCA. *Dotted line* indicating capsular insertion. *MFCA*: Medial Femoral Circumflex Artery

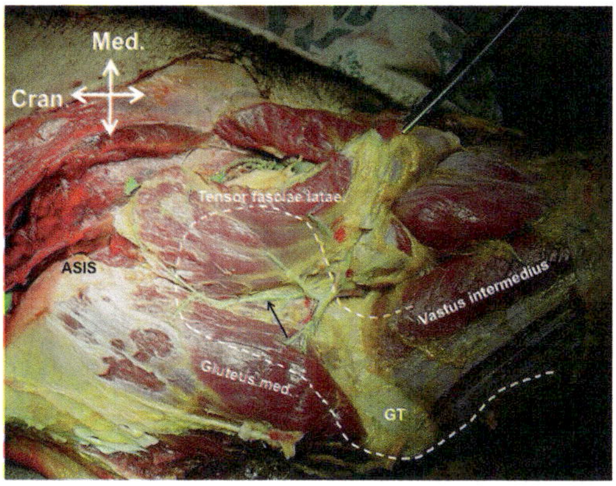

Fig. 1.4 Anterolateral aspect of right hip demonstrates vascularization of tensor and abductor muscles by LFCA. The tensor is flipped over to show its undersurface. *ASIS*: Anterior superior iliac spine. *GT*: Greater trochanter

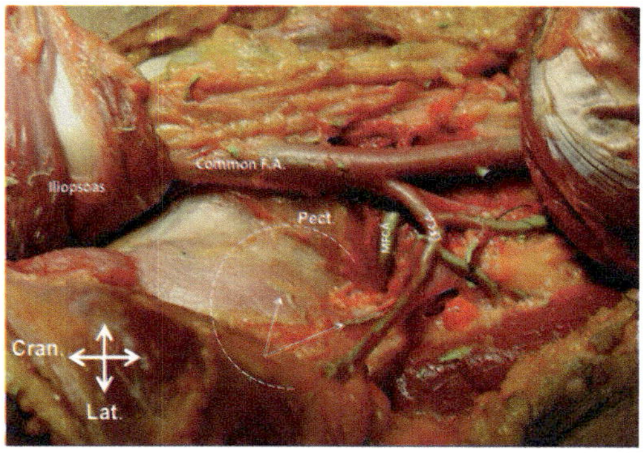

Fig. 1.6 Anterior aspect of right hip after proximal retraction of iliopsoas muscle to show the anatomic position of circumflex femoral arteries. *Arrows* indicating capsular branches of LFCA. *Broken circular line*: femoral head. *Pect.*: pectineus muscle. *MFCA*: Medial Femoral Circumflex Artery; *LFCA*: Lateral Femoral Circumflex Artery; *Common F.A.*: Common femoral artery

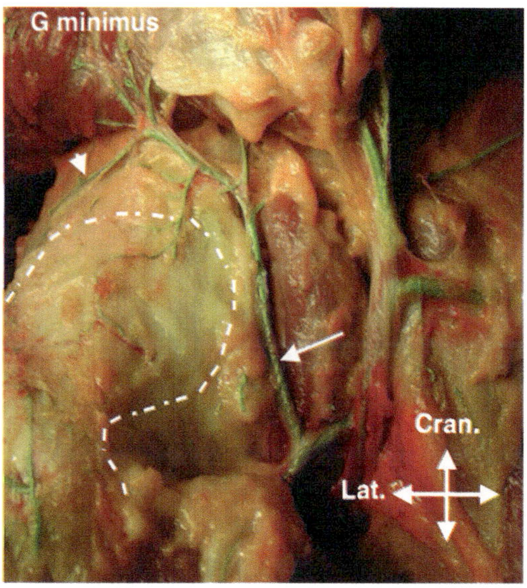

Fig. 1.5 Anterolateral surface of right hip to demonstrate the anastomosis between ascending branch of LFCA (*long arrow*) and supra-acetabular branch of SGA (*short arrow*). *G minimums*.: Gluteus minimus

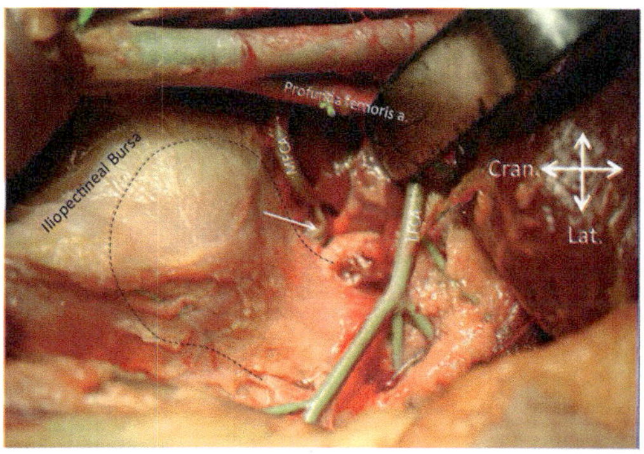

Fig. 1.7 *Arrow* shows the medial retinacular artery branching off from MFCA before capsulotomy. *MFCA*: Medial Femoral Circumflex Artery; *LFCA*: Lateral Femoral Circumflex Artery; *Profunda femoris a.*: Profunda femoris artery

femoral head (Fig. 1.6). The first femoral head-supplying artery pierces the medial capsule near its femoral attachment to enter the joint (Fig. 1.7).

On the posterior aspect of the hip joint the MFCA courses laterally toward the greater trochanter running along the inferior border of the obturator externus muscle to emerge between the quadratus femoris muscle and obturator externus tendon near their attachments to the greater trochanter (Fig. 1.8). After giving off the trochanteric branch, the artery crosses the obturator externus tendon in close contact posteriorly and runs superomedially to enter the joint (Fig. 1.9).

1.3.2.2 Intra-Capsular Course

The terminal branch of MFCA perforates the femoral attachment of the capsule in the posterolateral aspect of the hip joint between the capsular attachment of obturator externus and conjoint tendon (Fig. 1.9). After entry into the joint it divides

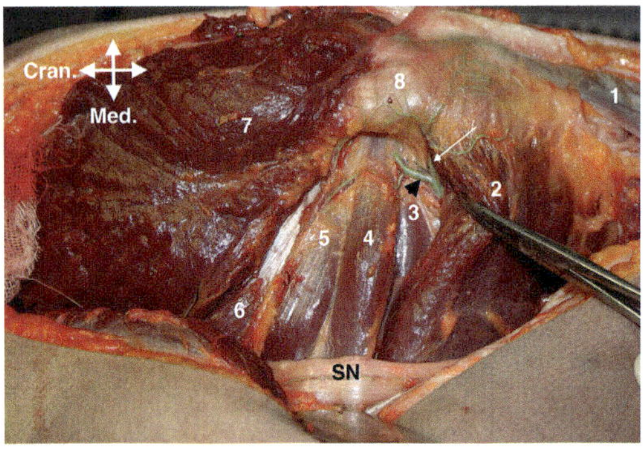

Fig. 1.8 Posterior aspect of right hip to show the deep branch of the MFCA before entry into the joint (*black arrow*). *White arrow* pointing toward the origin of trochanteric branch. *SN*: sciatic nerve; 1. vastus lateralis; 2. quadratus femoris; 3. obturator externus; 4. gemellus inferior; 5. gemellus superior; 6. piriformis; 7. gluteus medius; 8. greater trochanter

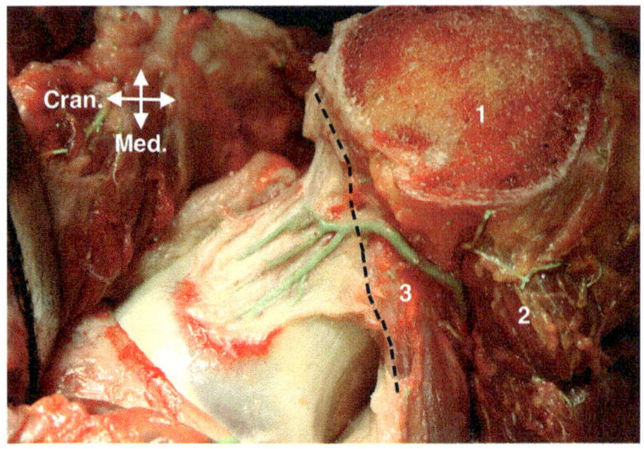

Fig. 1.10 Posterior aspect of hip after capsulotomy to demonstrate the terminal branches of the MFCA after entry into the joint. *Broken line*: imprint of capsular attachment. 1. greater trochanter (osteotomized); 2. quadratus femoris; 3. obturator externus

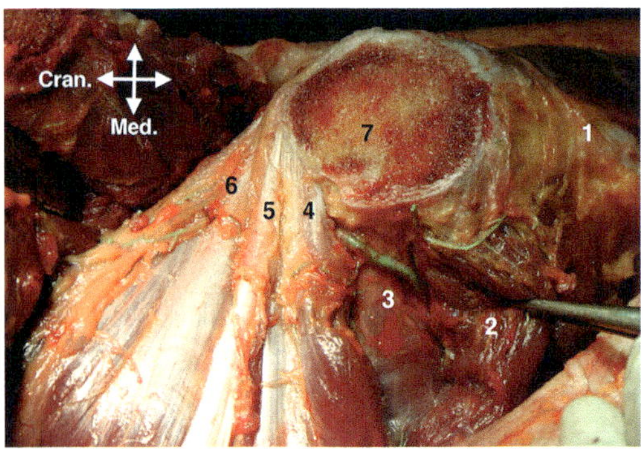

Fig. 1.9 The same as Fig. 1.8 after removal of gluteus medius and vastus lateralis. 1. vastus lateralis; 2. quadratus femoris; 3. obturator externus; 4. conjoint tendon of triceps coxae; 5. piriformis; 6. gluteus minimus; 7. greater trochanter

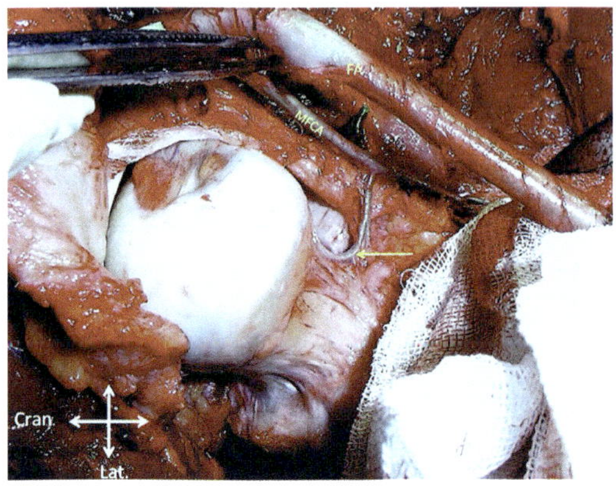

Fig. 1.11 Anteromedial aspect of hip joint to demonstrate the medial retinacular artery on top of Weitbrecht's ligament (*arrow*). *MFCA*: Medial Femoral Circumflex Artery; *FA*: Femoral Artery. Adapted with permission from [11]

into 2–6 branches running on the posterolateral surface of the neck toward the femoral head while covered and fixed by the retinaculum (Fig. 1.10).

In the inferomedial aspect of the joint the first retinacular artery, a branch of the MFCA pierces the femoral attachment of the capsule to enter the joint. Inside the joint it lies on the medial or posteromedial aspect of the neck as inferior retinacular artery and runs toward the head in a fold of a relatively mobile retinaculum called Weitbrecht's ligament (Fig. 1.11). This relative mobility allows the artery to escape from being damaged in some femoral neck fractures. Mobilization of this artery during intra-articular procedures is much easier than the superior retinacular arteries. It also provides blood supply to the Pipkin fractures in femoral head fracture dislocations. Unlike what is frequently mentioned in the literature a sub-capital and basal neck vascular ring rarely is seen inside the capsule.

1.4 Course and Distribution of the Obturator and Gluteal Arteries

The superior gluteal, inferior gluteal, and obturator arteries have intra-pelvic origin and branching off from the internal iliac artery.

1.4.1 SGA: Superior Gluteal Artery

Underlying the gluteus maximus and medius muscles, the SGA emerges from the pelvis at the uppermost part of the sciatic notch and proximal to the piriformis muscle (Fig. 1.12). The artery turns anteriorly and laterally and ramifies to supply the gluteal muscles and the acetabular bone by its muscular and periosteal branches, respectively. The most prominent periosteal branch is the supra-acetabular artery; it is protected and covered by the gluteus minimus muscle along its course from the posteromedial to the anterolateral aspect of the acetabulum. Its terminal 1/2 is periosteal and underlies the gluteus minimus muscle. The supra-acetabular branch gives multiple small arteries toward the hip capsule and finally anastomose with the ascending branch of LFCA (Fig. 1.13). Variable anastomoses can be found between the intra-pelvic and extra-pelvic vascular system in the area between and around the iliac spines.

1.4.2 IGA: Inferior Gluteal Artery

Branching off from the internal iliac artery the IGA courses distally along the sciatic nerve and posteromedial to it (Fig. 1.14). It supplies the short hip external rotators and the periacetabular

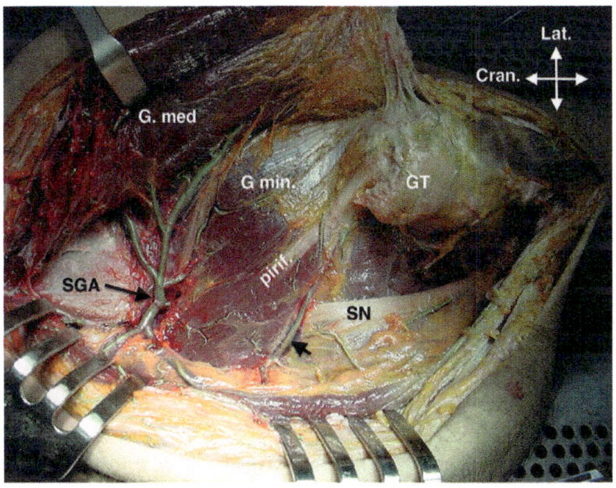

Fig. 1.12 Posterior aspect of right hip after retraction of gluteus medius and maximus to show the distribution of the SGA (*long arrow*). *Short arrow* indicating branch of the IGA. *SGA*: Superior Gluteal Artery; *IGA*: Inferior Gluteal Artery *SN*: sciatic nerve; *GT*: Greater trochanter; *G.med*: gluteus medius; *G.min*: gluteus minimus; *GT*: greater trochanter; *piri*: piriformis; *Cran.*: cranial; *Lat.*: lateral

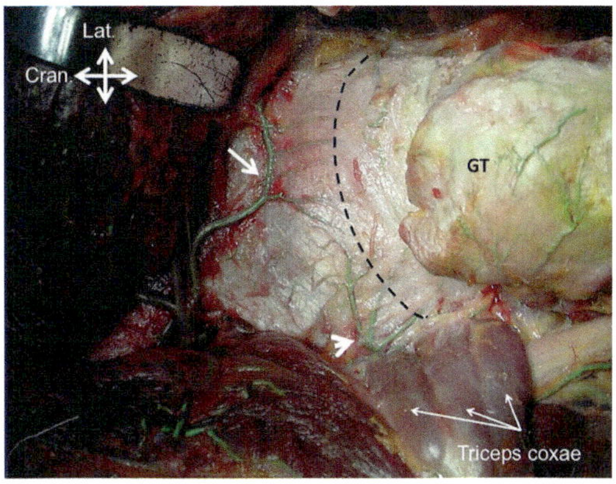

Fig. 1.13 Posterior aspect of hip joint after reflection of short hip rotators and gluteal muscles to expose the supra-acetabular branch of the SGA (*arrow*). *Arrowhead* indicates the acetabular branch of IGA. *Thin arrows* indicating the reflected triceps coxae muscles. *Broken line*: acetabular capsular attachment; *GT*: Greater trochanter. Adapted with permission from [11]

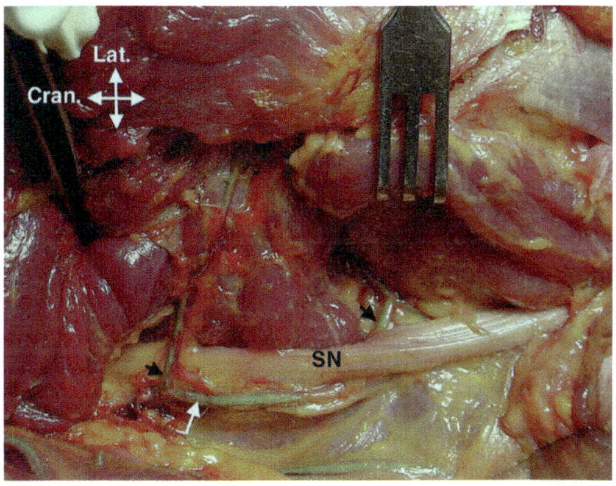

Fig. 1.14 Posterior aspect of hip joint to demonstrate the course and branches of the IGA (*arrows*) relative to sciatic nerve and short rotators. The hook is retracting the quadratus femoris muscle. *SN*: sciatic nerve

bone by its muscular and periosteal branches that leave the artery superficial or deep to the sciatic nerve. The IGA consistently contributes to the perfusion of the femoral head by a branch anastomosing with the MFCA in the area of the short hip external rotators. This anastomotic branch most often originates from the deep acetabular branch in the area between gemellus inferior and quadratus femoris muscles (Fig. 1.15), but less often from the muscular branches crossing the proximal short rotators superficially to reach the deep branch of MFCA.

As an important anatomic variation, in about 15% of hips the IGA is the main supplier of the femoral head from the posterior aspect, while the MFCA is then accessory. The femoral head-supplying artery usually branches off from the IGA at the level of the lesser sciatic notch or ischial tuberosity and lies usually deep to the sciatic nerve. It runs anteriorly and laterally, first between gemellus inferior and quadratus femoris, and then between conjoint and obturator externus tendon (Fig. 1.16). It never crosses the tendon of obturator externus as the deep branch of MFCA does. It finally perforates the capsule in immediate vicinity to the capsular attachment of the conjoint tendon as well as the deep branch of MFCA.

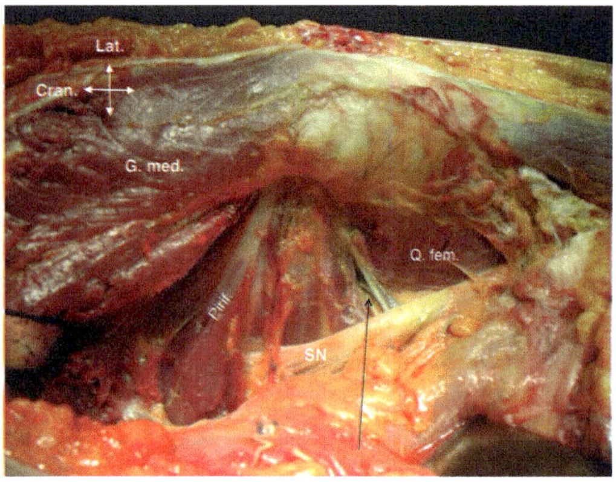

Fig. 1.15 Posterior aspect of hip joint to show the distal acetabular branch of the IGA (*arrow*) contributing to the circulation of the femoral head. *Pirif*: piriformis; *Q. fem.*: quadratus femoris; *G. med.*: gluteus medius; *SN*: sciatic nerve

1.4.3 OA: Obturator Artery

The OA has an intra-pelvic course along with the obturator nerve. Principally it supplies the hamstring and adductor muscles after exiting the pelvis through the obturator foramen. By its acetabular branch the OA contributes to the vascularization of the acetabulum (Fig. 1.17). Its contribution to the femoral head circulation via the ligamentous teres is not significant in adults. In spherical acetabular osteotomies, which are placed very near to the acetabulum, this artery remains one of the main suppliers of the acetabular fragment.

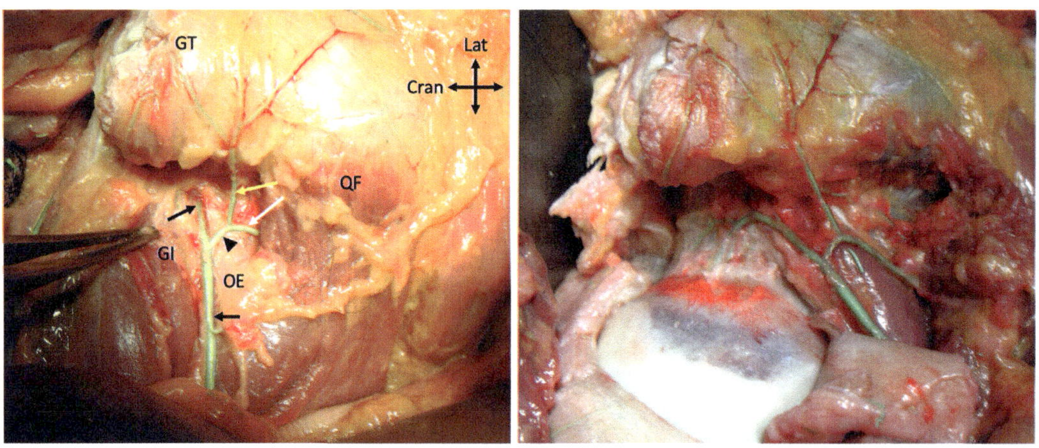

Fig. 1.16 Posterior aspect of right hip to show the dominance of the IGA over the MFCA in perfusion of the femoral head as an anatomic variation. **Left**: *black arrow* pointing to branch of the IGA. *White arrow* pointing to the deep branch of the MFCA; *Yellow arrow* pointing to the trochanteric branch; *Black arrowhead* pointing to the anastomosis between the two. **Right**: After removal of the external rotators except obturator externus, the IGA branch continues directly into the retinacular vessels while the deep branch of the MFCA is a small guage anastomosis. *GT*: greater trochanter. *QF*: quadratus femoris. *OE*: obturator externus; *GI*: gemellus inferior

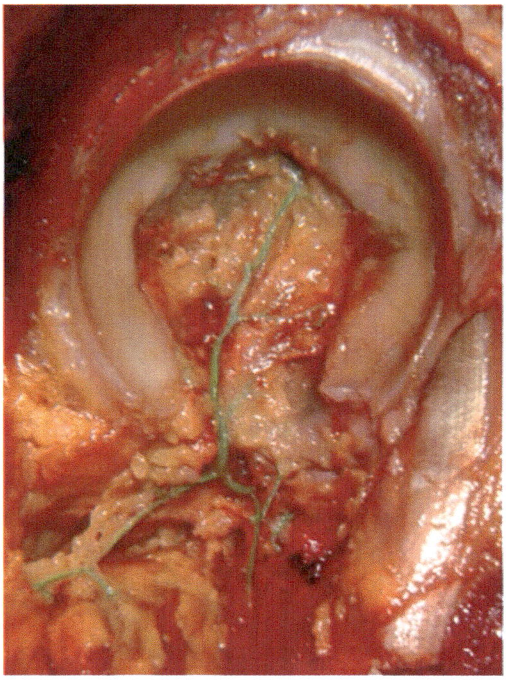

Fig. 1.17 Acetabular artery mainly fed by the obturator artery

1.5 Periacetabular Vascular Ring

Underlying the gluteal and short external rotator muscles and running on the external iliac surface exists a network of periosteal vessels originating principally from the gluteal arteries (Fig. 1.18).

Vessels derived from SGA form the superior part of this periosteal network. The most prominent periosteal branch of the SGA is the supra-acetabular branch. Arterial branches derived from IGA form the distal part of this network. Anastomoses between periosteal branches of the gluteal arteries in one side and between gluteal and circumflex femoral arteries in the other side configure the so-called periacetabular vascular ring. The ring receives also contributions from intra-pelvic periosteal vessels in the anterior and medial aspect of the acetabulum. The periacetabular vascular ring supplies the acetabular bone, capsule, and labrum.

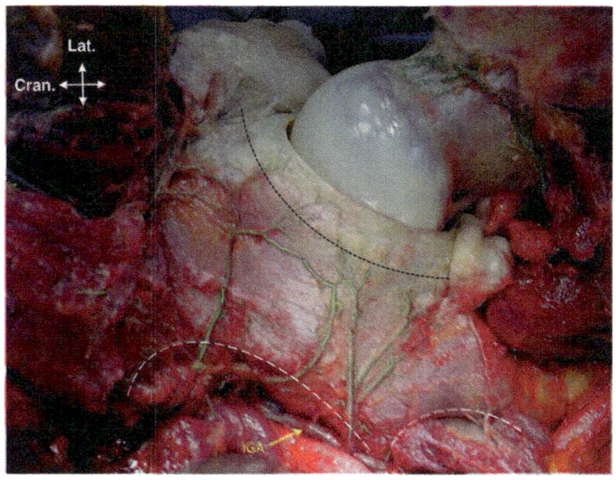

Fig. 1.18 Posterior aspect of right hip to demonstrate parts of the periacetabular periosteal ring formed by both gluteal arteries. *Dotted black line*: capsular imprint. *Broken white lines*: greater and lesser sciatic notch. *IGA*: inferior gluteal artery. Adapted with permission from [11]

1.6 Blood Supply to Capsule and Labrum

The hip capsule receives its blood from three sources: Vessels coming from the acetabular side originating principally from the periacetabular vascular ring, vessels coming from the femoral side originating from the circumflex femoral arteries, and perforating vessels from overlying muscles and tendons (Fig. 1.19). All these vessels enter to the non-articular surface of the capsule and make variable numbers of anastomoses with each other. Capsular vessels communicate with the acetabular bone through the vessels running superficially on the non-articular surface of the capsule; this contribution however only exists as long as the overlying muscles are not dissected from the capsule for exposure.

The acetabular labrum receives its blood supply exclusively from radial arteries originating from periacetabular periosteal ring (Fig. 1.20). Number and size of these vessels are highly variable in different parts of the labrum but are more concentrated in the posterior and superior aspect of the joint. After traversing the capsule subperiosteally

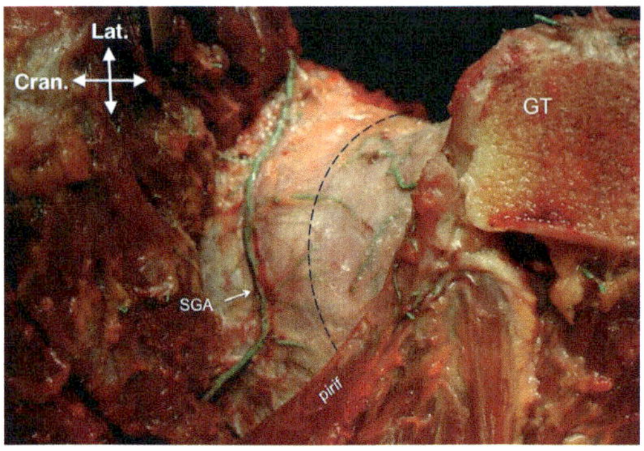

Fig. 1.19 Superior part of the vascular ring fed by the acetabular branch of the superior gluteal artery (*arrow*). *Broken line*: capsular imprint. *GT*: greater trochanter. *Pirif*: piriformis. *SGA*: superior gluteal artery

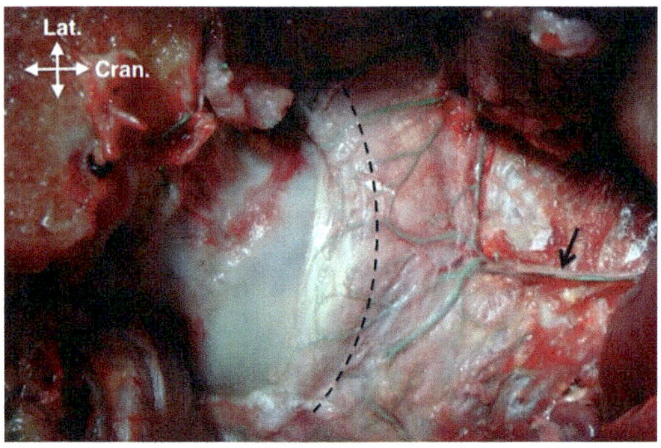

Fig. 1.20 Vascular ring in the superior aspect fed by the supra-acetabular branch of the SGA (*arrow*). Also, the picture shows vascularization of labrum by periosteal vessels traversing the capsule (*broken curve line* shows the acetabular attachment of the capsule). Adapted with permission from [12]

they reach the non-articular surface of the labrum, covered by synovial tissue, which is in continuation with the synovial layer of the capsule. In contrast to the results of previous studies, the capsule, synovium, and the bony acetabulum have no direct role in the perfusion of the labrum.

1.7 Vascularization of the Acetabulum

The acetabulum receives its blood supply from intraosseous and extraosseous sources. Nutrient arteries provide the intraosseous supply through vascular foramina. They enter the bone from internal or external surface of the pelvis. Number and size of these vessels are highly variable. The most prominent nutrient artery is derived from the iliolumbar artery, which enters the internal aspect of iliac bone distal to the SI joint and anterior or posterior to the pelvic brim. The extraosseous blood supply to the acetabulum is provided by the acetabular branch of the OA, by the periosteal arteries originating from the periacetabular vascular ring and by variable contributions provided by the anastomotic vessels running between capsule and periacetabular bone.

1.8 Vascularization of the Acetabulum After Periacetabular Osteotomy and Acetabular Fracture

Depending on the distance between osteotomy and capsule, the periacetabular cuts of the different procedures may be associated with varying rate of decrease in acetabular perfusion. In juxtacapsular periacetabular osteotomies through posterior and lateral approaches, nearly all intra- and extraosseous blood supply to the acetabulum are liable to damage except the acetabular branch of the OA. The closer the osteotomy to the capsule, the higher the risk of iatrogenic osteonecrosis would be (Fig. 1.21). Vascular communications between the hip capsule and peri-capsular tissues is established through the vessels running superficially on muscular surface of the capsule. These vessels are subject to damage during capsular exposure, therefore capsular contribution to the acetabular circulation cannot be expected following periacetabular osteotomies. The same is true for acetabular wall fragments in case of wide capsular exposure. With the Bernese PAO, executed via a modified anterior Smith-Petersen approach [18] and with abductor sparing technique [19], the extraosseous source of supply can partly be preserved in addition to the acetabular branch of the OA (Fig. 1.21). The anterior approach helps to preserve the capsular contribution to the acetabular perfusion running on the posterior and posterolateral surface. Since the osteotomy is performed with a distance from the

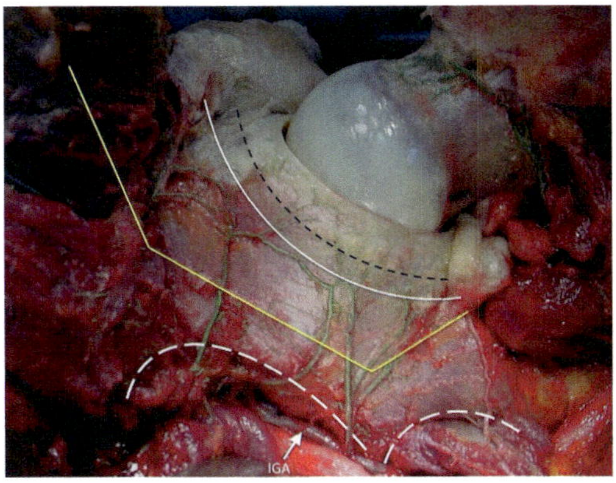

Fig. 1.21 Supra- and retro-acetabular periosteal blood supply. *Broken black line* representing the line of capsular attachment; *white line* representing the level of spherical osteotomies inside the vascular ring; *yellow line* representing the level of PAO outside the vascular ring; *white broken lines* representing greater and lesser sciatic notches; *IGA*: inferior gluteal artery. Adapted with permission from [11]

capsule, that part of the periosteal supply derived from the supra-acetabular branch of the SGA can also be preserved, provided the gluteus minimus muscle is tunnelled subperiosteally for soft tissue protection during the first branch of the supra- and retro-acetabular osteotomy.

1.9 Effect of Capsulotomy on Femoral Head and Acetabular Circulation

All femoral head-supplying vessels enter the joint via distal or femoral attachment of the capsule. The two main and consistent entry points are inferomedial and posterolateral. Insignificant contributions enter from anterior and rarely from posterior femoral attachments of the capsule. Any shape and extent of capsulotomy can be safe unless it violates the arterial entry points. Anterior and posterior longitudinal capsulotomies along femoral neck axis are safe. Also, a proximal transverse capsulotomy, whether partial or circumferential, has little or no effect on the femoral head blood supply. Distal transverse capsulotomy near the femoral attachment of the capsule carries a significant risk unless it avoids the inferomedial and posterolateral areas. A Z-shaped capsulotomy is harmless provided its distal transverse limb avoids the arterial entry points.

Capsular exposure, not necessarily capsulotomy, may affect the circulation of periacetabular bone by disrupting the communicating vessels running superficially between the capsule and pericapsular bone. This can have an effect in periacetabular osteotomy and acetabular fracture surgery when the circulation of the fragment is compromised.

1.10 Discussion

Successful results in preserving hip surgeries, especially with recently developed intra-articular procedures are directly dependent on the protection of the blood supply to the femoral head and acetabulum. Knowledge of the MFCA in its extracapsular course has led to development of safe surgical hip dislocation nearly 20 years ago [8]. Protection of the intra-capsular or retinacular vessels using the extended retinacular flap [17] has led to development of surgical techniques to directly manage the femoral head and neck deformities (Figs. 1.10, 1.11 and 1.22).

MFCA provides the main blood supply to the femoral head by the inferomedial and posterolateral retinacular arteries. The medial retinacular artery runs toward the head on the medial aspect of the femoral neck in a fold of retinaculum called Weitbrecht's ligament. This ligament is only fixed to the neck at its two ends. Thanks to this mobility the inferomedial retinacular artery is likely to remain intact in some femoral neck fractures. Pipkin fractures are usually pedicled by this ligament and its enfolded artery. Protection of this artery during fixation of Pipkin fractures can help to keep the fragment alive. In the posterior aspect of the greater trochanter, the deep branch of MFCA lies in intimate relationship with the tendon of obturator externus muscle. In its way toward the hip capsule, it lies between conjoint tendon and obturator externus tendon. Finally, it perforates the capsule at anterior margin of piriformis fossa while partially covered by the capsular attachment of the conjoint tendon. Whether normal or anatomic variation, the main vessels supplying the

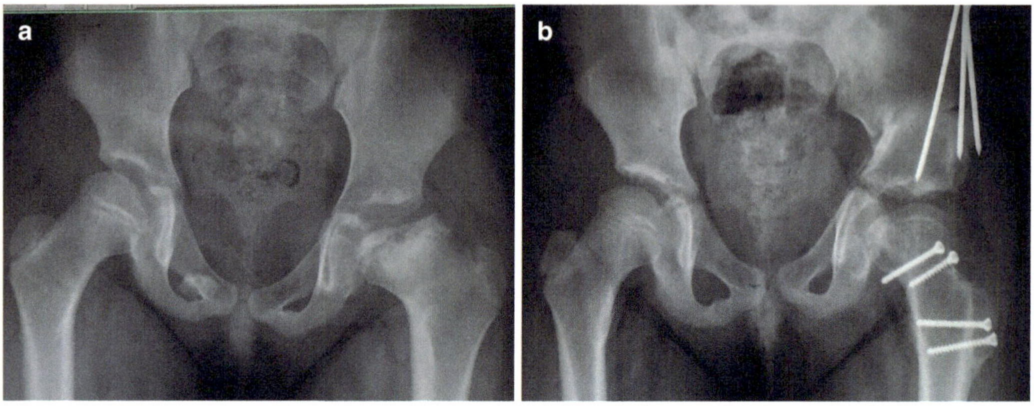

Fig. 1.22 (**a**) Morbus Perthes with hinged abduction and secondary adaptation of the acetabular roof. (**b**) One-year result after surgical dislocation, relative neck lengthening, femoral head reduction osteotomy, and PAO. Well contained femoral head with reasonable sphericity

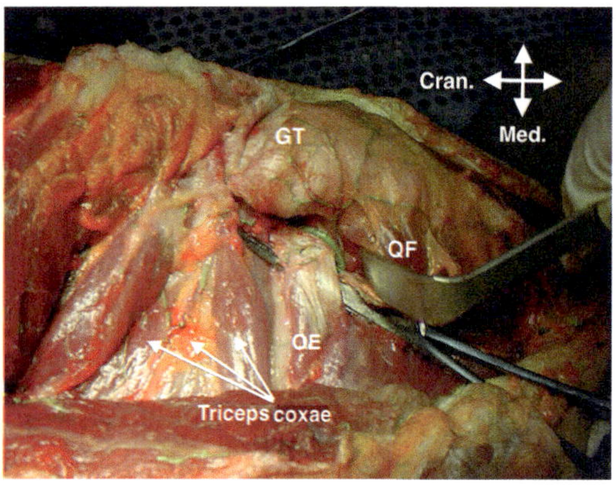

Fig. 1.23 Trochanteric area with upper border of quadratus femoris muscle retracted and obturator externus tendon lifted. Possible tenotomy of external rotators including obturator externus and conjoint tendon of triceps coxae during Kocher Langenbeck approach would interrupt the blood supply to the femoral head. *GT*: greater trochanter. *QF*: quadratus femoris. *OE*: obturator externus

femoral head are located in the area between the gemellus inferior and the quadratus femoris muscle. As a result, iatrogenic or traumatic injuries of short external rotators near their attachments to the greater trochanter carry a significant risk of femoral head AVN as seen frequently in acetabular fractures when fixed via a Kocher Langenbeck approach. This is especially true after tenotomy of the obturator externus and conjoint tendon close to their capsular attachments (Fig. 1.23). If such tenotomy is essential, a distance of at least 2 cm. from posterior border of the greater trochanter is needed to minimize the risk of vascular injury. On the other side, integrity of muscle and both attachments of the obturator externus are indicative for an intact femoral head perfusion in traumatic hip dislocation [7].

Capsulotomy per se, has little or no detrimental impact on vascularity of the femoral head, unless the entry points for nutrient arteries at femoral attachment of the capsule are invaded.

Retinacular vessels running on posterolateral and posteromedial aspect of the neck are identifiable after capsulotomy. The posterolateral retinacular arteries are the main blood carrying vessels to the femoral head. They are fixed to the neck by the retinaculum. They can only be mobilized from their distal side by extracapsular and subperiosteal extension of an extended retinacular flap (Fig. 1.24). The posteromedial retinacular artery usually runs in a fold of retinaculum, which is relatively mobile and easier to mobilize (Fig. 1.11).

Studies of the pelvic blood supply confirmed the safety of the Bernese periacetabular osteotomy [19] with regard to fragment perfusion [9]. Osteonecrosis after Bernese periacetabular osteotomy is anecdotal; the external vessels may be stretched during fragment correction (Fig. 1.25), but perfusion returns to normal after a few minutes [20]. It has been postulated that capsulotomy

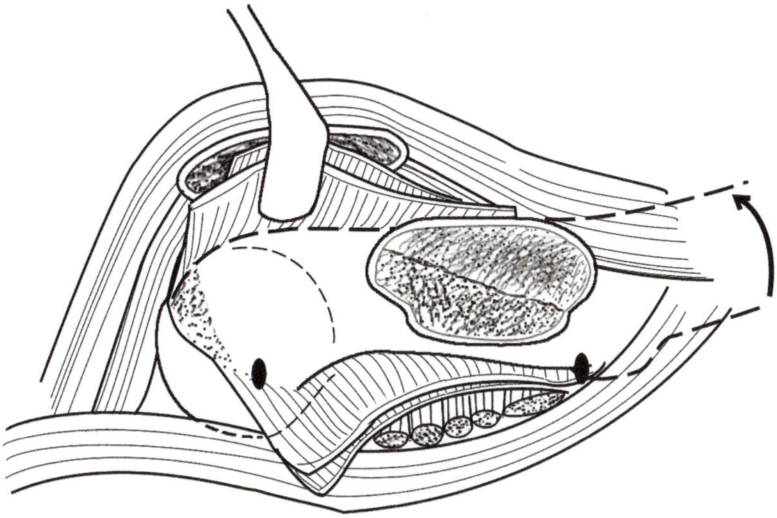

Fig. 1.24 Extended retinacular soft tissue flap containing the blood vessels to the femoral head. Black points indicate the length of the flap from the lesser trochanter to the insertion at the head-neck junction—Modified from Ganz et al. [17]

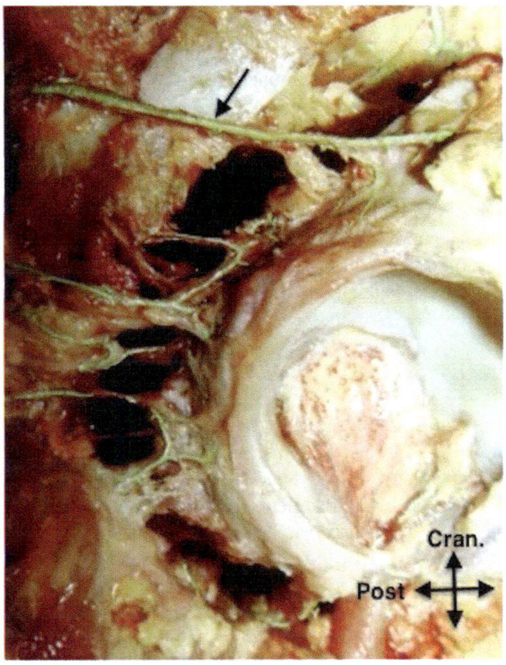

Fig. 1.25 Periacetabular vascular ring after Bernese PAO to show the functioning periacetabular vessels. Correction of the acetabular fragment may temporarily stretch the periosteal vessels; however, perfusion of the fragment returns after few minutes [18]. These vessel branches remain intact when the posterior cortex is broken rather than cut. *Arrow* shows the supra-acetabular artery

during PAO may further affect the compromised circulation of the acetabulum [21, 22]. Similarly, preserving capsular attachment to the acetabular wall fragment can keep the fragment alive during fracture surgery [23]. Considering the anatomic pattern of capsular vessels, it is the capsular exposure, not capsulotomy per se, that may interrupt the capsular contribution to acetabular perfusion [12]. This can specifically affect vascularity of the acetabulum through posterior and lateral approaches.

Refixation or repair of the acetabular labrum is a new trend in hip preserving surgery [24–26]. Labral blood supply has extra-articular origin. Terminal arteries originating from periacetabular periosteal network traverse the capsule subperiosteally to enter the non-articular surface of the labrum while covered by a layer of synovium continuous with synovial layer of the capsule [12]. Femoroacetabular impingement secondary to the altered femoral head morphology is the most frequent cause of labral tear. The majority of these labral tears begin from articular side; the vascular side remains intact. This can preserve the healing potential of torn labrum. Whether such a tear should be repaired after unloading the labrum by correction of the offending structural abnormalities, is an additional controversy.

Complete surgical detachment of the labrum to trim the osseous rim is a common treatment aspect of the impinging hip [24]. Such detachment deprives the labral sector from perfusion [12]. Reperfusion and healing following repair may be facilitated by the neighboring capsule but with more scar and adhesion leading to a frequently seen obliteration of the recess between the two structures. As a consequence, the mobility of the labrum goes with the capsule instead of the head. This pathophysiology may be the reason for recurrence of pain, frequently observed after a free period of 6–8 weeks. Future research may look for a way of labrum refixation from the articular side, leaving the capsular side of the labrum untouched.

References

1. Gray H. Anatomy of the human body. 20th ed. Philadelphia: Lea & Febiger; 1918.
2. Hollinshead WH. Anatomy for surgeons. In: The back and limbs, vol. 3. London: Harper & Row; 1969. p. 637–9.
3. Anderson JE. Grant's atlas of anatomy. 8th ed. Baltimore: Williams & Wilkins; 1983.
4. Tucker FR. Arterial supply to the femoral head and its clinical importance. J Bone Joint Surg Br. 1949;31B:82–93.
5. Howe WW, Lacey T, Schwartz RP. A study of the gross anatomy of the arteries supplying the proximal portion of the femur and the acetabulum. J Bone Joint Surg Am. 1950;32 A:856–66.
6. Trueta J, Harrison MH. The normal vascular anatomy of the femoral head in adult man. J Bone Joint Surg Br. 1953;35-B:442–61.
7. Gautier E, Ganz K, Krügel N, et al. Anatomy of the medial femoral circumflex artery and its surgical implications. J Bone Joint Surg Br. 2000;82:679–83. https://doi.org/10.1302/0301-620x.82b5.10426.
8. Ganz R, Gill TJ, Gautier E, et al. Surgical dislocation of the adult hip. A technique with full access to the femoral head and acetabulum without the risk of avascular necrosis. J Bone Joint Surg Br. 2001;83:1119–24. https://doi.org/10.1302/0301-620x.83b8.11964.
9. Beck M, Leunig M, Ellis T, et al. The acetabular blood supply: implications for periacetabular osteotomies. Surg Radiol Anat. 2003;25:361–7. https://doi.org/10.1007/s00276-003-0149-3.
10. Grose AW, Gardner MJ, Sussmann PS, et al. The surgical anatomy of the blood supply to the femoral head: description of the anastomosis between the medial femoral circumflex and inferior gluteal arteries at the hip. J Bone Joint Surg Br. 2008;90:1298–303. https://doi.org/10.1302/0301-620X.90B10.20983.
11. Kalhor M, Beck M, Huff TW, Ganz R. Capsular and pericapsular contributions to acetabular and femoral head perfusion. J Bone Joint Surg Am. 2009;91:409–18. https://doi.org/10.2106/JBJS.G.01679.
12. Kalhor M, Horowitz K, Beck M, et al. Vascular supply to the acetabular labrum. J Bone Joint Surg Am. 2010;92:2570–5. https://doi.org/10.2106/JBJS.I.01719.
13. Sussmann PS, Ranawat AS, Shehaan M, et al. Vascular preservation during arthroscopic osteoplasty of the femoral head-neck junction: a cadaveric investigation. Arthroscopy. 2007;23:738–43. https://doi.org/10.1016/j.arthro.2007.01.025.
14. Khan A, Lovering AM, Bannister GC, et al. The effect of a modified posterior approach on blood flow to the femoral head during hip resurfacing. Hip Int. 2009;19:52–7.
15. Kalhor M, Horowitz K, Gharehdaghi J, et al. Anatomic variations in femoral head circulation. Hip Int. 2012;22:307–12. https://doi.org/10.5301/HIP.2012.9242.
16. Leunig M, Slongo T, Ganz R. Subcapital realignment in slipped capital femoral epiphysis: surgical hip dislocation and trimming of the stable trochanter to protect the perfusion of the epiphysis. Instr Course Lect. 2008;57:499–507.
17. Ganz R, Huff TW, Leunig M. Extended retinacular soft-tissue flap for intra-articular hip surgery: surgical technique, indications, and results of application. Instr Course Lect. 2009;58:241–55.
18. Ganz R, Klaue K, Vinh TS, Mast JW. A new periacetabular osteotomy for the treatment of hip dysplasias. Technique and preliminary results. Clin Orthop Relat Res. 1988;232:26–36.
19. Murphy SB, Millis MB. Periacetabular osteotomy without abductor dissection using direct anterior exposure. Clin Orthop Relat Res. 1999;364:92–8. https://doi.org/10.1097/00003086-199907000-00013.
20. Hempfing A, Leunig M, Nötzli HP, et al. Acetabular blood flow during Bernese periacetabular osteotomy: an intraoperative study using laser Doppler flowmetry. J Orthop Res. 2003;21:1145–50. https://doi.org/10.1016/S0736-0266(03)00083-4.
21. Hsieh P-H, Shih C-H, Lee P-C, et al. A modified periacetabular osteotomy with use of the transtrochanteric exposure. J Bone Joint Surg Am. 2003;85:244.
22. Ko J-Y, Wang C-J, Lin C-FJ, Shih C-H. Periacetabular osteotomy through a modified Ollier transtrochanteric approach for treatment of painful dysplastic hips. J Bone Joint Surg Am. 2002;84:1594.
23. Johnson EE, Matta JM, Mast JW, Letournel E. Delayed reconstruction of acetabular fractures 21-120 days following injury. Clin Orthop Relat Res. 1994;305:20–30.
24. Espinosa N, Rothenfluh DA, Beck M, et al. Treatment of femoro-acetabular impingement: preliminary results of labral refixation. J Bone Joint Surg Am. 2006;88:925. https://doi.org/10.2106/JBJS.E.00290.
25. Kelly BT, Weiland DE, Schenker ML, Philippon MJ. Arthroscopic labral repair in the hip: surgical technique and review of the literature. Arthroscopy. 2005;21:1496–504. https://doi.org/10.1016/j.arthro.2005.08.013.
26. Murphy KP, Ross AE, Javernick MA, Lehman RA. Repair of the adult acetabular labrum. Arthroscopy. 2006;22:567.e1–3. https://doi.org/10.1016/j.arthro.2005.07.033.

Femoro-Acetabular Impingement: History, Concept, and Treatment

2

Reinhold Ganz

2.1 History

In the past, osteoarthritis of the hip (OA) was understood as the result of static, mostly eccentric overload or of an intrinsic abnormality of the joint cartilage [1, 2]. Despite intensive genetic and molecular biological research, intrinsic factors could not be established as causing coefficient, nor could body weight be identified to be an influencing factor for the hip as it has been proven for the knee [3]. A typical and frequent morphology with eccentric overload and structural instability is residual acetabular dysplasia [4]; together with other established patho-morphologies, e.g., after Morbus Perthes or SCFE osteoarthritic changes are named secondary. When no morphological abnormalities could be identified, and this was the case in about 70% of the hips, OA was called primary [5, 6].

Five decades ago, Murray speculated about an influence of a frequent minor deformity of the head-neck junction on OA [6]. This "tilt" was further investigated by Solomon [7] and Harris [8]; it was then called "pistol grip" deformity [9] which was also related to a silent SCFE [9, 10]. With this interpretation, the incidence of primary or idiopathic OA has dramatically dropped to about 10% [11]. Although the hypothesis made sense, the patho-mechanical explanation remained unclear. Reduction of contact area and overload is a valid explanation for the joint deterioration in residual acetabular dysplasia; however, it can hardly explain the cartilage destruction in the presence of a subtle deformity and a rather large and congruent loading area. It was finally the impingement concept which allowed to confirm Murrays hypothesis [11, 12].

R. Ganz (✉)
Faculty of Medicine, University of Bern,
Bern, Switzerland

2.2 Concept

The impingement mechanism could only be studied with safe surgical hip dislocation, a technique which was developed in the 1990s [13] based on detailed vascular studies of the proximal femur [14, 15]. On the open joint, details of stability–instability and dislocation–relocation of the femoral head could be studied as well as it was possible to observe how impingement between head and acetabulum takes place during different ranges of motion. With routine use of surgical dislocation varying impingement pattern have been identified and finally a concept of femoro-acetabular impingement (FAI) could be formulated and validated [11, 12]. The perception was that even minor morphological irregularities like reduced wasting of the head-neck junction but also local or global acetabular over-coverage could lead to intraarticular impingement followed by damage of the adjacent acetabular cartilage and labrum. In contrast, the cartilage of the femoral head in its weight bearing area

R. Ganz (ed.), *Modern Hip Preservation*, https://doi.org/10.1007/978-3-030-91967-2_2

remains intact until the corresponding acetabular cartilage is destroyed [11]. Thereafter the head migrates into the acetabular cartilage defect, an aspect which is hardly visible on standard radiographies but may be demonstrated on MRI with a slightly larger posterior joint space. The velocity of the impact plays an important role for amount and progression of the cartilage destruction. Impingement can be followed by instability and subluxation of the femoral head on the opposite side of the joint. Impingement is believed to be the primary mechanism of traumatic and recurrent hip dislocation [16, 17].

The terms cam and pincer impingement were used primarily [11, 12] (Fig. 2.1).

Today the terms inclusive and impacting impingement are favored [18]. Inclusive impingement is more often seen in male patients while female patients suffer more from impacting impingement and have a deep socket [19]. Major deformities as seen after severe chronic SCFE may lead to inclusive and impacting impingement depending on femoral rotation [20]. The progression of cartilage damage is faster with inclusive impingement, but less painful while the impacting impingement is more benign and more painful [21]. It is known that often more than one morphological malformation per case is present, eventually becoming relevant only after removal of the leading deformity [22]. While the joint damage starts at the acetabular side, the femoral cartilage becomes involved after a substantial amount of acetabular cartilage is abraded, allowing the head to migrate into the deficient area. Only thereafter OA may become visible with radiographic narrowing of the antero-superior joint space, a situation which is consistent with advanced cartilage destruction.

The impingement concept has precursors. In 1891, a saddle-like extension of the anterolateral head-neck contour was described in the French literature [23]. Shortly after, Poirier [24] interpreted it as reactive indentation produced by the opposite iliac bone with repetitive flexion and called it "emprinte iliacque." A picture in Lane's book on the operative treatment of fractures from 1905 is indicative of the same mechanism [25]. Recently, this interpretation was re-discussed as sub-spine impingement [26]. In 1907, Preiser showed in cadaver studies that a mal-oriented acetabular opening was related with OA [27] and in 1913, the same author published observations that patients with limited internal rotation later often developed OA [28].

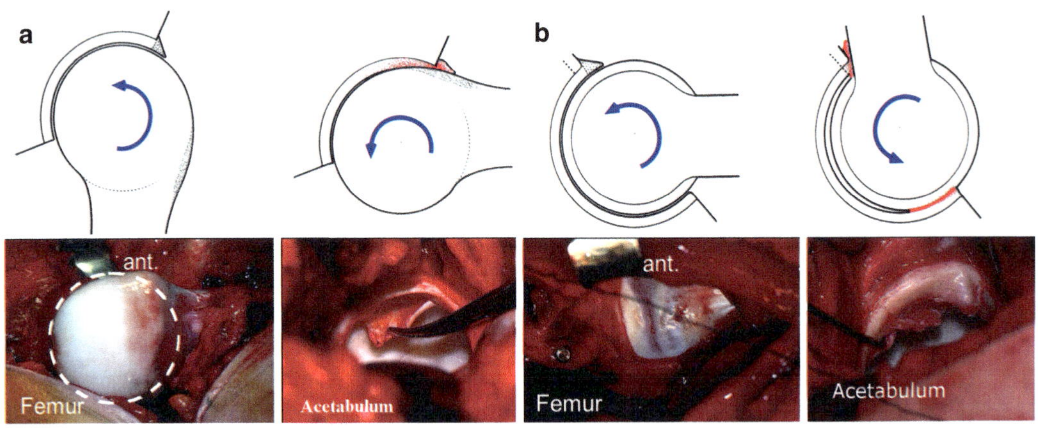

Fig. 2.1 (Modified from Ganz et al. [11]) Impingement types (**a**) Cam impingement. When a hip with a non-spherical sector of the femoral head is flexed, this area will be jammed into the socket leading to abrasion of the acetabular cartilage near the rim or even to outside-in avulsion of the cartilage from the labrum. The labrum itself is primarily not affected. (**b**) Pincer impingement. When a hip with local or general over-coverage of the head is flexed, the head-neck junction hits against the acetabular rim with a linear contact. The direct injury leads to an indentation line at the head-neck junction. Chronic pincer impingement leads to a destruction of the labrum itself while the adjacent cartilage remains intact. Repetitive pincer impingement leads to cartilage abrasion of the postero-inferior acetabular cartilage

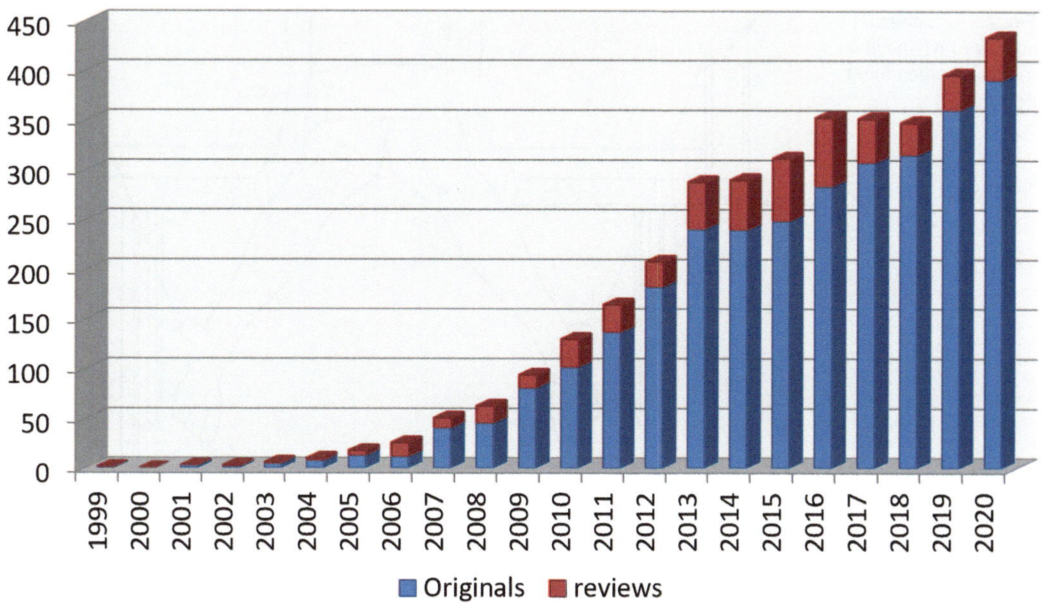

Fig. 2.2 Increase of publications about FAI since first article in 1999

In 1903, von Mikulicz [29] had described how to resect a head-neck prominence limiting abduction and internal rotation, a method which was later taken over by Vulpius and Stoffel [30] and again by Heyman et al. [31] for resection of anterolateral metaphyseal bumps in severe SCFE limiting flexion and internal rotation. Smith-Petersen had similar ideas by resecting parts of the osteophytic overgrowth of the anterior acetabular wall together with an excavation of the anterior head-neck junction to improve motion in ankylosing OA [32]. Rab was the first to demonstrate that SCFE hips produce contact between the prominent anterolateral metaphysis and the acetabular cartilage; however, his computer simulation did not include motion and therefore he did not speculate much on consequences for the cartilage [33]. In 1970, Teinturier [34] confirmed the observation of Preiser [27] that OA was correlated with abnormal version of the acetabulum. He enlarged the spectrum by adding reduced femoral version as contributing factor, which was later confirmed by Tönnis and Heinecke [35]. Our first attention on impingement was focused in the early 1990s when analyzing a small series of femoral neck fractures healed in slight retro tilt. This produced a painful anterior conflict with the acetabular rim in flexion and internal rotation; however, we did not think about the damaging influence on the acetabular cartilage [36].

FAI was observed for the first time intraoperatively in 1996 thanks to the technique of surgical dislocation of the hip. In the following years the mechanism was communicated by several publications [11, 12, 21, 37–50] and meanwhile was repeatedly confirmed worldwide by independent centers [51–60]. Smaller pieces are continuously added to the mosaic [22, 26, 61, 62] and the overall literature on FAI is still exponentially increasing (Fig. 2.2). Although FAI can take place everywhere around the hip joint, the most common site is anterolateral and is produced during internal rotation in flexion. This led to an impingement test and the predictive character of limited internal rotation in hip flexion was validated with a special examination chair (Fig. 2.3) [12, 47, 48].

2.3 FAI Treatment

Aggressive conservative treatment, e.g., stretching is contra-productive. Reduction or modification of physical activity can alleviate the

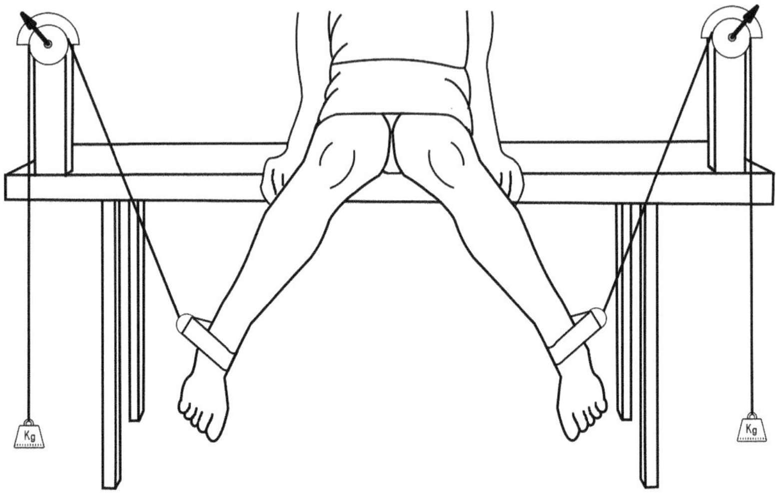

Fig. 2.3 Examination chair for FAI-specific internal rotation in 90° flexion [63]

symptoms. NSAIDs may decrease pain but also its protective function. For the younger patient with significant deformities and high physical demands, surgery may be considered when thorough clinical and radiographic evaluation including MRI has brought forward the specific patho-morphologies. Surgical treatment can be performed by different surgical techniques; however, the type of underlying abnormality and consecutive pathology should be considered when selecting the most appropriate surgical technique. Surgical hip dislocation (Fig. 2.4) allows to follow a causal treatment strategy including necessary extensions. Such a strategy was established simultaneously together with the process of formulating the impingement process. It was refined over time and has been reported in several articles [64–67]. Basically, it is a femoral osteochondroplasty to re-establish a spherical head contour and/or a sufficient head-neck offset. Transparent templates help to define border and extension of the area to be shaped. On the acetabular side the osseous rim is trimmed down to the necessary level, which was estimated on radiographies and controlled intraoperatively with repeated testing of impingement-free motion; in deep sockets this could even be circumferential. The labrum is refixed whenever possible (Fig. 2.5) with the aim of re-establishing a seal and better load distribution [68–71]. In selected cases even allograft reconstruction has been executed [72]. Reversed PAO to treat acetabular retroversion was successfully performed in young patients with only little or no damage to the acetabular cartilage and a posterior rim running medial of the center of the head [73]. When femoral version loomed and is substantial, it should be corrected additionally [22, 62]. Others have treated anterior cam impingement with an anterior mini incision eventually with arthroscopic assistance and report about promising early results [74]. Computer assistance with fluoroscopic control of the osteochondroplasty has also been tested [75]. Finally, hip arthroscopy has adopted the FAI treatment, which became one of its largest fields of activity. It is reflected by numerous publications resumed in two most recently published textbooks [76, 77]. Although refinement of the arthroscopic techniques is constantly advancing, the execution of therapeutic hip arthroscopy is technically challenging and needs a thorough understanding of the spectrum of FAI pathology. It has its limitations for some intracapsular comorbidities and cannot treat extra-articular components of the individual FAI pathology. Best indication is the isolated anterior impingement. When all aspects of standard FAI surgery including refixation of the labrum are to be fulfilled, the arthroscopic surgery may take longer than the open procedure with dislocation of the femoral head and has a higher risk of col-

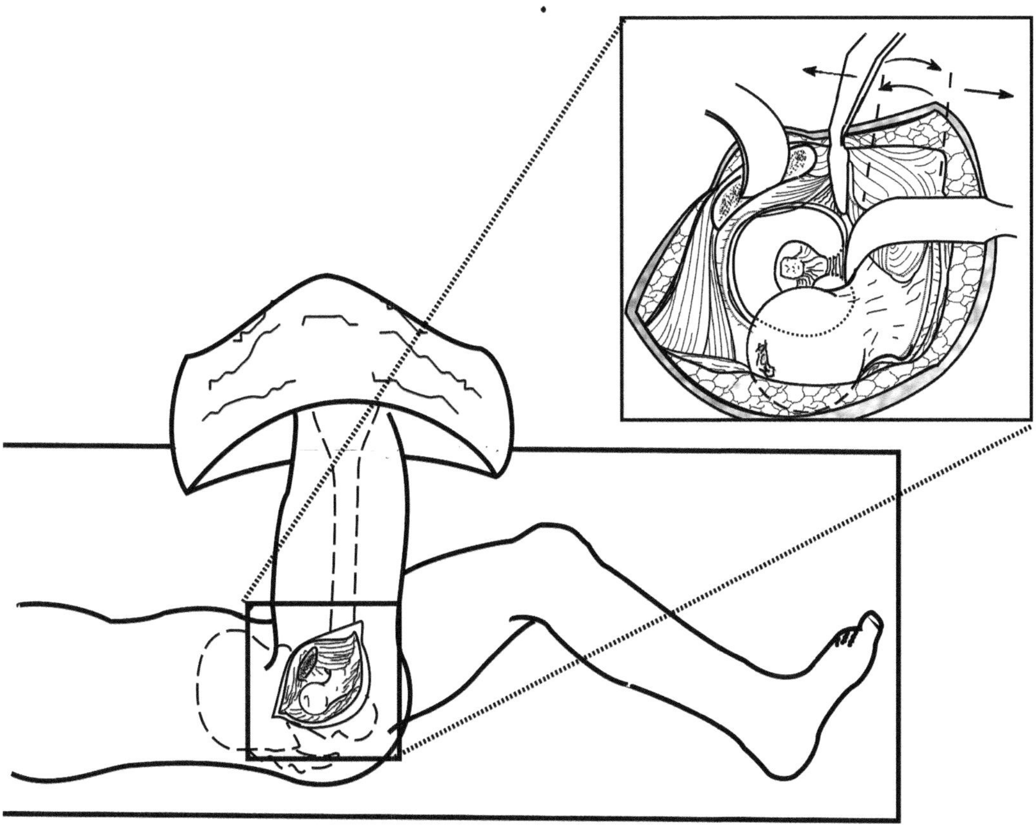

Fig. 2.4 (Modified from Ganz et al. [13]) Safe surgical hip dislocation allowing to view 360° of the acetabulum and nearly 360° of the femoral head

lateral damages especially of the femoral cartilage. Failure to address all underlying patho-morphology is not rare, likely leading to continued symptoms, revision surgery, and poor outcome [78, 79].

Extra-articular impingement can create a recurrent destabilization or even joint subluxation on the opposite side of the impingement area [62]. Such impingement is mainly seen in hips with a short neck and/or a large and high riding greater trochanter with abduction but also with external rotation in different positions of flexion. Typical example is the deformity after Legg–Calvé–Perthes disease. Classic trochanteric advancement may improve abduction in extension but has little influence on rotation because the trochanteric base will continue to impinge. True femoral neck lengthening procedures [80] lateralize the shaft; without tapering of the metaphyseal area of the remaining base of the trochanter, posterior extra-articular impingement will continue. After additional intertrochanteric osteotomy metaphyseal trimming may jeopardize the perfusion of the largely denuded metaphysis. The technique of relative neck lengthening after a trochanteric flip osteotomy however can include a reduction of the residual trochanteric bone down to the level and contour of the neck. The trimming must result in a strictly subperiosteal dissection of the retinacular flap containing the vessels to the head, while the perfusion of the metaphysis comes from the femoral diaphysis. This technique increases the superior, posterior, and anterior femoro-acetabular clearance without the risk of femoral head/

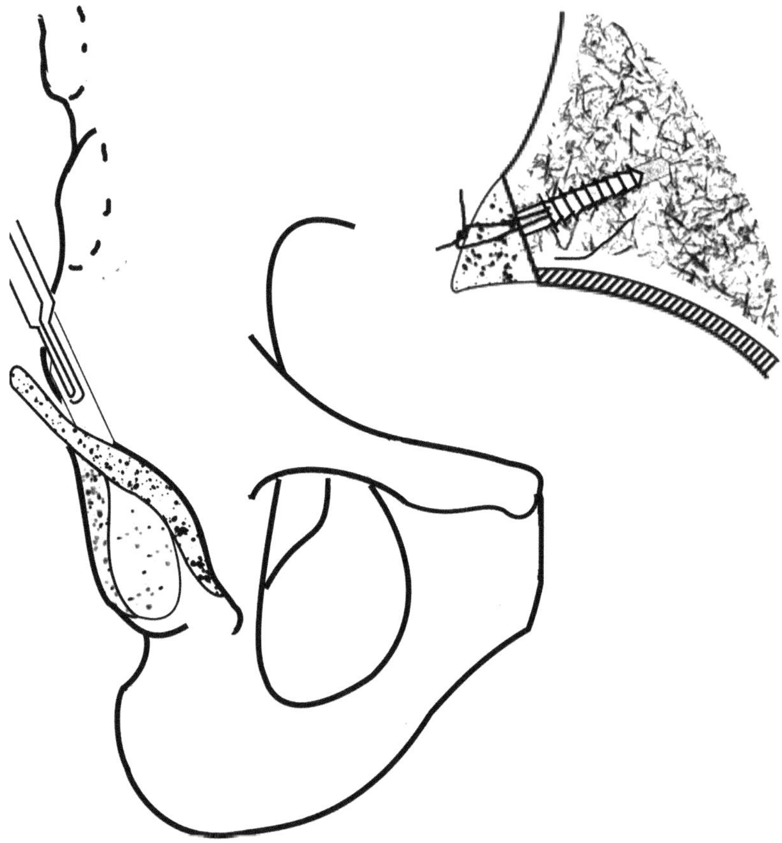

Fig. 2.5 (Modified from Leunig et al. [19]) Rim trimming and labrum refixation using anchors

neck necrosis, while the distance between the calcar femoris and the pelvis remains unchanged. At the end of the procedure the trochanteric fragment with the muscular insertions is advanced distally according to the needs of the individual hip. Relative lengthening can be an autonomous procedure to treat extra-articular impingement but can also be combined with other techniques (Fig. 2.6). In one hip the femoral neck broke as a result of a fall in the immediate postoperative phase resulting in a THR. Performed since 1998, the extended retinacular soft tissue flap quickly rendered greater importance as necessary step for a new class of safe intracapsular surgery beyond classic osteotomies [81].

All in all, the concept of FAI is still relatively new. Besides some fascinating recognitions and promising treatment approaches, so far, our experience relies on short and midterm follow-up with 68–96% good results. Nevertheless, so far, no necrosis of the femoral head has been reported [82].

15 years after surgery, the patient remains pain free. ROM is nearly symmetrical. She gave birth to 2 children and works full time as hairdresser. The leg length discrepancy is not a problem for her; at work she wears shoes with length compensation. All in all, she is very happy with the result and denies the need for metal removal or a surgical procedure for leg lengthening.

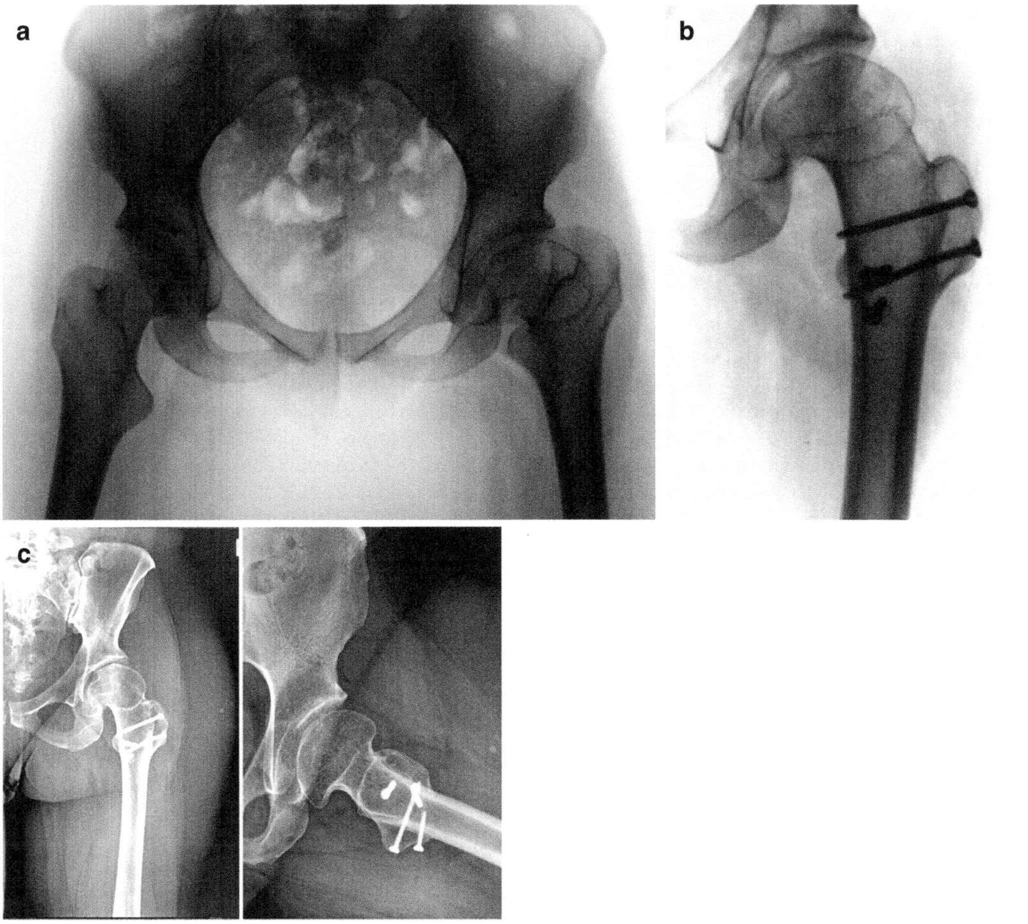

Fig. 2.6 (**a**) Perthes deformity with intra- and extra-articular impingement including impingement between lesser trochanter and ischium. (**b**) Result after shaping of the head, relative lengthening the neck with distal advancement of greater and lesser trochanter. (**c**) Radiological result 15 years after surgery without morphological changes since postoperative appearance

References

1. Pauwels F. Biomechanics of the normal and diseased hip: theoretical foundation, technique and results of treatment an atlas. Berlin: Springer; 1976.
2. Solomon L, Schnitzler CM, Browett JP. Osteoarthritis of the hip: the patient behind the disease. Ann Rheum Dis. 1982;41:118–25. https://doi.org/10.1136/ard.41.2.118.
3. Oliveria SA, Felson DT, Cirillo PA, et al. Body weight, body mass index, and incident symptomatic osteoarthritis of the hand, hip, and knee. Epidemiology. 1999;10:161–6. https://doi.org/10.1097/00001648-199903000-00013.
4. Ganz R, Leunig M. Hip dysplasia overview. In: Callaghan JJ, Clohisy JC, Beaule P, et al., editors. The adult hip + the adult hip - hip preservation surgery: arthroplasty and its alternatives. 3rd ed. Lippincott Williams & Wilkins; 2015.
5. Morscher E. Die intertrochantäre Osteotomie bei Coxarthrose: Multizentrische Nachuntersuchung von 2251 intertrochantären Osteotomien bei Coxarthrose. Bern: Huber; 1971. p. 56–96.
6. Murray RO. The aetiology of primary osteoarthritis of the hip. Br J Radiol. 1965;38:810–24. https://doi.org/10.1259/0007-1285-38-455-810.
7. Solomon L. Geographical and anatomical patterns of osteoarthritis. Br J Rheumatol. 1984;23:177–80. https://doi.org/10.1093/rheumatology/23.3.177.
8. Harris WH. Etiology of osteoarthritis of the hip. Clin Orthop Relat Res. 1986;213:20–33.
9. Stulberg SD. Unrecognized childhood hip disease: a major cause of idiopathic osteoarthritis of the hip. The

hip: proceedings of the third open scientific meeting of the hip society, 1975. St Louis: CV Mosby; 1975.
10. Goodman DA, Feighan JE, Smith AD, et al. Subclinical slipped capital femoral epiphysis. Relationship to osteoarthrosis of the hip. J Bone Joint Surg Am. 1997;79:1489–97. https://doi.org/10.2106/00004623-199710000-00005.
11. Ganz R, Leunig M, Leunig-Ganz K, Harris WH. The etiology of osteoarthritis of the hip: an integrated mechanical concept. Clin Orthop Relat Res. 2008;466:264. https://doi.org/10.1007/s11999-007-0060-z.
12. Ganz R, Parvizi J, Beck M, et al. Femoroacetabular impingement: a cause for osteoarthritis of the hip. Clin Orthop Relat Res. 2003;417:112–20. https://doi.org/10.1097/01.blo.0000096804.78689.c2.
13. Ganz R, Gill TJ, Gautier E, et al. Surgical dislocation of the adult hip. A technique with full access to the femoral head and acetabulum without the risk of avascular necrosis. J Bone Joint Surg Br. 2001;83:1119–24. https://doi.org/10.1302/0301-620x.83b8.11964.
14. Ganz K, Krügel N. The medial femoral circumflex artery. Topographical course and anastomoses. Doctoral thesis, Department of Orthopedic Surgery, University of Bern; 1997.
15. Gautier E, Ganz K, Krügel N, et al. Anatomy of the medial femoral circumflex artery and its surgical implications. J Bone Joint Surg Br. 2000;82:679–83. https://doi.org/10.1302/0301-620x.82b5.10426.
16. Manner HM, Mast NH, Ganz R, Leunig M. Potential contribution of femoroacetabular impingement to recurrent traumatic hip dislocation. J Pediatr Orthop B. 2012;21:574–8. https://doi.org/10.1097/BPB.0b013e328357bf04.
17. Steppacher SD, Albers CE, Siebenrock KA, et al. Femoroacetabular impingement predisposes to traumatic posterior hip dislocation. Clin Orthop Relat Res. 2013;471:1937–43. https://doi.org/10.1007/s11999-013-2863-4.
18. Tibor LM, Ganz R. Hip osteoarthritis: definition and etiology Chapter 9. In: Nho S, Leunig M, Kelly B, et al., editors. Hip arthroscopy and hip joint preservation surgery. New York, NY: Springer Science & Business Media; 2015. p. 177–88.
19. Leunig M, Ganz R. The evolution and concepts of joint-preserving surgery of the hip. Bone Joint J. 2014;96-B:5–18. https://doi.org/10.1302/0301-620X.96B1.32823.
20. Ganz R, Aprato A, Mazziotta G, Pignatti G. Joint instability after anatomic reconstruction of severe, chronic slipped capital femoral epiphysis: a report of 3 cases, with high femoral anteversion in 1 and adaptive acetabular roof deformation in 3. JBJS Case Connect. 2016;6:e50. https://doi.org/10.2106/JBJS.CC.15.00149.
21. Beck M, Kalhor M, Leunig M, Ganz R. Hip morphology influences the pattern of damage to the acetabular cartilage: femoroacetabular impingement as a cause of early osteoarthritis of the hip. J Bone Joint Surg Br. 2005;87:1012–8. https://doi.org/10.1302/0301-620X.87B7.15203.
22. Tibor LM, Liebert G, Sutter R, et al. Two or more impingement and/or instability deformities are often present in patients with hip pain. Clin Orthop Relat Res. 2013;471:3762–73. https://doi.org/10.1007/s11999-013-2918-6.
23. Bertaux TA. Humerus and femur. Reflexions on species and human races regarding gender and age. Doctoral thesis, Le Bigot Frères; 1891.
24. Poirier P. Traité d'anatomie humaine, vol. 1. Embryologie (Prenant A.) Ostéologie et Arthologie. Masson; 1895.
25. Lane WA. The operative treatment of fractures. London: Medical Publishing Company; 1905.
26. Hetsroni I, Poultsides L, Bedi A, et al. Anterior inferior iliac spine morphology correlates with hip range of motion: a classification system and dynamic model. Clin Orthop Relat Res. 2013;471:2497–503. https://doi.org/10.1007/s11999-013-2847-4.
27. Preiser G. Arthritis of the hip and its relation with abnormal version of the acetabulum. Dtsch Zeitschr Chirurg. 1907;89:541.
28. Preiser G. Statische Gelenkerkrankungen. Stuttgart: F. Enke; 1911.
29. von Mikulicz J. In: von Bergmann E, von Bruns P, von Mikulicz J, editors. Handbuch der praktischen Chirurgie, Bd IV, Chirurgie der Extremitäten. Stuttgart: Enke; 1903. p. 600.
30. Vulpius O, Stoffel A. Orthopadische Operationslehre: mit 627 zum teil farbigen abbildungen. 3rd ed. Stuttgart: F. Enke; 1913.
31. Heyman CH, Herndon CH. Slipped femoral epiphysis with severe displacement: a conservative operative treatment. J Bone Joint Surg Am. 1957;39:293–303.
32. Smith-Petersen MN. Treatment of malum coxae senilis, old slipped upper femoral epiphysis, intrapelvic protrusion of the acetabulum, and coxa plana by means of acetabuloplasty. J Bone Joint Surg Am. 1936;18:869–80.
33. Rab GT. The geometry of slipped capital femoral epiphysis: implications for movement, impingement, and corrective osteotomy. J Pediatr Orthop. 1999;19:419–24.
34. Teinturier P. Abnormal orientation of the femur neck and acetabulum. Statistical study of 200 centered arthrosic hips. Rev Chir Orthop Reparatrice Appar Mot. 1970;56:219–30.
35. Tönnis D, Heinecke A. Diminished femoral antetorsion syndrome: a cause of pain and osteoarthritis. J Pediatr Orthop. 1991;11:419–31. https://doi.org/10.1097/01241398-199107000-00001.
36. Ganz R, Bamert P, Hausner P, et al. Cervicoacetabular impingement after femoral neck fracture. Unfallchirurg. 1991;94:172–5.
37. Beck M, Leunig M, Clarke E, Ganz R. Femoroacetabular impingement as a factor in the development of nonunion of the femoral neck: a report of three cases. J Orthop Trauma. 2004;18:425–30.

38. Ito K, Leunig M, Ganz R. Histopathologic features of the acetabular labrum in femoroacetabular impingement. Clin Orthop Relat Res. 2004;429:262–71.
39. Ito K, Minka-II M-A, Leunig M, et al. Femoroacetabular impingement and the cam-effect. J Bone Joint Surg. 2001;83-B:171–6. https://doi.org/10.1302/0301-620X.83B2.0830171.
40. Leunig M, Beck M, Dora C, Ganz R. Femoroacetabular impingement: etiology and surgical concept. Oper Tech Orthop. 2005;15:247–55. https://doi.org/10.1053/j.oto.2005.06.005.
41. Leunig M, Beck M, Kalhor M, et al. Fibrocystic changes at anterosuperior femoral neck: prevalence in hips with femoroacetabular impingement. Radiology. 2005;236:237–46. https://doi.org/10.1148/radiol.2361040140.
42. Leunig M, Casillas MM, Hamlet M, et al. Slipped capital femoral epiphysis: early mechanical damage to the acetabular cartilage by a prominent femoral metaphysis. Acta Orthop Scand. 2000;71:370–5. https://doi.org/10.1080/000164700317393367.
43. Leunig M, Podeszwa D, Beck M, et al. Magnetic resonance arthrography of labral disorders in hips with dysplasia and impingement. Clin Orthop Relat Res. 2004;418:74–80.
44. Meyer DC, Beck M, Ellis T, et al. Comparison of six radiographic projections to assess femoral head/neck asphericity. Clin Orthop Relat Res. 2006;445:181–5. https://doi.org/10.1097/01.blo.0000201168.72388.24.
45. Nötzli HP, Wyss TF, Stoecklin CH, et al. The contour of the femoral head-neck junction as a predictor for the risk of anterior impingement. J Bone Joint Surg. 2002;84-B:556–60. https://doi.org/10.1302/0301-620X.84B4.0840556.
46. Reichenbach S, Jüni P, Werlen S, et al. Prevalence of cam-type deformity on hip magnetic resonance imaging in young males: a cross-sectional study. Arthritis Care Res. 2010;62:1319–27. https://doi.org/10.1002/acr.20198.
47. Reichenbach S, Leunig M, Werlen S, et al. Association between cam-type deformities and magnetic resonance imaging-detected structural hip damage: a cross-sectional study in young men. Arthritis Rheum. 2011;63:4023–30. https://doi.org/10.1002/art.30589.
48. Siebenrock KA, Wahab KHA, Werlen S, et al. Abnormal extension of the femoral head epiphysis as a cause of cam impingement. Clin Orthop Relat Res. 2004;418:54–60.
49. Wagner S, Hofstetter W, Chiquet M, et al. Early osteoarthritic changes of human femoral head cartilage subsequent to femoro-acetabular impingement. Osteoarthr Cartil. 2003;11:508–18. https://doi.org/10.1016/S1063-4584(03)00075-X.
50. Werlen S, Leunig M, Ganz R. Magnetic resonance arthrography of the hip in femoroacetabular impingement: technique and findings. Oper Tech Orthop. 2005;15:191–203. https://doi.org/10.1053/j.oto.2005.07.007.
51. Armfield DR, Towers JD, Robertson DD. Radiographic and MR imaging of the athletic hip. Clin Sports Med. 2006;25:211–39. https://doi.org/10.1016/j.csm.2005.12.009.
52. Beall DP, Sweet CF, Martin HD, et al. Imaging findings of femoroacetabular impingement syndrome. Skelet Radiol. 2005;34:691–701. https://doi.org/10.1007/s00256-005-0932-9.
53. Beaulé PE, Zaragoza E, Motamedi K, et al. Three-dimensional computed tomography of the hip in the assessment of femoroacetabular impingement. J Orthop Res. 2005;23:1286–92. https://doi.org/10.1016/j.orthres.2005.03.011.1100230608.
54. Blankenbaker DG, Tuite MJ. The painful hip: new concepts. Skelet Radiol. 2006;35:352–70. https://doi.org/10.1007/s00256-006-0105-5.
55. Bredella MA, Stoller DW. MR imaging of femoroacetabular impingement. Magn Reson Imaging Clin N Am. 2005;13:653–64. https://doi.org/10.1016/j.mric.2005.08.001.
56. Jäger M, Wild A, Westhoff B, Krauspe R. Femoroacetabular impingement caused by a femoral osseous head–neck bump deformity: clinical, radiological, and experimental results. J Orthop Sci. 2004;9:256–63. https://doi.org/10.1007/s00776-004-0770-y.
57. Kassarjian A, Yoon LS, Belzile E, et al. Triad of MR Arthrographic findings in patients with cam-type femoroacetabular impingement. Radiology. 2005;236:588–92. https://doi.org/10.1148/radiol.2362041987.
58. Tanzer M, Noiseux N. Osseous abnormalities and early osteoarthritis: the role of hip impingement. Clin Orthop Relat Res. 2004;429:170–7. https://doi.org/10.1097/01.blo.0000150119.49983.ef.
59. Wenger DE, Kendell KR, Miner MR, Trousdale RT. Acetabular labral tears rarely occur in the absence of bony abnormalities. Clin Orthop Relat Res. 2004;426:145–50. https://doi.org/10.1097/01.blo.0000136903.01368.20.
60. Wisniewski SJ, Grogg B. Femoroacetabular impingement: an overlooked cause of hip pain. Am J Phys Med Rehabil. 2006;85:546–9. https://doi.org/10.1097/01.phm.0000219148.00549.e8.
61. Leunig M, Jüni P, Werlen S, et al. Prevalence of cam and pincer-type deformities on hip MRI in an asymptomatic young Swiss female population: a cross-sectional study. Osteoarthr Cartil. 2013;21:544–50. https://doi.org/10.1016/j.joca.2013.01.003.
62. Tibor LM, Ganz R, Leunig M. Case reports: anteroinferior acetabular rim damage due to femoroacetabular impingement. Clin Orthop Relat Res. 2013;471:3781–7. https://doi.org/10.1007/s11999-013-2921-y.
63. Reichenbach S, Jüni P, Nüesch E, et al. An examination chair to measure internal rotation of the hip in routine settings: a validation study. Osteoarthr Cartil. 2010;18:365–71. https://doi.org/10.1016/j.joca.2009.10.001.
64. Eijer H, Podeszwa DA, Ganz R, Leunig M. Evaluation and treatment of young adults with femoro-

acetabular impingement secondary to Perthes disease. Hip Int. 2006;16:273–80. https://doi.org/10.5301/HIP.2008.4906.
65. Kim YJ, Ganz R, Murphy SB, et al. Hip joint-preserving surgery: beyond the classic osteotomy. Instr Course Lect. 2006;55:145–58.
66. Leunig M, Parvizi J, Ganz R. Nonarthroplasty surgical treatment of hip osteoarthritis. Instr Course Lect. 2006;55:159–66.
67. Peters CL, Erickson JA. Treatment of femoro-acetabular impingement with surgical dislocation and débridement in young adults. J Bone Joint Surg Am. 2006;88:1735–41. https://doi.org/10.2106/JBJS.E.00514.
68. Crawford MJ, Dy CJ, Alexander JW, et al. The 2007 Frank Stinchfield award: the biomechanics of the hip labrum and the stability of the hip. Clin Orthop Relat Res. 2007;465:16–22. https://doi.org/10.1097/BLO.0b013e31815b181f.
69. Ferguson SJ, Bryant JT, Ganz R, Ito K. The acetabular labrum seal: a poroelastic finite element model. Clin Biomech. 2000;15:463–8. https://doi.org/10.1016/S0268-0033(99)00099-6.
70. Ferguson SJ, Bryant JT, Ganz R, Ito K. An in vitro investigation of the acetabular labral seal in hip joint mechanics. J Biomech. 2003;36:171–8. https://doi.org/10.1016/S0021-9290(02)00365-2.
71. Ferguson SJ, Bryant JT, Ganz R, Ito K. The influence of the acetabular labrum on hip joint cartilage consolidation: a poroelastic finite element model. J Biomech. 2000;33:953–60. https://doi.org/10.1016/S0021-9290(00)00042-7.
72. Rocha PC, Klingenstein G, Ganz R, et al. Circumferential reconstruction of severe acetabular labral damage using hamstring allograft: surgical technique and case series. Hip Int. 2013;23:42–53. https://doi.org/10.5301/HIP.2013.11662.
73. Siebenrock KA, Schoeniger R, Ganz R. Anterior femoro-acetabular impingement due to acetabular retroversion : treatment with periacetabular osteotomy. J Bone Joint Surg Am. 2003;85:278–86.
74. Clohisy JC, McClure JT. Treatment of anterior femoroacetabular impingement with combined hip arthroscopy and limited anterior decompression. Iowa Orthop J. 2005;25:164–71.
75. Ecker TM, Puls M, Steppacher SD, et al. Computer-assisted femoral head-neck osteochondroplasty using a surgical milling device: an in vitro accuracy study. J Arthroplast. 2012;27:310–6. https://doi.org/10.1016/j.arth.2011.03.048.
76. Byrd JWT. Operative hip arthroscopy. New York, NY: Springer; 2012.
77. Safran M, Ranawat A, Sekiya J. Techniques in hip arthroscopy and joint preservation surgery: with expert consult access. Philadelphia, PA: Saunders/Elsevier; 2011.
78. Heyworth BE, Shindle MK, Voos JE, et al. Radiologic and intraoperative findings in revision hip arthroscopy. Arthroscopy. 2007;23:1295–302. https://doi.org/10.1016/j.arthro.2007.09.015.
79. May O, Matar WY, Beaulé PE. Treatment of failed arthroscopic acetabular labral debridement by femoral chondro-osteoplasty. J Bone Joint Surg Br. 2007;89-B:595–8. https://doi.org/10.1302/0301-620X.89B5.18753.
80. Wagner H. Femoral osteotomies for congenital hip dislocation. In: Weil UH, editor. Acetabular dysplasia. Berlin: Springer; 1978. p. 85–105.
81. Ganz R, Huff TW, Leunig M. Extended retinacular soft-tissue flap for intra-articular hip surgery: surgical technique, indications, and results of application. Instr Course Lect. 2009;58:241–55.
82. Clohisy JC, St John LC, Schutz AL. Surgical treatment of femoroacetabular impingement: a systematic review of the literature. Clin Orthop Relat Res. 2010;468:555–64. https://doi.org/10.1007/s11999-009-1138-6.

3 Overview on Developmental Dysplasia of the Hip

Alessandro Aprato, Laura Ravera, and Alessandro Massè

3.1 Introduction

Developmental dysplasia of the hip (DDH) is an important cause of childhood disability. This disorder underlies up to 9% of all primary hip replacements and up to 29% of those in people aged 60 years and younger [1].

DDH encompasses a spectrum of physical and imaging findings, ranging from mild temporary instability to frank dislocation. The child's hip will not develop normally if it remains unstable and anatomically abnormal by walking age. Therefore, careful physical examination of all infants to diagnose and treat significant DDH is critical to provide the best possible functional outcome.

Historically the most commonly used term for this condition was the acronym CDH: congenital dislocation (or dysplasia) of the hip [2]. Since clinical screening for neonatal hip abnormalities began in the 1950s, it has been recognized that this disorder is not always congenital. Although widespread use of the older term CDH continued until the mid-1990s [3], the term DDH is now routinely used. "Developmental" has replaced "congenital" in recognition of the fact that this disorder has a variable presentation. "Dysplasia" is a more appropriate term than "dislocation" since the spectrum of pathology ranges from acetabular dysplasia with enlocated, stable hips to complete dislocation. The precise definition of DDH is itself controversial and it has been defined in both a clinical and imaging context. Developmental dysplasia of the hip includes frank dislocation (luxation), partial dislocation (subluxation), instability wherein the femoral head comes in and out of the socket, and an array of radiographic abnormalities that reflects inadequate formation of the acetabulum [4].

Despite a normal newborn and infant hip examination, a late-onset hip dislocation still occurs in approximately 1 in 5000 infants as well as dysplasia in young adults [5].

3.2 Incidence

The incidence of DDH varies from 1.5 to 25.0 per 1000 live births, depending on the criteria used for diagnosis, the population studied, and the method of screening [5].

The prevalence of DDH varies between populations. This may be secondary to genetic or environmental factors, or a combination of both. Most notably it is rarely seen in the African population, with Bantu Africans having a prevalence of almost zero [6]. The prevalence in the USA is quoted as 1.5–15 per 1000 live births, with the African American subgroup as 0.46 per 1000 live births. The higher prevalence among African Americans compared with native Africans is possibly secondary to the effects of environmental factors in the USA and/or genetic heterogeneity

A. Aprato (✉) · L. Ravera · A. Massè
University of Turin, Turin, Italy

R. Ganz (ed.), *Modern Hip Preservation*, https://doi.org/10.1007/978-3-030-91967-2_3

[7]. DDH is more common in ethnic groups where swaddling of infants with the hips extended and adducted has been especially prevalent including the Navajo Indian population [8, 9], Saudi Arabia [10], Turkey [11], and Japan [12].

Relative risk rates are stated in the American Academy of Pediatrics' (AAP) 2000 clinical practice guidelines, and the overall DDH risk is about 1 per 1000 [5].

DDH is unilateral in approximately 80% of cases and bilateral in the remainder [13]. In cases of unilateral DDH, the left hip is affected four times more commonly than the right. This is thought to be related to intrauterine positioning where the fetus more commonly lies with his or her left side against the maternal sacrum, resulting in adduction of the left hip [3, 13]. It is clinically more difficult to diagnose a bilateral DDH and as a result is more commonly diagnosed later than unilateral DDH [7].

3.3 Risk Factors

A number of fetal and maternal factors are widely accepted as being associated with a higher risk of DDH. Female gender, breech positioning at delivery and family history of DDH have been most consistently shown, in both case control and observational studies, to be associated with DDH [4]. A number of other risk factors for DDH have been reported including oligohydramnios, primiparity, high birthweight, post maturity and infant swaddling, environmental factors [4, 5].

Breech presentation is probably the most important single risk factor, with DDH reported in 2% to 20% of male and female infants presenting in the breech position [5].

Breech presentation is known to put the fetus at increased risk of DDH, with reported odds ratios (OR) ranging from 9.65 to 10.03 [14, 15]. Chan et al. [14] found that the mode of delivery further modified the risk of DDH associated with breech presentation. In their study of 1127 patients with DDH, they reported a significantly higher OR in those breech infants delivered vaginally (17.15) than by cesarean section (10.03), when compared with vertex presentation. No significant difference in risk was seen for vaginal delivery compared with cesarean section in the setting of vertex presentation. The authors concluded that although DDH is likely a deformation occurring later in gestation, it may be aggravated by passage through the birth canal in the breech position. The OR for breech presentation delivered by emergency cesarean section (13.19), usually performed after onset of labor, was higher than that for breech delivered by elective cesarean section (7.56), supporting the above conclusion.

Although the presence of these risk factors has been shown to confer an increased risk of DDH, most infants with DDH (73–90%) have no identifiable risk factors, with the exception of female gender, while the prevalence of DDH in infants with risk factors is 1–10%. Therefore, risk factors are considered a useful adjunct to but not a replacement for clinical examination.

Isolated DDH has repeatedly been shown to be more common in female than male infants, with reported ratios ranging from 2.4:1 to 9.2:1 [14–17]. In addition, abnormalities seen on neonatal hip US are less likely to spontaneously resolve in female than male infants [18]. Female susceptibility to DDH has not yet been entirely explained. Popular theories are mainly based on increased susceptibility of the female fetus and infant to the effects of maternal and fetal hormones, presumed to lead to increased ligamentous laxity.

Relaxin increases the secretion of collagenase and plasminogen activator, two important enzymes involved in collagenolysis. This results in a change in the cellular formation of the tissue, increasing cell extension and flexibility. These effects are important both to facilitate growth during pregnancy and to relax the maternal pelvic ligaments in preparation for the birth [19]. Studies have failed to show a positive correlation between cord blood relaxin concentration and neonatal hip abnormalities [14, 19] or indeed between relaxin concentration in female newborns with hip abnormalities when compared with concentrations in male newborns with hip abnormalities [19]. To date the role of expression of the relaxin receptor by the developing fetal hip joint has not been established.

Newborn infants have hip and knee flexion contractures because of their normal intrauterine position. These contractures resolve over time with normal developmental maturation. Animal studies have shown that forced hip and knee extension in the neonatal period leads to hip dysplasia and dislocation because of increased tension in the hamstring and iliopsoas muscles that stresses the hip capsule, which may have underlying laxity or instability [20].

Comprehensive ultrasound screening during the immediate newborn period has demonstrated hip laxity in approximately 15% of infants [21, 22]. The combination of capsular laxity and abnormal muscle tension is the most likely mechanism of DDH for infants who are maintained with the lower extremities extended and wrapped tightly together. In contrast, cultures that carry their children in the straddle or jockey position, common in warmer climates, have very low rates of hip dislocation compared with cultures that wrap their infants tightly with the lower limbs together and extended [23].

Family studies [17, 24–26] have shown that the concordance of DDH is much higher in monozygotic compared with dizygotic twins. In addition, they have demonstrated a significantly higher prevalence of DDH in siblings (4.3–14%) and parents (1.6–2.3%) of affected infants than in the general population. A slightly increased relative risk (RR) has also been seen in infants with a first cousin affected with DDH (RR 1.7) [27]. It should be noted that data regarding parental prevalence of DDH from many of the earlier family studies are of limited value due to the fact that the majority of cases of DDH were diagnosed late in the era before clinical screening became widely practiced. In addition, the degree of disability caused by late diagnosis often meant that people with severe DDH did not have children of their own [25].

A number of other fetal and/or maternal factors have been shown to confer an increased risk of DDH including: oligohydramnios (OR 3.97) [14], primiparity (OR 1.71–2.19) [14, 15, 27], high birthweight (>4000 g, OR 1.55–24,15,17; >4500 g OR 2.6715), and post maturity (OR 1.48–2.09) [14, 15].

Prematurity appears to protect against DDH with gestation less than 37 weeks having an OR of 0.10 when compared with gestation 37–41 weeks [15], supporting the theory that DDH arises in later intrauterine life [28, 29] and may be due in part to reduced intrauterine mechanical stress on smaller infants.

Swaddling, an old tradition in certain ethnic groups, has become popular practice in recent years in many developed countries due to its benefits in terms of promoting infant sleep [30].

However, studies have shown that swaddling an infant so that the legs are kept extended and adducted promotes hip dysplasia [11, 20]. The physiologic hip position in a newborn infant is flexion and abduction. This aids hip development in enlocated hips by maintaining contact between the femoral head and the acetabulum. Although most acetabular dysplasia seen on neonatal hip US resolves spontaneously [21, 31], swaddling of such infants may exacerbate the dysplasia and alter the natural course of hip development [30]. DDH is more prevalent in populations where swaddling is commonly used.

3.4 Associated Abnormalities

Where congenital torticollis is associated with a clinically and sonographically evident mass within the sternocleidomastoid muscle, it is known as congenital muscular torticollis (CMT). Where there is torticollis but no mass or tightening within the sternocleidomastoid muscle, the term congenital postural torticollis is used. DDH has been reported as being present in 11.6–17% patients with CMT [32–34]. Von Heideken et al. [32] found that male infants with CMT were almost five times more likely to have DDH than female infants with CMT. Postural muscular torticollis has not been found to be associated with a higher risk of DDH. In one study where CMT was graded according to the degree of deficit of passive rotation of the neck, the incidence of DDH was found to correlate with the severity of deficit of neck rotation. It is proposed that infants with CMT be screened both clinically and with hip US for DDH [34].

Traditionally congenital talipes equinovarus (TEV) has been considered an indication for hip US screening for DDH, included in the UK screening guidelines [35]. However, recent studies have failed to show a higher prevalence of DDH in infants with TEV of either the congenital (fixed) or postural type [36, 37]. DDH has been shown to be more common in infants with congenital talipes calcaneus valgus (4–6.5%) and in metatarsus adductus (4%) [36], suggesting that infants with either of these two foot deformities be screened for DDH.

3.5 Normal Hip Development

The formation of the hip joint begins at the seventh week of gestation. The acetabulum and the femoral head develop from the same group of mesenchymal stem cells [38–40]. At the seventh week of gestation, a cleft develops in the precartilaginous cells. This cleft defines the acetabulum from the femoral head. By the 11th week of gestation, the hip joint is fully formed, but acetabular development continues throughout intrauterine life, particularly by means of growth and development of the labrum [39–41].

In the normal hip at birth, the femoral head is deeply seated in the acetabulum and held within the confines of the acetabulum by the surface tension of the synovial fluid. It is extremely difficult to dislocate a normal infant hip, even after incising the hip joint capsule [42, 43]. Hips in newborns with developmental dysplasia are not just normal hips with capsular laxity; they are structurally abnormal. In the infant, the entire proximal end of the femur, including the greater trochanter, the intertrochanteric zone, and the proximal femur, is composed of cartilage. Between the fourth and seventh months of life, the proximal femoral ossification center appears. The bony centrum and its anlage continue to enlarge until adulthood. The proximal femur and the trochanter enlarge by appositional cartilage cell proliferation [44].

The growth areas in the proximal femur are the physeal plate, the growth plate of the greater trochanter, and the femoral neck isthmus [44]. A balance among the growth rates of these centers accounts for the normal configuration of the proximal femur, the relationship between the proximal femur and the greater trochanter, and the overall width of the femoral neck. Growth of the proximal femur is affected by the pull of muscles inserting on the proximal femur, forces being transmitted across the hip joint with weightbearing, normal joint nutrition, normal joint circulation, and normal muscle tone [44–47]. Normal development and subsequent functioning of the hip joint requires a balanced growth of the acetabular and triradiate cartilages as well as a concentrically reduced femoral head. Experimental animal studies and clinical findings in humans with unreduced hip dislocations suggest that the main stimulus for the concave shape of the acetabulum is the presence of a spherical femoral head [48, 49]. Harrison [49] and co-workers determined that the acetabulum failed to deepen in area and depth after femoral head excision in rats. He also demonstrated atrophy and degeneration of the acetabular cartilage [48].

The acetabulum is deepened by the natural pressure from the developing femoral head on the acetabulum [48–51]. The depth of the acetabulum is further enhanced at puberty by the development of three secondary ossification centers [43, 49, 52].

The os acetabulum develops in the thick cartilage that separates the acetabular cavity from the pubis. The os acetabulum is the epiphysis of the pubis and forms the anterior wall of the acetabulum. The epiphysis of the ilium, the acetabular epiphysis, forms a major portion of the superior edge of the acetabulum. A third small epiphysis also forms in the ischial region and contributes to its normal growth.

3.6 Natural History of DDH

The natural history of mild dysplasia and instability noted in the first few weeks of life is typically benign, with up to 88% resolving by 8 weeks of age [53]. However, the natural history of a child's hip that remains subluxated or dislocated by walking age is poor. Normal development of the hip joint depends on a femoral head that is stable and concentrically reduced in the acetabulum, a requirement for both to form spherically. Looseness or laxity within the acetabulum is termed instability. A nonconcentric position is termed subluxation. The deformity of the femoral head and acetabulum is termed dysplasia. With dislocation or severe subluxation, during the second half of infancy and beyond, limited hip abduction occurs, which the parent may notice during diaper change. As the child reaches walking age, a limp and lower-limb-length discrepancy may be apparent.

With maturity and later in adulthood, patients may develop pain and degenerative arthritis in the hip, knee, and low back. Hip dysplasia, subluxation, and dislocation each have their own natural history. Subluxation may not be as well tolerated as dislocation if arthritis develops in early adulthood from excessive cartilage contact pressure. A completely dislocated hip with the femoral head located in the soft tissue may not cause functional problems other than knee or back pain or limp with limb-length discrepancy if the dislocation is unilateral. Completely dislocated hips, if bilateral with the femoral heads located in the soft tissues, may lead to severe waddling gait but can likewise be surprisingly pain free. Dislocated hips in which the femoral head cartilage is in contact with the bony pelvis may develop early arthritis by the fourth or later decades because of excessive wear of the femoral head cartilage on the pelvic bone. When arthritis develops in early adulthood, the burden of disability is high, with many requiring complex hip replacement at an early age. Over time, other diseases of the hip may occur and confound the natural history and outcome. These diseases include trauma to the hip, infection, sickle cell disease, Perthes disease, slipped capital femoral epiphysis, and tuberculosis in resource-poor countries [54].

According to the Center for Disease Control, 25% of Americans will experience symptomatic hip arthritis during their lifetimes, and it has been estimated that 20% to 50% of disease burden is secondary to acetabular dysplasia.

Hip dysplasia refers to an abnormality in development, such as in size, shape, or organization, of the femoral head, acetabulum, or both [55]. These changes may lead to increased contact pressures on the joint and ultimately to hip arthritis [3, 56–59]. However, before the development of frank degenerative changes, many patients become symptomatic secondary to abnormal hip biomechanics, hip instability, impingement, or labral and chondral pathologies [3, 56–58]. These processes arise from increased and abnormal forces across the joint with resultant shear forces causing pathologic changes. Changes classically appear at the anterolateral region of the acetabulum, the posterior region of the femoral head, or the femoral head and neck junction [56].

Eventually, the mechanical hip dysfunction from dysplasia leads to early hip degeneration and osteoarthritis [59]. It has been suggested that there is a direct correlation between the onset of radiographically determined degenerative joint disease and the amount of acetabular dysplasia present [56, 60]. Neonatal hip instability has been associated with a 2.6 times increased risk for total hip replacement in young adulthood in comparison to stable hips [61]. And, one quarter of hip replacements performed in patients aged 40 years or younger are due to underlying hip dysplasia [62].

Studies have demonstrated that acetabular dysplasia leads to degenerative changes over time, likely secondary to mechanical factors and related to increased contact stresses [63–67]. Reduced acetabular size and obliquity create shearing forces on the articular cartilage. These forces lead to chronic overload of the anterior and anterolateral acetabular rim. Eventually, the articular cartilage of the anterior acetabulum and the femoral head fail. Previous reports demonstrate that radiographic degenerative joint disease correlates with the magnitude and length of the excessive pressure [66, 68].

In 2011, Ross [69] and colleagues published their results of arthroscopy in 73 dysplastic hips undergoing periacetabular osteotomies. A labral tear or chondral degeneration was found in 86%

of hips, and 63% of hips demonstrated a hypertrophied labrum. Only 7% of hips were without intra-articular pathology. Labral disease was most common in the anterior (81%) and superolateral (67%) labrochondral junctions. Over two-thirds of patients were found to have acetabular chondromalacia. Acetabular chondral lesions were primarily located at the anterior (76%) and superolateral (84%) labrochondral junctions. Femoral head chondromalacia was seen in only 11% of hips. Sixty-three percent of patients were found to have intra-articular pathology sufficient to require surgical treatment [69].

While there is considerable evidence that radiographic acetabular dysplasia leads to secondary degenerative joint disease [70, 71], there are no predictive radiographic parameters. Cooperman and associates [66] studied 32 dysplastic hips with lateral center edge angles of less than 20° for more than 20 years in order to determine the natural history of acetabular dysplasia. The investigators found that all patients eventually developed radiographic evidence of degenerative joint disease. Moreover, they determined that none of the conventional radiographic parameters used to describe hip dysplasia were able to predict the rate of the degenerative joint disease [66].

3.7 Anatomy in Skeletally Mature Patient

Dysplastic hips often share anatomic abnormalities. The classic dysplastic acetabulum is typically shallow, lateralized, and anteverted [23, 56, 72–76]. The coverage is typically deficient anteriorly, laterally, and superiorly. In some cases, the entire pelvis may be underdeveloped. The dysplastic femur has a small femoral head with excessive femoral neck anteversion and a short neck with an increased neck shaft angle [56, 77–79]. The greater trochanter is often displaced posteriorly and the lesser trochanter assumes a relatively more anterior position. The femoral canal is usually narrow and has been described as a "pipe stem" femur.

As these bony changes develop, the soft tissues also become abnormal. The abductor muscles become oriented more transversely and therefore function less efficiently. The psoas tendon hypertrophies and the hip capsule thickens. In addition, the hamstrings, adductors, and rectus femoris muscles all shorten. These pathologic changes result in abnormalities within the hip joint. As the hip joint becomes less stable, the acetabular labrum initially hypertrophies in an attempt to maintain the femoral head within the acetabulum [3]. Similarly, the ligamentum teres hypertrophies. If chronic shear stress persists, the labral soft tissue compensation will likely fail, and the labrum can be torn away from the acetabular rim, resulting in increased contact forces on the cartilage surfaces [3, 58, 80–84]. Ultimately, these pathologic processes lead to decreased contact area between the femoral head and the acetabulum and lateralization of the center of rotation of the hip. This results in an increased body-weight arm and resultant higher forces transmitted through a smaller surface area, culminating in degenerative hip changes.

3.8 Physical Examination in the Newborn and Infant

A proper examination of infants includes observation for lower-limb-length discrepancy, asymmetric thigh or gluteal folds, Ortolani sign or maneuver, and limited or asymmetric abduction [85]. The Ortolani maneuver, in which a subluxated or dislocated femoral head is gently reduced into the acetabulum with hip abduction by the examiner, is the most important clinical test for detecting dysplasia in the newborn [86]. The Ortolani maneuver is a continuous smooth examination starting with the hip flexed and adducted with gentle anterior pressure on the trochanter followed by gently abducting the hip while sensing whether the hip slips into the acetabulum over the hypertrophied articular cartilage. It answers the essential question: Is the femoral head dislocated and can it be reduced into the acetabulum? The examiner should not forcefully attempt to dislocate the femoral head. Although the Ortolani sign represents the palpable sensation of the femoral head moving into the acetabulum over the hypertrophied rim of the acetabular cartilage (termed the neolimbus), isolated high-pitched clicks represent the movement of myofascial tissues from the trochanter, knee, or other soft tissue [87].

By about 3 months of age, a dislocated hip may become less mobile on physical examination, thus limiting the usefulness and sensitivity of the Ortolani maneuver. However, currently, restricted, asymmetric hip abduction becomes an important finding of hip dysplasia. Diagnosing bilateral DDH in older infants can be difficult because of the symmetry present when there is bilateral limited hip abduction. Other signs of a dislocated hip that are noticeable as infants reach walking age are a proximal thigh crease, a positive Galeazzi sign (in which the hips and knees are flexed 90° and the knee on the dislocated side appears lower), a wider-appearing perineum, a more prominent hip curvature, and a more proximally located posterior knee crease. By walking age, infants may have a delay in walking, a Trendelenburg limp, and a bilateral waddling gait if both hips are dislocated. On the other hand, mild hip dysplasia may have no symptoms or physical findings in infants or older children.

3.9 Physical Examination in Skeletally Mature Patient

Patients who present with hip pain require a thorough history and physical examination to elucidate the source of their symptoms. Patient factors, including age, overall health, activity level, occupation, and illicit habits, should be identified. In addition, a specific hip history should be taken, including family history of hip problems, any known previous hip disease, and any history of prior hip surgery.

Previous hip disease or related treatments, such as childhood and adolescent hip problems, previous hip surgery, hip trauma, and osteonecrosis, may indicate a secondary dysplasia. Pain characteristics need to be thoroughly evaluated. Patients with hip dysplasia may initially present with mild peritrochanteric pain reflecting abductor fatigue, an almost universal finding in prearthritic hip dysplasia in the mature adult [88]. Commonly, patients with dysplasia will have groin pain in the affected hip that is worsened with activity [88]. Similarly, the pattern of symptoms may help elucidate the nature of the dysplasia. Pain worse with weightbearing and activity may indicate underlying joint pathology. Pain with flexion positions or prolonged periods of sitting may commonly be associated with femoroacetabular impingement (FAI). The sensation of locking or catching in the affected joint may indicate intra-articular mechanical problems, such as labral tear, chondral flap, or loose body.

Nunley [89] and colleagues examined 57 patients with known hip dysplasia. Ninety-seven percent of their patients reported an insidious onset of hip pain without an inciting event. Seventy-two percent of these patients localized their pain to the groin. Eighty-eight percent of patients noted activity-related pain with 81% reporting that their symptoms were exacerbated by walking and 80% while running. At least one mechanical symptom was reported by 80% of their patients. Almost half of the studied patients reported a limp. Night pain was also found in more than half of the patients [89].

The physical examination of the patient with suspected hip dysplasia should consider general condition and body habitus, the patient's sitting posture, and their gait pattern. It is also important to assess for a leg length discrepancy. Standing measurements will allow an assessment of pelvic balance and are therefore considered the best way to assess a leg length discrepancy [88, 90].

Resting lower extremity rotation should be assessed with the patient lying supine on the exam table. Normal lower extremity rotation is between 10° and 30° of external rotation. Abnormal rotation may result from abnormal acetabular version, abnormal femoral version, or femoral head-neck abnormalities [88].

Hip range of motion testing is essential for not only diagnosis but also for pre-procedure planning [91]. The examiner should steady the pelvis with one hand while performing range of motion testing, including hip flexion and internal and external rotation both in 90° of flexion and full extension.

In contrast to classic FAI, which may demonstrate restricted hip flexion and internal rotation, patients with classic dysplasia will generally demonstrate normal hip flexion and normal internal rotation [81, 92, 93].

Some special tests may help elucidate the nature of the hip pathology. The anterior impingement test is a special maneuver that is indicative of disorders of the anterior acetabular rim [94, 95]. It is very sensitive for a range of anterior hip lesions, including labral tears and rim fractures, but fairly non-specific for intra-articular disease and joint irritability [94]. The patient is placed supine, and the affected extremity is passively flexed, adducted and internally rotated. The test is considered positive if this maneuver reproduces the patient's pain. Nunley reported that 97% of the patients in his study had a positive impingement sign [89]. The apprehension test is another special maneuver that is useful to assess for anterior hip instability, though it may be positive in patients with labral lesions as well. It is performed by having the patient lie supine on the table. The affected extremity is extended and rapidly externally rotated. The test is considered positive if it elicits apprehension or anterior hip pain.

Finally, patients should be assessed for hip abductor weakness. The Trendelenburg sign is elicited if the patient leans away from the affected extremity during single legged stance on the affected extremity. Nunley reported that 38% of patients in his study had a positive Trendelenburg sign [89]. Alternatively, abductor strength can be tested by having the patient lie on his unaffected side and asking him to abduct the leg against resistance.

3.10 Imaging of DDH in the Newborn and Infant

Plain radiography becomes most useful by 4 to 6 months of age, when the femoral head's secondary center of ossification (ossific nucleus) forms, a finding that occurs earlier in female infants [96]. A single anteroposterior (AP) view of the entire pelvis is obtained, with positioning of the pelvis without rotation. Acetabular dysplasia, subluxation, and dislocation are easily detected on the radiographs if taken after the femoral head's ossific nucleus has appeared. If subluxation or dislocation is noted, an AP view of the pelvis with the hips abducted can be done to document hip reducibility. However, there is debate whether minor radiographic variability in young infants (increased acetabular index) constitutes actual disease [97]. Radiographic hip screening is traditionally indicated for infants with risk factors, such as a history of breech presentation or an abnormal physical examination at 4 months of age [85, 98–100]. An AP radiograph of the pelvis is obtained in newborns or infants if other conditions, such as congenital short femur, proximal focal femoral deficiency, septic hip infection, or coxa vara, are suspected.

The American Institute of Ultrasound in Medicine (AIUM) and the American College of Radiology (ACR) have published a joint guideline for the standardized performance of the infantile hip ultrasound [101]. Ultrasonography can provide detailed static and dynamic imaging of the hip before femoral head ossification. Ultrasound hip imaging can be universal for all infants or selective for those at risk for having DDH. Because disease prevalence is low at 1% to 2%, universal ultrasound screening is not generally practiced in North America or in countries with limited resources. Many barriers to successful ultrasound screening programs in the United States include expense, lack of availability, lack of trained personnel to assure quality imaging and interpretation, inconvenience, subjectivity, a high false-positive rate, and controversy about effectiveness.

Universal ultrasound screening of all infants is practiced in many European countries, with programs typically showing a decrease in the number of hips needing surgical reduction after their programs were begun. Most recently, a large randomized controlled study of universal or selective ultrasound screening in Norway that was compared with a well-done physical examination showed higher treatment rates but no significant decrease in late cases of DDH [102]. This same group of patients who underwent ultrasound screening and were followed to skeletal maturity did not have less acetabular dysplasia or degenerative change, although there was also no increased rate of avascular necrosis [102]. Despite this screening program for DDH, 92% of young adults with hip dysplasia who required a total hip arthroplasty were not detected at birth [61]. Results of these quality studies indicate that a well-performed physical examination in infants is the most important means of detecting instability; however, dysplasia is currently undetectable at birth for many adults.

In countries with very limited resources, even selective ultrasound screening is not typically available. The lack of ultrasound screening in low-income countries does not necessarily restrict the delivery of quality care for detecting and treating DDH. In these countries, primary prevention through education about proper swaddling, early detection with a properly performed physical examination by trained health care workers, and early safe conservative treatment are the basis of an effective DDH program. Despite successful early prevention, undetected genetically determined acetabular dysplasia may still present in the young adult [9].

Ultrasound screening should not be performed before 3 to 4 weeks of age in infants with clinical signs or risk factors for DDH because of the normal physiologic laxity that typically resolves by 6 weeks of age [101]. Most minor sonographic hip anomalies seen at 4 weeks to 4 months of age will resolve spontaneously. These anomalies include minor changes in morphology and subluxation (uncoverage) with stress maneuvers. Proper timing, performance, and interpretation of infantile hip ultrasound imaging per the guidelines of the AIUM and the ACR are critical to avoid undertreatment or overtreatment.

If available, ultrasound imaging can be used to guide the reduction of a dislocated hip in infants who are being treated in a Pavlik harness or other hip abduction orthosis. With the current medicolegal climate that fosters defensive medicine, widespread ultrasonography has become the default ordered test, resulting in excessive referral and treatment as well as poor use of limited resources for infants with very mild dysplasia or laxity [103, 104]. Developing local/regional criteria for screening imaging and referral based on best resources, especially for ultrasonography, should promote more uniform and cost-effective treatment.

3.11 Screening for Developmental Dysplasia of the Hip

Screening for DDH is important because the condition may be initially occult, is easily treated when caught early, but difficult to treat later. When detected late, it may lead to long-term disability. Although detection in the neonatal period is ideal, a reasonable goal is to detect the subluxated or dislocated hip by 6 months of age. The physical examination is by far the most important means of detection. Radiography or sonography imaging should be used to confirm the suspicion of DDH. Despite all current methods of screening for DDH, most young adults with dysplasia who require a hip arthroplasty are not detected at birth [61].

3.12 Imaging of DDH in in Skeletally Mature Patient

The evaluation of a patient with suspected hip dysplasia is confirmed with imaging. The radiographic features of adult hip dysplasia may range from subtle acetabular dysplasia to complete dislocation of the femoral head from the native acetabulum. The goals of imaging are to assess the structural anatomy of the hip, determine the congruency of the articulation, examine the integrity of the joint space, and to assess the soft tissues [93].

The anterior-posterior (AP) view of the pelvis is the single most important view for defining acetabular coverage of the femoral head, femoral head sphericity [105], the contour of the femoral head-neck junction, the height of the greater trochanter, position of the joint center, the joint space, and Shenton's line.

Lateral radiographs allow better definition of the osseous anatomy of the proximal femur, anterior and posterior joint spaces, and the acetabular rim. Lateral radiographs include the cross table lateral and frog lateral. Also, among the lateral views is the false profile view [106]. This image is obtained by having the patient stand with their foot parallel to the radiographic plate and their pelvis rotated 65° relative to the film. This view constitutes a true lateral view of the acetabulum. It allows measurement of the anterior coverage of the acetabulum and may also allow better detection of the degenerative changes that tend to begin at the anterior aspect of the joint.

Computer tomography (CT) is a complementary study in evaluating hip dysplasia when dysplastic signs have been recognized on plain films and surgical correction is anticipated. It allows reliable measurements of acetabular coverage, femoral neck anteversion, and the appearance and position of the femoral head [107]. It also allows better characterization of osseous impingement lesions [59, 93].

Magnetic resonance imaging (MRI) is not routinely necessary in hips with obvious structural abnormalities. It may assist in the evaluation of a painful hip in the absence of structural osseous abnormalities and can be useful in the diagnosis of osteonecrosis of the femoral head, stress fracture, neoplasm, or infection. MRI and MRI arthrogram are useful adjuvants to evaluate the labrum and should be obtained in patients with mechanical symptoms.

3.13 Treatment

The earlier DDH is detected, the simpler and more effective the treatment is. The type of treatment is dependent upon the age of diagnosis. When detected early, non-surgical treatment with a harness or cast is possible. The primary aim of this treatment is to achieve a stable concentric reduction of the hip to enable normal joint development. A harness dynamically positions the hips in flexion and abduction while allowing motion. A complication of this non-surgical treatment is avascular necrosis of the hip (AVN). When DDH is detected late, it can be necessary to consider reorientation acetabular or combined femoral and acetabular osteotomies. If DDH is not treated it may lead to juvenile arthritis and lifelong gait problems, in those stages a total hip replacement should be considered.

References

1. Furnes O, Lie SA, Espehaug B, et al. Hip disease and the prognosis of total hip replacements. A review of 53,698 primary total hip replacements reported to the Norwegian Arthroplasty Register 1987-99. J Bone Joint Surg Br. 2001;83:579–86. https://doi.org/10.1302/0301-620x.83b4.11223.
2. Klisic PJ. Congenital dislocation of the hip--a misleading term: brief report. J Bone Joint Surg Br. 1989;71:136.
3. Aronsson DD, Goldberg MJ, Kling TF, Roy DR. Developmental dysplasia of the hip. Pediatrics. 1994;94:201–8.
4. Bracken J, Tran T, Ditchfield M. Developmental dysplasia of the hip: controversies and current concepts. J Paediatr Child Health. 2012;48:963–72; quiz 972–973. https://doi.org/10.1111/j.1440-1754.2012.02601.x.
5. Schwend RM, Shaw BA, Segal LS. Evaluation and treatment of developmental hip dysplasia in the newborn and infant. Pediatr Clin N Am. 2014;61:1095–107. https://doi.org/10.1016/j.pcl.2014.08.008.
6. Roper A. Hip dysplasia in the African Bantu. J Bone Joint Surg Br. 1976;58:155–8.
7. Haasbeek JF, Wright JG, Hedden DM. Is there a difference between the epidemiologic characteristics of hip dislocation diagnosed early and late? Can J Surg. 1995;38:437–8.
8. Pratt WB, Freiberger RH, Arnold WD. Untreated congenital hip dysplasia in the Navajo. Clin Orthop Relat Res. 1982;162:69–77.
9. Schwend RM, Pratt WB, Fultz J. Untreated acetabular dysplasia of the hip in the Navajo. A 34 year case series followup. Clin Orthop Relat Res. 1999;364:108–16. https://doi.org/10.1097/00003086-199907000-00015.
10. Kremli MK, Alshahid AH, Khoshhal KI, Zamzam MM. The pattern of developmental dysplasia of the hip. Saudi Med J. 2003;24:1118–20.
11. Kutlu A, Memik R, Mutlu M, et al. Congenital dislocation of the hip and its relation to swaddling used in Turkey. J Pediatr Orthop. 1992;12:598–602.
12. Ishida K. Prevention of the development of the typical dislocation of the hip. Clin Orthop Relat Res. 1977;126:167–9.
13. Cady RB. Developmental dysplasia of the hip: definition, recognition, and prevention of late

sequelae. Pediatr Ann. 2006;35:92–101. https://doi.org/10.3928/0090-4481-20060201-09.
14. Chan A, McCaul KA, Cundy PJ, et al. Perinatal risk factors for developmental dysplasia of the hip. Arch Dis Child Fetal Neonatal Ed. 1997;76:F94–100. https://doi.org/10.1136/fn.76.2.f94.
15. Yiv BC, Saidin R, Cundy PJ, et al. Developmental dysplasia of the hip in South Australia in 1991: prevalence and risk factors. J Paediatr Child Health. 1997;33:151–6. https://doi.org/10.1111/j.1440-1754.1997.tb01019.x.
16. Leck I. An epidemiological assessment of neonatal screening for dislocation of the hip. J R Coll Physicians Lond. 1986;20:56–62.
17. Tachdjian MO. Tachdjian's pediatric orthopaedics. Philadelphia: WB Saunders Company; 2002.
18. Bache CE, Clegg J, Herron M. Risk factors for developmental dysplasia of the hip: ultrasonographic findings in the neonatal period. J Pediatr Orthop B. 2002;11:212–8.
19. Forst J, Forst C, Forst R, Heller KD. Pathogenetic relevance of the pregnancy hormone relaxin to inborn hip instability. Arch Orthop Trauma Surg. 1997;116:209–12. https://doi.org/10.1007/bf00393711.
20. Yamamuro T, Ishida K. Recent advances in the prevention, early diagnosis, and treatment of congenital dislocation of the hip in Japan. Clin Orthop Relat Res. 1984;184:34–40.
21. Rosendahl K, Markestad T, Lie RT. Ultrasound screening for developmental dysplasia of the hip in the neonate: the effect on treatment rate and prevalence of late cases. Pediatrics. 1994;94:47–52.
22. US Preventive Services Task Force. Screening for developmental dysplasia of the hip: recommendation statement. Pediatrics. 2006;117:898–902. https://doi.org/10.1542/peds.2005-1995.
23. Salter RB. Etiology, pathogenesis and possible prevention of congenital dislocation of the hip. Can Med Assoc J. 1968;98:933–45.
24. Wynne-Davies R. Acetabular dysplasia and familial joint laxity: two etiological factors in congenital dislocation of the hip. A review of 589 patients and their families. J Bone Joint Surg Br. 1970;52:704–16.
25. Wynne-Davies R. A family study of neonatal and late-diagnosis congenital dislocation of the hip. J Med Genet. 1970;7:315–33.
26. Czeizel A, Szentpétery J, Tusnády G, Vizkelety T. Two family studies on congenital dislocation of the hip after early orthopaedic screening Hungary. J Med Genet. 1975;12:125–30.
27. Stevenson DA, Mineau G, Kerber RA, et al. Familial predisposition to developmental dysplasia of the hip. J Pediatr Orthop. 2009;29:463–6. https://doi.org/10.1097/BPO.0b013e3181aa586b.
28. Bjerkreim I, van der Hagen CB. Congenital dislocation of the hip joint in Norway. V. Evaluation of genetic and environmental factors. Clin Genet. 1974;5:433–48.
29. Dunn PM. Congenital postural deformities. Br Med Bull. 1976;32:71–6. https://doi.org/10.1093/oxfordjournals.bmb.a071327.
30. Mahan ST, Kasser JR. Does swaddling influence developmental dysplasia of the hip? Pediatrics. 2008;121:177–8. https://doi.org/10.1542/peds.2007-1618.
31. Shipman SA, Helfand M, Moyer VA, Yawn BP. Screening for developmental dysplasia of the hip: a systematic literature review for the US Preventive Services Task Force. Pediatrics. 2006;117:e557–76. https://doi.org/10.1542/peds.2005-1597.
32. von Heideken J, Green DW, Burke SW, et al. The relationship between developmental dysplasia of the hip and congenital muscular torticollis. J Pediatr Orthop. 2006;26:805–8. https://doi.org/10.1097/01.bpo.0000235398.41913.51.
33. Tien YC, Su JY, Lin GT, Lin SY. Ultrasonographic study of the coexistence of muscular torticollis and dysplasia of the hip. J Pediatr Orthop. 2001;21:343–7.
34. Cheng JC, Tang SP, Chen TM. Sternocleidomastoid pseudotumor and congenital muscular torticollis in infants: a prospective study of 510 cases. J Pediatr. 1999;134:712–6. https://doi.org/10.1016/s0022-3476(99)70286-6.
35. Screening for the detection of congenital dislocation of the hip. Arch Dis Child. 1986;61:921–6. https://doi.org/10.1136/adc.61.9.921.
36. Paton RW, Choudry Q. Neonatal foot deformities and their relationship to developmental dysplasia of the hip: an 11-year prospective, longitudinal observational study. J Bone Joint Surg Br. 2009;91:655–8. https://doi.org/10.1302/0301-620X.91B5.22117.
37. Westberry DE, Davids JR, Pugh LI. Clubfoot and developmental dysplasia of the hip: value of screening hip radiographs in children with clubfoot. J Pediatr Orthop. 2003;23:503–7.
38. Lee J, Jarvis J, Uhthoff HK, Avruch L. The fetal acetabulum. A histomorphometric study of acetabular anteversion and femoral head coverage. Clin Orthop Relat Res. 1992;281:48–55.
39. Strayer LM. The embryology of the human hip joint. Yale J Biol Med. 1943;16:13–26.6.
40. Strayer LM. Embryology of he human hip joint. Clin Orthop Relat Res. 1971;74:221–40.
41. Watanabe RS. Embryology of the human hip. Clin Orthop Relat Res. 1974;98:8–26. https://doi.org/10.1097/00003086-197401000-00003.
42. Dunn PM. The anatomy and pathology of congenital dislocation of the hip. Clin Orthop Relat Res. 1976;119:23–7.
43. Ponseti IV. Morphology of the acetabulum in congenital dislocation of the hip. Gross, histological and roentgenographic studies. J Bone Joint Surg Am. 1978;60:586–99.
44. Siffert RS. Patterns of deformity of the developing hip. Clin Orthop Relat Res. 1981;160:14–29.
45. Gage JR, Cary JM. The effects of trochanteric epiphyseodesis on growth of the proximal end of

the femur following necrosis of the capital femoral epiphysis. J Bone Joint Surg Am. 1980;62:785–94.
46. Osborne D, Effmann E, Broda K, Harrelson J. The development of the upper end of the femur, with special reference to its internal architecture. Radiology. 1980;137:71–6. https://doi.org/10.1148/radiology.137.1.7422864.
47. Sugano N, Noble PC, Kamaric E, et al. The morphology of the femur in developmental dysplasia of the hip. J Bone Joint Surg Br. 1998;80:711–9. https://doi.org/10.1302/0301-620x.80b4.8319.
48. Harrison TJ. The influence of the femoral head on pelvic growth and acetabular form in the rat. J Anat. 1961;95:12–24.2.
49. Harrison TJ. The growth of the pelvis in the rat—a mensural and morphological study. J Anat. 1958;92:236–260.3.
50. Coleman CR, Slager RF, Smith WS. The effect of environmental influence on acetabular development. Surg Forum. 1958;9:775–80.
51. Smith WS, Ireton RJ, Coleman CR. Sequelae of experimental dislocation of a weight-bearing ball-and socket joint in a young growing animal; gross alterations in bone and cartilage. J Bone Joint Surg Am. 1958;40-A:1121–7.
52. Weinstein SL. Natural history of congenital hip dislocation (CDH) and hip dysplasia. Clin Orthop Relat Res. 1987;225:62–76.
53. Barlow TG. Early diagnosis and treatment of congenital dislocation of the hip. J Bone Joint Surg Br. 1962;44-B:292–301. https://doi.org/10.1302/0301-620X.44B2.292.
54. Oniankitan O, Kakpovi K, Fianyo E, et al. Risk factors of hip osteoarthritis in Lomé, Togo. Med Trop (Mars). 2009;69:59–60.
55. Guille JT, Pizzutillo PD, MacEwen GD. Development dysplasia of the hip from birth to six months. J Am Acad Orthop Surg. 2000;8:232–42.
56. Sanchez-Sotelo J, Trousdale RT, Berry DJ, Cabanela ME. Surgical treatment of developmental dysplasia of the hip in adults: I. Nonarthroplasty options. J Am Acad Orthop Surg. 2002;10:321–33.
57. Felson DT. Risk factors for osteoarthritis: understanding joint vulnerability. Clin Orthop Relat Res. 2004;427(Suppl):S16–21. https://doi.org/10.1097/01.blo.0000144971.12731.a2.
58. Wenger DE, Kendell KR, Miner MR, Trousdale RT. Acetabular labral tears rarely occur in the absence of bony abnormalities. Clin Orthop Relat Res. 2004;426:145–50. https://doi.org/10.1097/01.blo.0000136903.01368.20.
59. Clohisy JC, Beaulé PE, O'Malley A, et al. AOA symposium. Hip disease in the young adult: current concepts of etiology and surgical treatment. J Bone Joint Surg Am. 2008;90:2267–81. https://doi.org/10.2106/JBJS.G.01267.
60. Murphy SB, Ganz R, Müller ME. The prognosis in untreated dysplasia of the hip. A study of radiographic factors that predict the outcome. J Bone Joint Surg Am. 1995;77:985–9. https://doi.org/10.2106/00004623-199507000-00002.
61. Engesaeter IØ, Lie SA, Lehmann TG, et al. Neonatal hip instability and risk of total hip replacement in young adulthood: follow-up of 2,218,596 newborns from the medical birth registry of Norway in the Norwegian Arthroplasty Register. Acta Orthop. 2008;79:321–6. https://doi.org/10.1080/17453670710015201.
62. Engesæter IØ, Lehmann T, Laborie LB, et al. Total hip replacement in young adults with hip dysplasia. Acta Orthop. 2011;82:149–54. https://doi.org/10.3109/17453674.2011.566146.
63. Milgram JW. Morphology of untreated bilateral congenital dislocation of the hips in a seventy-four-year-old man. Clin Orthop Relat Res. 1976;119:112–5.
64. Fairbank JC, Howell P, Nockler I, Lloyd-Roberts GC. Relationship of pain to the radiological anatomy of the hip joint in adults treated for congenital dislocation of the hip as infants: a long-term follow-up of patients treated by three methods. J Pediatr Orthop. 1986;6:539–47. https://doi.org/10.1097/01241398-198609000-00004.
65. Malvitz TA, Weinstein SL. Closed reduction for congenital dysplasia of the hip. Functional and radiographic results after an average of thirty years. J Bone Joint Surg Am. 1994;76:1777–92. https://doi.org/10.2106/00004623-199412000-00004.
66. Cooperman DR, Wallensten R, Stulberg SD. Acetabular dysplasia in the adult. Clin Orthop Relat Res. 1983;175:79–85.
67. Harris WH. Etiology of osteoarthritis of the hip. Clin Orthop Relat Res. 1986;213:20–33.
68. Wiberg G Studies on dysplastic acetabula and congenital subluxation of the hip joint with special reference to the complication of osteoarthritis. Exp., Norstedt; 1939.
69. Ross JR, Zaltz I, Nepple JJ, et al. Arthroscopic disease classification and interventions as an adjunct in the treatment of acetabular dysplasia. Am J Sports Med. 2011;39(Suppl):72S–8S. https://doi.org/10.1177/0363546511412320.
70. Hoaglund FT, Healey JH. Osteoarthrosis and congenital dysplasia of the hip in family members of children who have congenital dysplasia of the hip. J Bone Joint Surg Am. 1990;72:1510–8.
71. Hoaglund FT, Yau AC, Wong WL. Osteoarthritis of the hip and other joints in southern Chinese in Hong Kong. J Bone Joint Surg Am. 1973;55:545–57.
72. Salter RB. Role of innominate osteotomy in the treatment of congenital dislocation and subluxation of the hip in the older child. J Bone Joint Surg Am. 1966;48:1413–39.
73. Lloyd-Roberts GC, Harris NH, Chrispin AR. Anteversion of the acetabulum in congenital dislocation of the hip: a preliminary report. Orthop Clin North Am. 1978;9:89–95.

74. Murphy SB, Kijewski PK, Millis MB, Harless A. Acetabular dysplasia in the adolescent and young adult. Clin Orthop Relat Res. 1990;261:214–23.
75. Wientroub S, Boyde A, Chrispin AR, Lloyd-Roberts GC. The use of stereophotogrammetry to measure acetabular and femoral anteversion. J Bone Joint Surg Br. 1981;63-B:209–13.
76. Mast JW, Brunner RL, Zebrack J. Recognizing acetabular version in the radiographic presentation of hip dysplasia. Clin Orthop Relat Res. 2004;418:48–53. https://doi.org/10.1097/00003086-200401000-00009.
77. Doudoulakis JK, Cavadias A. Open reduction of CDH before one year of age. 69 hips followed for 13 (10-19) years. Acta Orthop Scand. 1993;64:188–92. https://doi.org/10.3109/17453679308994568.
78. Sanchez-Sotelo J, Berry DJ, Trousdale RT, Cabanela ME. Surgical treatment of developmental dysplasia of the hip in adults: II. Arthroplasty options. J Am Acad Orthop Surg. 2002;10:334–44.
79. Perry KI, Berry DJ. Femoral considerations for total hip replacement in hip dysplasia. Orthop Clin North Am. 2012;43:377–86. https://doi.org/10.1016/j.ocl.2012.05.010.
80. Beck M, Kalhor M, Leunig M, Ganz R. Hip morphology influences the pattern of damage to the acetabular cartilage: femoroacetabular impingement as a cause of early osteoarthritis of the hip. J Bone Joint Surg Br. 2005;87:1012–8. https://doi.org/10.1302/0301-620X.87B7.15203.
81. Beck M, Leunig M, Parvizi J, et al. Anterior femoroacetabular impingement: part II. Midterm results of surgical treatment. Clin Orthop Relat Res. 2004;418:67–73.
82. Ito K, Leunig M, Ganz R. Histopathologic features of the acetabular labrum in Femoroacetabular impingement. Clin Orthop Relat Res. 2004;429:262–71.
83. Harris WH, Bourne RB, Oh I. Intra-articular acetabular labrum: a possible etiological factor in certain cases of osteoarthritis of the hip. J Bone Joint Surg Am. 1979;61:510–4.
84. McCarthy JC, Noble PC, Schuck MR, et al. The Otto E. Aufranc award: the role of labral lesions to development of early degenerative hip disease. Clin Orthop Relat Res. 2001;393:25–37. https://doi.org/10.1097/00003086-200112000-00004.
85. Clinical practice guideline: early detection of developmental dysplasia of the hip. Committee on Quality Improvement, Subcommittee on Developmental Dysplasia of the Hip. American Academy of Pediatrics. Pediatrics. 2000;105:896–905. https://doi.org/10.1542/peds.105.4.896.
86. Lipton GE, Guille JT, Altiok H, et al. A reappraisal of the Ortolani examination in children with developmental dysplasia of the hip. J Pediatr Orthop. 2007;27:27–31. https://doi.org/10.1097/BPO.0b013e31802b70e5.
87. Bond CD, Hennrikus WL, DellaMaggiore ED. Prospective evaluation of newborn soft-tissue hip "clicks" with ultrasound. J Pediatr Orthop. 1997;17:199–201. https://doi.org/10.1097/00004694-199703000-00011.
88. Sierra RJ, Trousdale RT, Ganz R, Leunig M. Hip disease in the young, active patient: evaluation and nonarthroplasty surgical options. J Am Acad Orthop Surg. 2008;16:689–703.
89. Nunley RM, Prather H, Hunt D, et al. Clinical presentation of symptomatic acetabular dysplasia in skeletally mature patients. J Bone Joint Surg Am. 2011;93(Suppl 2):17–21. https://doi.org/10.2106/JBJS.J.01735.
90. Sabharwal S, Kumar A. Methods for assessing leg length discrepancy. Clin Orthop Relat Res. 2008;466:2910–22. https://doi.org/10.1007/s11999-008-0524-9.
91. Sankar WN, Laird CT, Baldwin KD. Hip range of motion in children: what is the norm? J Pediatr Orthop. 2012;32:399–405. https://doi.org/10.1097/BPO.0b013e3182519683.
92. Ganz R, Parvizi J, Beck M, et al. Femoroacetabular impingement: a cause for osteoarthritis of the hip. Clin Orthop Relat Res. 2003;417:112–20. https://doi.org/10.1097/01.blo.0000096804.78689.c2.
93. Clohisy JC, Keeney JA, Schoenecker PL. Preliminary assessment and treatment guidelines for hip disorders in young adults. Clin Orthop Relat Res. 2005;441:168–79. https://doi.org/10.1097/01.blo.0000193511.91643.2a.
94. Hananouchi T, Yasui Y, Yamamoto K, et al. Anterior impingement test for labral lesions has high positive predictive value. Clin Orthop Relat Res. 2012;470:3524–9. https://doi.org/10.1007/s11999-012-2450-0.
95. Clohisy JC, Knaus ER, Hunt DM, et al. Clinical presentation of patients with symptomatic anterior hip impingement. Clin Orthop Relat Res. 2009;467:638–44. https://doi.org/10.1007/s11999-008-0680-y.
96. Scoles PV, Boyd A, Jones PK. Roentgenographic parameters of the normal infant hip. J Pediatr Orthop. 1987;7:656–63.
97. Mladenov K, Dora C, Wicart P, Seringe R. Natural history of hips with borderline acetabular index and acetabular dysplasia in infants. J Pediatr Orthop. 2002;22:607–12.
98. Imrie M, Scott V, Stearns P, et al. Is ultrasound screening for DDH in babies born breech sufficient? J Child Orthop. 2010;4:3–8. https://doi.org/10.1007/s11832-009-0217-2.
99. Karmazyn BK, Gunderman RB, Coley BD, et al. ACR appropriateness criteria® on developmental dysplasia of the hip—child. J Am Coll Radiol. 2009;6:551–7. https://doi.org/10.1016/j.jacr.2009.04.008.

100. Schwend RM, Schoenecker P, Richards BS, et al. Screening the newborn for developmental dysplasia of the hip: now what do we do? J Pediatr Orthop. 2007;27:607–10. https://doi.org/10.1097/BPO.0b013e318142551e.
101. American Institute of Ultrasound in Medicine, American College of Radiology. AIUM practice guideline for the performance of an ultrasound examination for detection and assessment of developmental dysplasia of the hip. J Ultrasound Med. 2009;28:114–9. https://doi.org/10.7863/jum.2009.28.1.114.
102. Laborie LB, Engesæter IØ, Lehmann TG, et al. Screening strategies for hip dysplasia: long-term outcome of a randomized controlled trial. Pediatrics. 2013;132:492–501. https://doi.org/10.1542/peds.2013-0911.
103. Elbourne D, Dezateux C, Arthur R, et al. Ultrasonography in the diagnosis and management of developmental hip dysplasia (UK hip trial): clinical and economic results of a multicentre randomised controlled trial. Lancet. 2002;360:2009–17. https://doi.org/10.1016/s0140-6736(02)12024-1.
104. Moore FH. Examining infants' hips--can it do harm? J Bone Joint Surg Br. 1989;71:4–5.
105. Eijer H, Myers SR, Ganz R. Anterior femoroacetabular impingement after femoral neck fractures. J Orthop Trauma. 2001;15:475–81. https://doi.org/10.1097/00005131-200109000-00003.
106. Lequesne M, de Seze. False profile of the pelvis. A new radiographic incidence for the study of the hip. Its use in dysplasias and different coxopathies. Rev Rhum Mal Osteoartic. 1961;28:643–52.
107. Klaue K, Wallin A, Ganz R. CT evaluation of coverage and congruency of the hip prior to osteotomy. Clin Orthop Relat Res. 1988;232:15–25.

4 Safe Surgical Dislocation of the Hip: Anatomic Preconditions, Technique, and Results

Reinhold Ganz and Antonio Campacci

4.1 Introduction

The premises of a well-functioning and long-lasting hip joint are based on its morphological geometry. Joint stability, as well as its shape, represent the conditions to allow infinite movement cycles without suffering a significant cartilage wear. While for insufficient coverage of the femoral head, overload is the damaging mechanism, in case of aberration of the head contour as well as with malorientation of proximal femur and acetabulum, motion is the damaging cause; chronicity and velocity of motion defines the speed of joint damage. The mechanism is called femoro-acetabular impingement (FAI). Adaptation to the anomalous kinematic conditions of the hip can further induce pain and morphological alterations both of tendons and muscular insertions around the hip. Understanding of FAI is the prerequisite to develop new surgical techniques but also to prevent early damage of the hip joint.

R. Ganz (✉)
Faculty of Medicine, University of Bern, Bern, Switzerland

A. Campacci
Dipartimento di ortopedia e traumatologia, Ospedale Sacro Cuore Don Calabria, Negrar (VR), Italy

4.2 Anatomic Preconditions

Beside THR, surgical dislocation of the hip was rarely executed and when, it was reported to be hazardous for avascular necrosis of the femoral head. Some favored a posterior approach as less dangerous [1, 2], in the experience of others the anterior approach was accompanied with a lower rate of necrosis [3]. The paper of Gautier et al. [4] based upon the doctoral thesis of Ganz and Krügel [5]. provided sufficient insights (Fig. 4.1) that a surgical dislocation of the hip could be executed safely [6], although the findings of the study were criticized as "perpetuated fallacies" [7].

It could be demonstrated that relatively peripheral anastomoses exist between the deep branch of the MFCA and the inferior and superior gluteal artery, which eventually could replace the supply coming from the deep branch (Fig. 4.2). These important findings may allow to save the natural hip joint in cases where the deep branch has to be sacrificed, e.g., for a radical tumor resection. Furthermore, the dissections demonstrated that the intact muscle and tendon of the obturator externus limit the distance of head dislocation and hereby protect the deep branch of the MFCA from being overstretched or even ruptured in case of dislocation [4] (Fig. 4.3).

More recent dissections revealed that variations in the blood supply to the femoral head exist in about 15% of the specimens. In addition, they highlighted the fact that the medial sector of the head has an independent and constant supply

R. Ganz (ed.), *Modern Hip Preservation*, https://doi.org/10.1007/978-3-030-91967-2_4

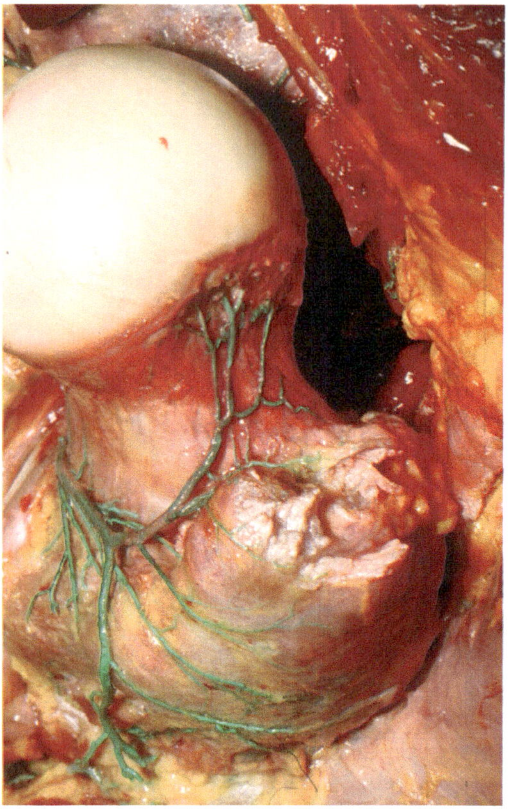

Fig. 4.1 (From Ganz K, Krügel N, 1997 [5]) Course of the deep branch of the MFCA along the intertrochanteric crest to the postero-superior neck where it arborizes into 3–5 retinacular branches which finally perforate the bone about 3–5 mm away from the femoral head cartilage

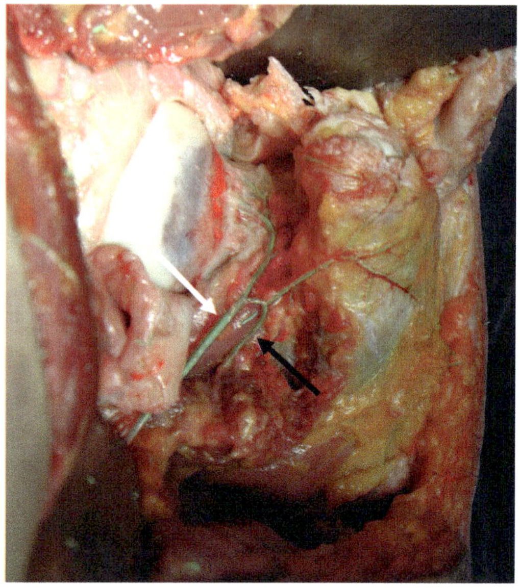

Fig. 4.2 Important anastomoses mainly from the inferior gluteal artery (*white arrow*) can replace the head perfusion from the deep branch (*black arrow*)

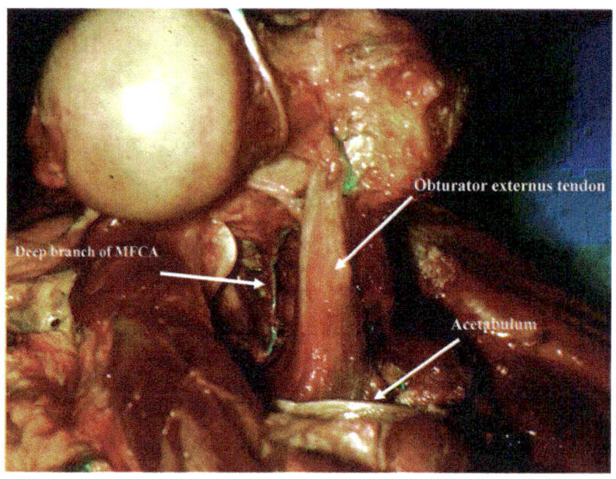

Fig. 4.3 Intact obturator externus muscle and tendon protect the deep branch of the MFCA (*Medial Femoral Circumflex Artery*) from being overstretched or ruptured during femoral head dislocation (*arrows*)

coming from a direct branch of the MFCA [8, 9]. This vessel runs on top of Weitbrecht's ligament and ensures for example the viability of a Pipkin femoral head fragment (Fig. 4.4).

Surgical hip dislocation is a trans-trochanteric flip approach to the joint followed by an anterior dislocation of the femoral head allowing visual control of 360° of the acetabulum and nearly 360° of the femoral head (Fig. 4.5). The dissection follows anatomical intervals and approach-related complications are rare [6, 10]; avascular necrosis was observed only anecdotally and could be explained with injury to the retinacular vessels due to a trochanteric osteotomy reaching into the superior neck contour [6, 10]. When trochanteric advancement is not required, a step osteotomy increases the stability of fixation and allows earlier full weight bearing [11, 12]. Surgical hip dislocation was the requisite to identify the morphological abnormalities and the mechanism of the intra-articular impact leading to the formulation of the femoro-acetabular impingement (FAI), which today is understood as a major initiator of OA besides residual acetabular dysplasia [13, 14]. In addition, surgical hip dislocation became the workhorse for a new generation of intracapsular osteotomies and other procedures [15–19], a quality which was already expressed as a desire in the foreword of Crock's book on the vascular anatomy of the skeleton and spinal cord, where in the prologue the following is mentioned: "Theoretically a method is required by which the human hip joint can be dislocated a-traumatically in the early phases of disease so that the blood supply of the upper end of the femur can be preserved. This would open the way… to treat significant intra-articular pathology, a treatment philosophy based on biologic and physiologic principles could be more routinely used" [20].

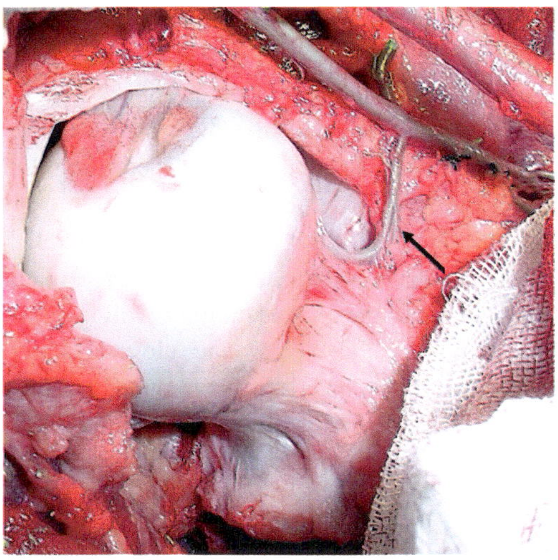

Fig. 4.4 Anterior branch of the MFCA on Weitbrecht's ligament (*black arrow*)

4.3 Surgical Technique

The patient is placed in lateral decubitus with mobile draping of the leg. Today we prefer a longitudinally incision centered on the greater trochanter instead of an angulated Kocher-Langenbeck incision (Fig. 4.6).

The gluteus maximus is not split but retracted posteriorly after release of its anterior border from the fascia lata. The gliding tissue over the

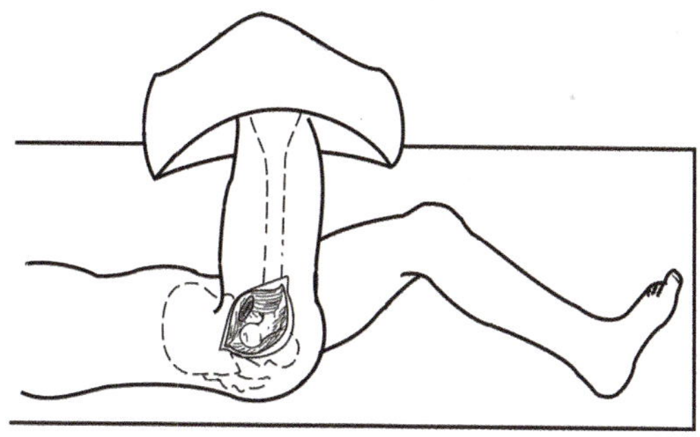

Fig. 4.5 (Modified from Ganz et al. [6]) Drawings showing the leg placed in a sterile bag on the opposite side of the table while acetabulum and femoral head can be inspected after dislocation

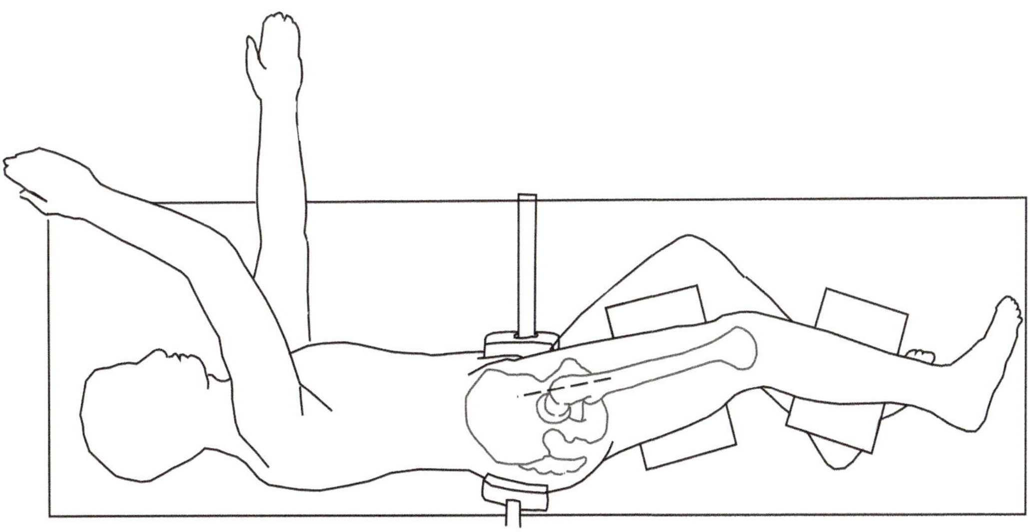

Fig. 4.6 Patients position on the table with the leg draped mobile for a straight (*broken line*) or angulated skin incision

greater trochanter is incised and retracted anteriorly and posteriorly allowing identification of the gluteus medius border and the trochanteric branch of the medial femoral circumflex artery (MFCA) (Fig. 4.7).

Next step is the digastric osteotomy of the greater trochanter resulting in a thickness of the mobile piece of about 1.5 cm and leaving all external rotators attached to the stable portion of the trochanter (Fig. 4.8). The trochanteric fragment is gradually mobilized anteriorly including the attached insertions of gluteus medius, vastus lateralis, and long tendon of gluteus minimus.

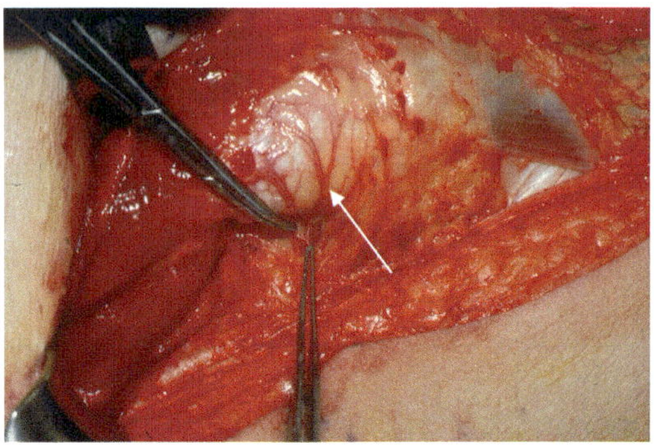

Fig. 4.7 The trochanteric arborization of the deep branch (*arrow*) allows to identify the level of the deep branch even when it is hidden behind fatty tissue

Exposure of the capsule between piriformis and gluteus minimus muscles does not interfere with the blood supply to the head (Fig. 4.9). After Z-shaped capsulotomy (right side) the femoral head can be sub-luxated using a hook around the calcar femoris. Throughout the capsulotomy care must be taken to preserve the integrity of the acetabular labrum. Joint subluxation allows the insertion of curved scissors to dissect the round ligament before full dislocation can be achieved. With the leg placed in a sterile bag on the opposite side of the table and three retractors placed against the acetabular rim, optimal access to acetabulum and femoral head is possible (Fig. 4.10).

Closure of the capsule should not be tight, a few stiches to re-adapt the flaps are sufficient. The trochanter is normally reattached using 2 or 3 3.5 mm or 4.5 mm screws, depending on the quality and size of the trochanteric fragment. If advancement is to be established, release of the long tendon of the gluteus minimus will facilitate the maneuver. Further wound closure is performed layer by layer with continuous or interrupted sutures; suction drainage is arbitrary.

The procedure allows several extensions: (1) When an additional periacetabular osteotomy is to be performed, the first ischial cut can be executed through the surgical dislocation approach.

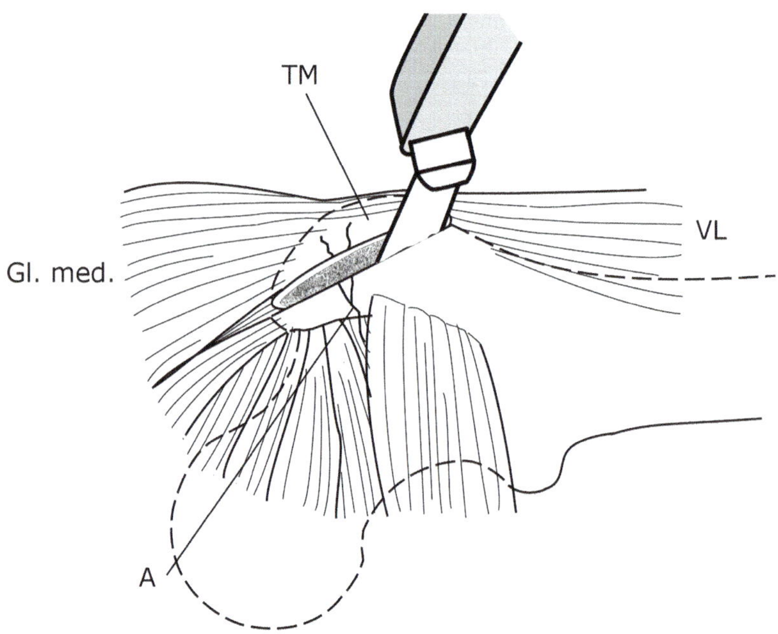

Fig. 4.8 (Modified from Ganz et al. [6]) The trochanteric osteotomy is called digastric although it also includes the long tendon of the gluteus minimus. The fragment should be about 1.5 cm thick. *TM*: Trochanter Major; *VL*: Vastus Lateralis; *Gl. med.*: Gluteus medius; *A*: Artery

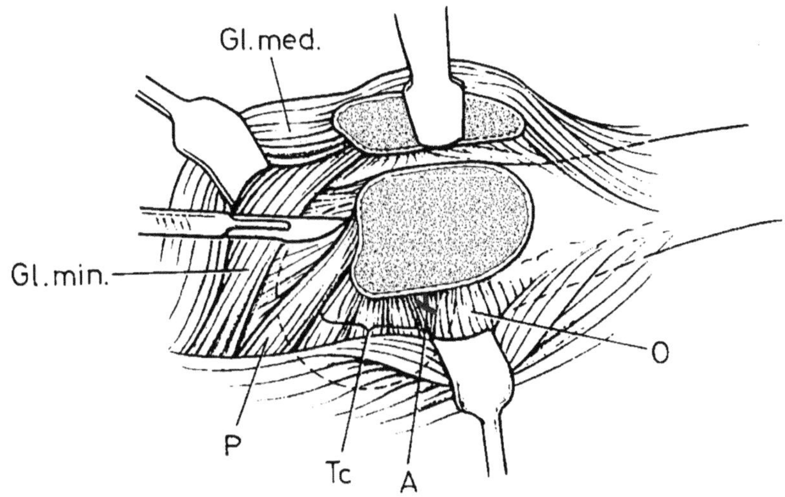

Fig. 4.9 The mobile trochanter is flipped anteriorly and the capsule is exposed between gluteus minimus and piriformis muscles and tendons. *Gl. med.*: Gluteus medius; *Gl.min.*: Gluteus minimus; *P*: Piriformis; *Tc*: Triceps coxae; *A*: Artery; *O*: Obturator Externus

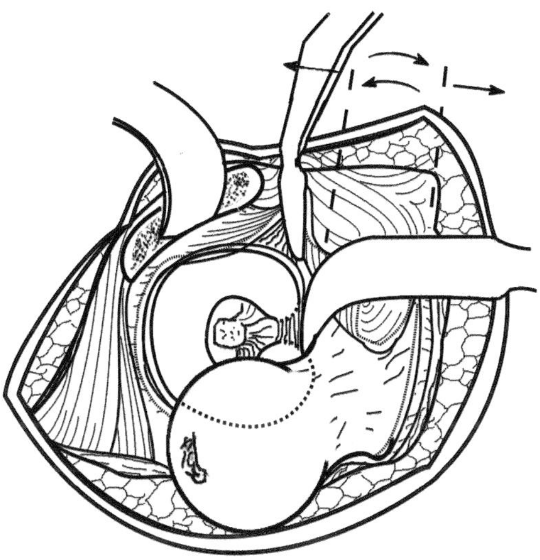

Fig. 4.10 (Modified from Ganz et al. [6]) Full exposure of acetabulum and nearly full exposure of the femoral head using three spiked retractors placed outside the labrum on the superior, anterior, and inferior acetabulum. Further view improvement with rotation of the femur (*arrows*)

The axilla between posterior acetabular lip and tuber ossis ischii is best palpated between gemellus inferior and quadratus femoris muscles. The area is freed from periosteum and the osteotomy performed under visual control of the sciatic nerve (Fig. 4.11) [16]. For better visual orientation of the muscle intervals, the osteotomy should be performed as first step of any procedure with the surgical dislocation approach. (2) Intertrochanteric osteotomy is rarely performed because the trochanteric osteotomy weakens the purchase of the blade of the classic 95° blade plate and application of the plate makes the dissection of the vastus lateralis origin necessary. (3) Sub-trochanteric rotational and/or shortening osteotomy is a frequently performed procedure together with a surgical dislocation [21]. Dissection of the vastus lateralis origin is not necessary; however, skin incision and anterior mobilization of its muscle belly must be more distally extended.

Aftertreatment is determined by the executed surgeries. If osteo-chondroplasty was the only procedure, a step osteotomy of the trochanter can be performed. When the quality of bone is good and the patient reliable, the use of two crutches for restricted weight bearing can be limited to 4 weeks; otherwise 6–8 weeks is the standard period. With individually adapted load restrictions rupture or non-union of the greater trochanter are rare. Routine prophylaxis of heterotopic ossification has also made this complication to be an exception [10].

4.4 Results

Results were reported for approaches and executed procedures. For the first 213 cases [6], the learning curve was short. Sink et al. [10] reported a low morbidity rate based on a multi-center

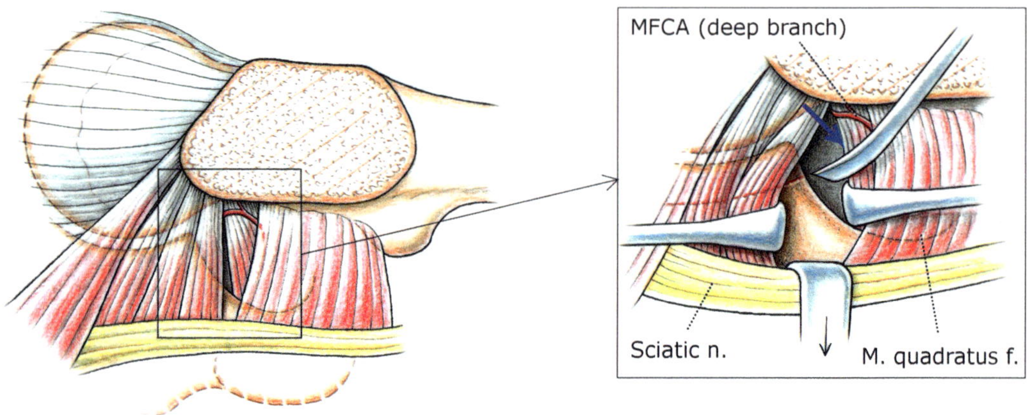

Fig. 4.11 Exposure of the ischial bone between gemellus inferior and quadratus femoris muscles for execution of the first ischial cut of a periacetabular osteotomy (PAO) under visual control of the sciatic nerve. The *blue arrow* points to the obturator externus muscle with the deep branch of the *MFCA* (Medial Femoral Circumflex Artery) which have a more medial course at this level. When approaching the infracotyloid groove the best way to avoid conflict with the vessel is to start the dissection of the gap posteriorly, close to the palpable ischial bone

study. The modification with a step osteotomy increased the stability of fixation, but was only feasible, when trochanter advancement was not necessary [12]. Meanwhile the approach has gained worldwide acceptance and the indication reaches from FAI-treatment in more complex cases [15, 18], relative neck lengthening to epiphyseal, sub capital- and true neck osteotomies [16, 19, 21]· and has gained appreciation for ORIF of femoral head fractures [22, 23].

References

1. Epstein HC. Posterior fracture-dislocations of the hip; long-term follow-up. J Bone Joint Surg Am. 1974;56:1103–27.
2. Epstein HC. Traumatic dislocations of the hip. Clin Orthop. 1973;(92):116–42. https://doi.org/10.1097/00003086-197305000-00011.
3. Swiontkowski MF, Thorpe M, Seiler JG, Hansen ST. Operative management of displaced femoral head fractures: case-matched comparison of anterior versus posterior approaches for Pipkin I and Pipkin II fractures. J Orthop Trauma. 1992;6:437–42.
4. Gautier E, Ganz K, Krügel N, et al. Anatomy of the medial femoral circumflex artery and its surgical implications. J Bone Joint Surg Br. 2000;82:679–83. https://doi.org/10.1302/0301-620x.82b5.10426.
5. Ganz K, Krügel N. The medial femoral circumflex artery. Topographical course and anastomoses. Doctoral thesis, Department of Orthopedic Surgery, University of Bern; 1997.
6. Ganz R, Gill TJ, Gautier E, et al. Surgical dislocation of the adult hip a technique with full access to the femoral head and acetabulum without the risk of avascular necrosis. J Bone Joint Surg Br. 2001;83:1119–24. https://doi.org/10.1302/0301-620x.83b8.11964.
7. Crock HV. Anatomy of the medial femoral circumflex artery and its surgical implications. J Bone Joint Surg Br. 2001:83-B:149–149. https://doi.org/10.1302/0301-620X.83B1.0830149.
8. Kalhor M, Horowitz K, Gharehdaghi J, et al. Anatomic variations in femoral head circulation. Hip Int. 2012;22:307–12. https://doi.org/10.5301/HIP.2012.9242.
9. Kalhor M, Beck M, Huff TW, Ganz R. Capsular and pericapsular contributions to acetabular and femoral head perfusion. J Bone Joint Surg Am. 2009;91:409–18. https://doi.org/10.2106/JBJS.G.01679.
10. Sink EL, Beaulé PE, Sucato D, et al. Multicenter study of complications following surgical dislocation of the hip. J Bone Joint Surg Am. 2011;93:1132–6. https://doi.org/10.2106/JBJS.J.00794.
11. Bastian JD, Wolf AT, Wyss TF, Nötzli HP. Stepped osteotomy of the trochanter for stable, anatomic refixation. Clin Orthop. 2009;467:732–8. https://doi.org/10.1007/s11999-008-0649-x.
12. Schoeniger R, LaFrance AE, Oxland TR, et al. Does trochanteric step osteotomy provide greater stability than classic slide osteotomy? A preliminary study. Clin Orthop. 2009;467:775–82. https://doi.org/10.1007/s11999-008-0668-7.
13. Ganz R, Leunig M, Leunig-Ganz K, Harris WH. The etiology of osteoarthritis of the hip: an integrated mechanical concept. Clin Orthop Relat Res. 2008;466:264. https://doi.org/10.1007/s11999-007-0060-z.
14. Ganz R, Parvizi J, Beck M, et al. Femoroacetabular impingement: a cause for osteoarthritis of the hip.

Clin Orthop Relat Res. 2003;(417):112–20. https://doi.org/10.1097/01.blo.0000096804.78689.c2.
15. Espinosa N, Rothenfluh DA, Beck M, et al. Treatment of femoro-acetabular impingement: preliminary results of labral refixation. J Bone Joint Surg Am. 2006;88:925. https://doi.org/10.2106/JBJS.E.00290.
16. Ganz R, Huff TW, Leunig M. Extended retinacular soft-tissue flap for intra-articular hip surgery: surgical technique, indications, and results of application. Instr Course Lect. 2009;58:241–55.
17. Ganz R, Slongo T, Siebenrock KA, et al. Surgical technique: the capsular arthroplasty: a useful but abandoned procedure for young patients with developmental dysplasia of the hip. Clin Orthop. 2012;470:2957–67. https://doi.org/10.1007/s11999-012-2444-y.
18. Lavigne M, Parvizi J, Beck M, et al. Anterior femoroacetabular impingement: part I. Techniques of joint preserving surgery. Clin Orthop. 2004;(418):61–6.
19. Leunig M, Slongo T, Kleinschmidt M, Ganz R. Subcapital correction osteotomy in slipped capital femoral epiphysis by means of surgical hip dislocation. Oper Orthop Traumatol. 2007;19:389–410. https://doi.org/10.1007/s00064-007-1213-7.
20. Crock HV. An atlas of vascular anatomy of the skeleton and spinal cord. London: Dunitz Martin Ltd; 1996.
21. Kamath AF, Ganz R, Zhang H, et al. Subtrochanteric osteotomy for femoral mal-torsion through a surgical dislocation approach. J Hip Preserv Surg. 2015;2:65–79. https://doi.org/10.1093/jhps/hnv011.
22. Massè A, Aprato A, Alluto C, et al. Surgical hip dislocation is a reliable approach for treatment of femoral head fractures. Clin Orthop. 2015;473:3744–51. https://doi.org/10.1007/s11999-015-4352-4.
23. Masse A, Aprato A, Rollero L, et al. Surgical dislocation technique for the treatment of acetabular fractures. Clin Orthop. 2013;471:4056–64. https://doi.org/10.1007/s11999-013-3228-8.

5 Extended Retinacular Flap for Intra-Articular Hip Surgery: Operative Technique and Indications

Reinhold Ganz and Michael Leunig

5.1 Introduction

Classic osteotomies of the proximal femur are executed at an inter- or subtrochanteric level. This is safe with regard to the femoral head perfusion; however, it is creating an undesired secondary deformity with a magnitude depending on the amount of correction and on the distance between osteotomy and joint [1]. An intra-articular osteotomy level could minimize or even avoid these side effects; however, fear of avascular necrosis of the femoral head has excluded this level from regular use in the adult hip. In children with epiphysiolysis and open physis anterior wedge osteotomy of the neck [2, 3], Sugioka's transtrochanteric osteotomy [4, 5] and Dunn's sub-capital realignment [6] have been performed; however, the published rate of necrosis, although small, has not led to a broader acceptance of these techniques [7, 8]. Due to better understanding of the vascular supply to the femoral head and of its extraosseous course [9, 10], safe surgical dislocation of the hip was possible [11] and has meanwhile reached international acceptance due to its versatility and low morbidity [12]. Only Dunn's technique comprises some active dissection of the retinaculum from the neck bone containing the terminal vessel branches of the medial femoral circumflex artery (MFCA) to the femoral head. However, the distance of dissection is limited by the greater trochanter and any manipulation in the very small gap can risk overstretching or even rupture of the retinaculum (Fig. 5.1).

The feasibility of a substantially longer flap opened up with the technique of relative neck lengthening to treat extraarticular impingement between the bone massif of the greater trochanter and the retro acetabular wall [13] (Fig. 5.2). With subperiosteal piece meal resection of the posterior trochanteric bone down to the level of the posterior neck, a flap could be developed containing all external rotators and the periosteum from postero-superior head-neck junction to the lesser trochanter. Further subperiosteal dissection exposes the posterior neck and together with medial subperiosteal dissection free access to the entire circumference of the neck is possible without interfering with the postero-medial and postero-lateral blood supply to the epiphysis.

5.2 Surgical Technique

First step of the procedure is a surgical hip dislocation [11]: In short, the patient is in a lateral decubitus; with a straight incision over the greater trochanter the fascia lata is divided anterior to the gluteus maximus. The muscle belly is retracted posteriorly to expose the posterior borders of

R. Ganz
Faculty of Medicine, University of Bern,
Bern, Switzerland

M. Leunig (✉)
Head of Hip Surgery, CMO, Schultess Klinik,
Zürich, Switzerland
e-mail: leunig.info@kws.ch

R. Ganz (ed.), *Modern Hip Preservation*, https://doi.org/10.1007/978-3-030-91967-2_5

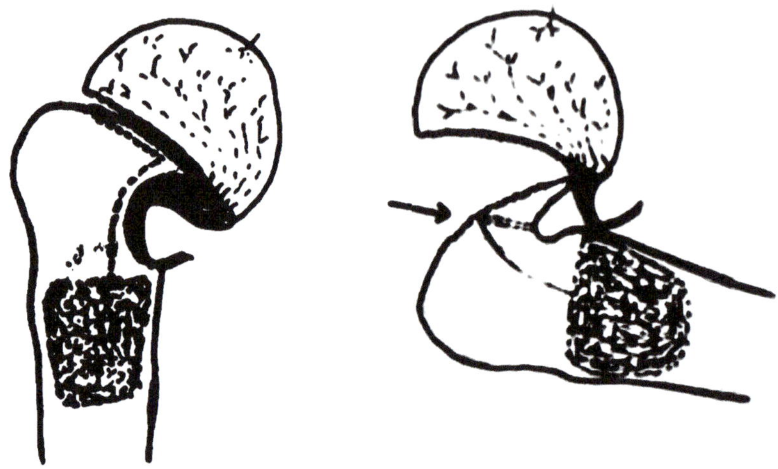

Fig. 5.1 Very short distance of retinacular dissection according to Dunn (from Dunn et al. [6])

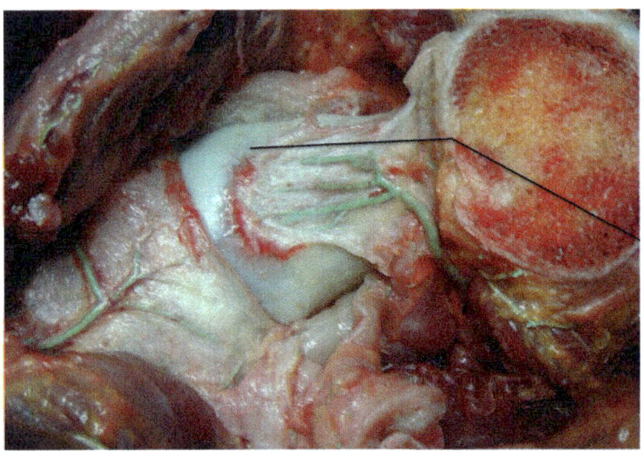

Fig. 5.2 Retinaculum and bone surface after trochanteric osteotomy. The *black line* shows where the preparation of the extended retinacular flap starts

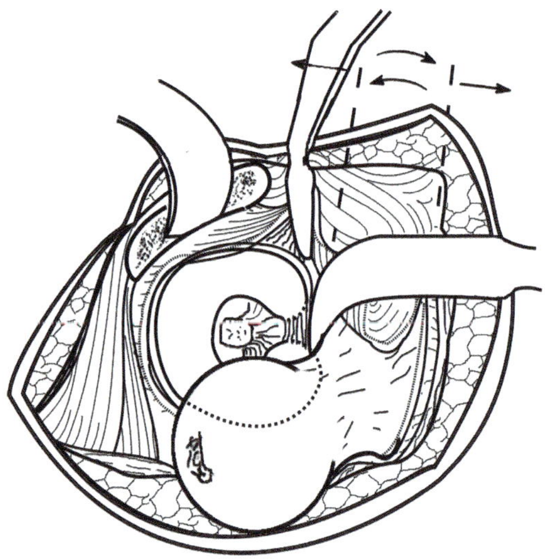

Fig. 5.3 (Modified from Ganz et al. [11]) Optimal view on acetabulum and femoral head with surgical hip dislocation and three retractors placed around the acetabular rim

vastus lateralis, greater trochanter, and gluteus medius muscle. It also allows inspection of the external rotators. A digastric trochanteric flip osteotomy allows exposure of the capsule between piriformis and gluteus minimus muscles. With a Z-shaped capsulotomy and after transection of the round ligament, the femoral head can be dislocated anteriorly. Optimal view of the joint is possible with the leg placed in a sterile bag on the opposite side of the table and three retractors placed around the acetabular rim (Fig. 5.3).

The postero-lateral retinacular flap is prepared with the femoral head reduced in the socket and the hip extended and slightly internally rotated. With a small straight osteotome and starting at the osteotomy surface of the stable trochanter 5 × 5 mm pieces of bone are cut out. The osteotome should not penetrate through the cortical side of the bone. Levering the osteotome should help to break the cortex. With a small bone clamp the mobilized fragment is turned in a way to allow subperiosteal dissection and removal. This maneuver is repeated until the level of the neck is reached. Multiple finger palpations allow to decide when the level of the neck is reached. Further dissection of the periosteum including the retinaculum is best performed with a sharp

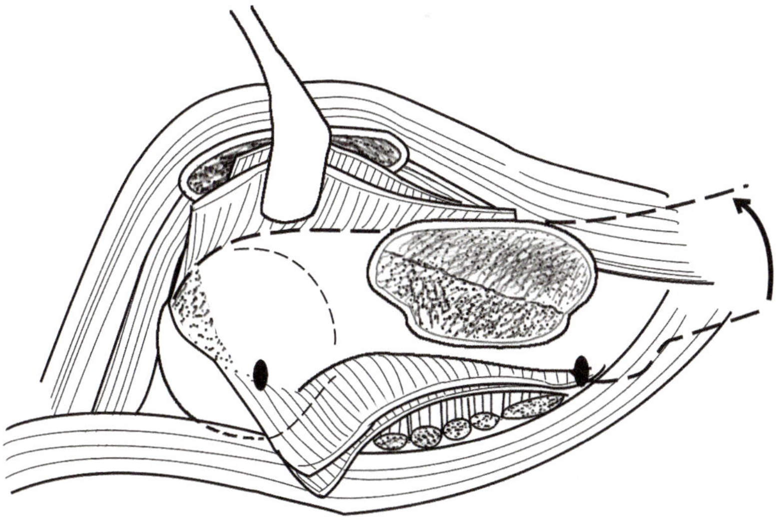

Fig. 5.4 (Modified from Ganz et al. [13]) Length of the extended retinacular flap from femoral head to lesser trochanter (*black arrows*)

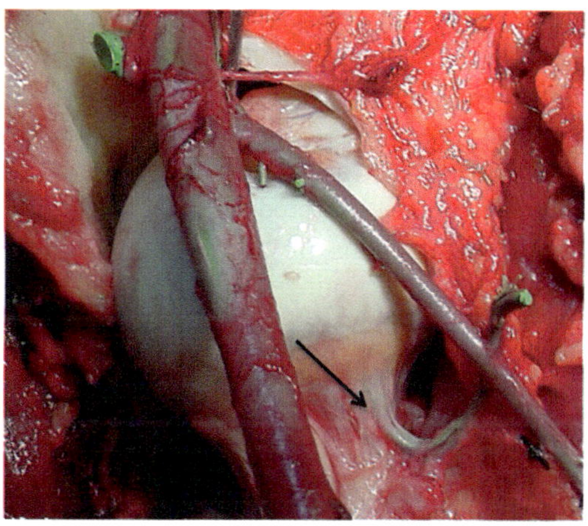

Fig. 5.5 Medial branch of the MFCA (Medial Femoral Circumflex Artery) running on Weitbrecht's ligament (*arrow*)

periosteal elevator. The end result is a continuous periosteal flap attached to the head-neck junction proximally and to the bone at the level of the lesser trochanter distally; it may reach a length of up to 12 cm (Fig. 5.4). Dissection of the medial periosteal flap is easier with the head dislocated and the femur slightly externally rotated. It is important to visualize Weitbrecht's ligament and include it into the flap because it carries the medial branch of the MFCA (Fig. 5.5). With a curved periosteal elevator inserted medially and/or laterally the posterior connection of both flaps is completed allowing full access to the circumference of the neck without interference with the blood supply to the head.

Dissection of the lateral periosteal flap only is indicated for relative lengthening of the femoral neck and for size reduction osteotomy of the head. Dissection of both, the lateral and the medial flap is necessary for neck osteotomy and sub-capital realignment but may also be useful for resection of exostoses or other tumors of the posterior neck [13, 14]. In severe chronic slips with ossified physis, the proximal insertion of the retinacular flap is ill defined, and the accessible part of the posterior neck is very short. For this condition an osteotomy into the head following the line of the posterior trochanteric resection is the method to overcome this difficult problem (Fig. 5.6) [15]. In case of a combination of a periacetabular osteotomy (PAO) together with a procedure necessitating a retinacular flap the ischial osteotomy of the PAO can be performed through the femoral approach but should be executed before the retinacular flap is dissected [13]. In the growing hip periosteum and retinaculum are thicker and therefore dissection from bone is easier; however, subperiosteal dissection at the level of the reduction of the trochanteric bone mass is easier in adults. During refixation of the greater

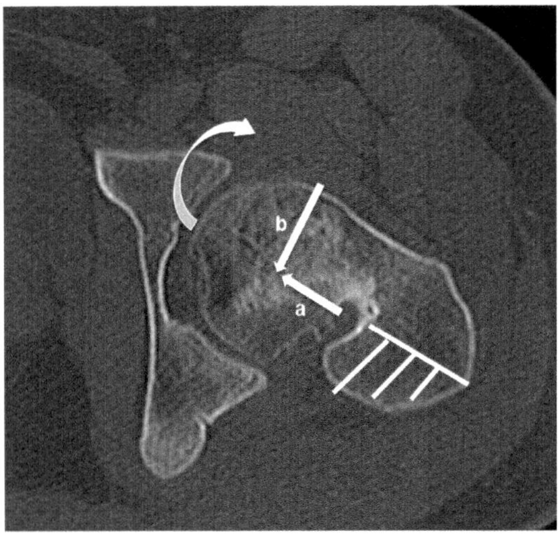

Fig. 5.6 In severe slips with fused growth plate, the posterior neck can be reduced to a small gap between head and greater trochanter. The entrance area of the retinacular vessels into the head may not be clearly defined. Therefore, the dissection of the retinaculum should not be propagated further towards the head, after the piece meal resection of the greater trochanter has reached the level of the neck (*scattered lines*). Using an oscillating saw, a cut is performed parallel to the anterior neck surface (*a*) to reach a second cut placed perpendicular to the first one at the anterior border of the head cartilage (*b*). This technique allows best protection of the perforation area of the retinacular vessels and a relatively long femoral neck

trochanter care must be taken to avoid compression of retinacular flap. One precaution is to perform a trochanteric advancement, which increases the space for the flap tissue and/or to interpose a bone wedge which brings the trochanter in a more vertical position (Fig. 5.7).

5.3 Clinical Relevance

The extended retinacular flap is an extension of the surgical dislocation approach, it allows to execute a number of osteotomies closer to the level of the joint. Such corrections are more powerful and at the same time minimize or even avoid negative side effects like leg shortening or impingement. Approach dependent avascular necrosis of the femoral head is extremely rare [13, 16, 17]. While it was first executed only on the growing hip, meanwhile it is also performed in young adults, e.g., when a unilateral varus osteotomy is indicated (Fig. 5.8). Executed on the neck level, it will produce substantially less leg shortening. Screw fixation is less prominent under the skin, creating less pain and allowing

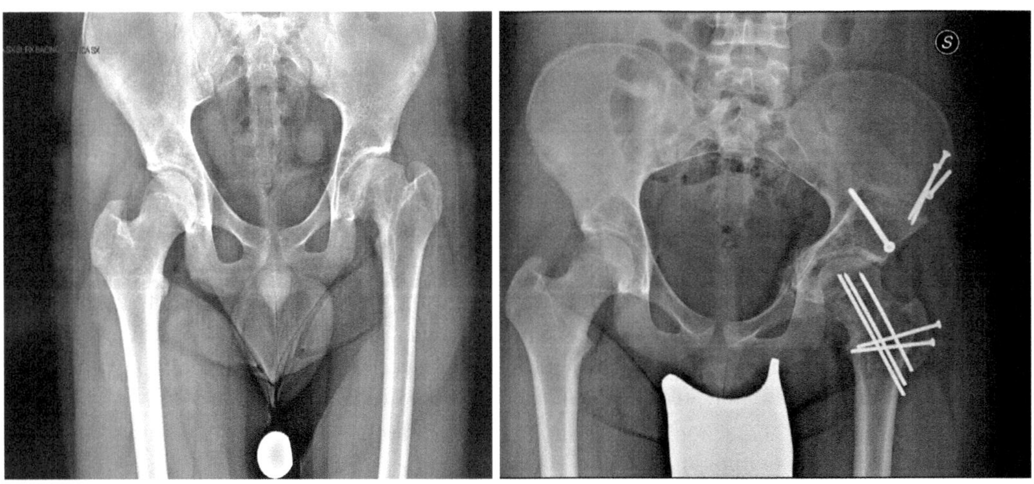

Fig. 5.7 Same case as in Fig. 5.6. Distal advancement of the trochanter allowed unfolding of the retinacular flap without compressing it during fixation. Acetabular adaptation has resulted in a flat roof making a periacetabular reorientation necessary to re-stabilize the femoral head in the socket

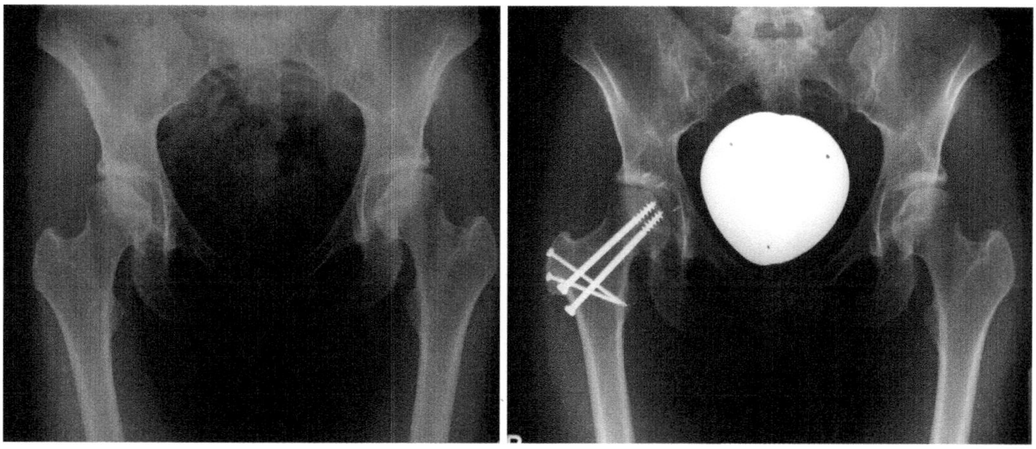

Fig. 5.8 Unilateral varus osteotomy at the neck level for high fovea leading to acceptable leg shortening. The bone anchors are for refixation of a partially disconnected labrum

easier and more complete abductor reinforcement compared to a blade- or screw plate fixation as normally used for intertrochanteric osteotomies.

References

1. Leunig M, Puloski S, Beck M, et al. Proximal femoral osteotomy: current indications and techniques. Semin Arthroplast. 2005;16:53–62. https://doi.org/10.1053/j.sart.2004.12.006.
2. Pearl AJ, Woodward B, Kellyrp. Cuneiform osteotomy in the treatment of slipped capital femoral epiphysis. J Bone Joint Surg Am. 1961;43-A:947–54.
3. Fish JB. Cuneiform osteotomy of the femoral neck in the treatment of slipped capital femoral epiphysis. A follow-up note. J Bone Joint Surg Am. 1994;76:46–59. https://doi.org/10.2106/00004623-199401000-00007.
4. Sugioka Y. Transtrochanteric rotational osteotomy in the treatment of idiopathic and steroid-induced femoral head necrosis, Perthes' disease, slipped capital femoral epiphysis, and osteoarthritis of the hip. Indications and results. Clin Orthop Relat Res. 1984;184:12–23.
5. Kramer WG, Craig WA, Noel S. Compensating osteotomy at the base of the femoral neck for slipped capital femoral epiphysis. J Bone Joint Surg Am. 1976;58:796–800.
6. Dunn DM, Angel JC. Replacement of the femoral head by open operation in severe adolescent slipping of the upper femoral epiphysis. J Bone Joint Surg Br. 1978;60-B:394–403.
7. Gage JR, Sundberg AB, Nolan DR, et al. Complications after cuneiform osteotomy for moderately or severely slipped capital femoral epiphysis. J Bone Joint Surg Am. 1978;60:157–65.
8. Diab M, Hresko MT, Millis MB. Intertrochanteric versus subcapital osteotomy in slipped capital femoral epiphysis. Clin Orthop Relat Res. 2004;427:204–12. https://doi.org/10.1097/01.blo.0000139252.09270.25.
9. Sevitt S, Thompson RG. The distribution and anastomoses of arteries supplying the head and neck of the femur. J Bone Joint Surg Br. 1965;47:560–73.
10. Gautier E, Ganz K, Krügel N, et al. Anatomy of the medial femoral circumflex artery and its surgical implications. J Bone Joint Surg Br. 2000;82:679–83. https://doi.org/10.1302/0301-620x.82b5.10426.
11. Ganz R, Gill TJ, Gautier E, et al. Surgical dislocation of the adult hip. A technique with full access to the femoral head and acetabulum without the risk of avascular necrosis. J Bone Joint Surg Br. 2001;83:1119–24. https://doi.org/10.1302/0301-620x.83b8.11964.
12. Glynn AA, Barattiero FY, Albers CE, et al. Surgical hip dislocation does not result in atrophy or fatty infiltration of periarticular hip muscles. J Hip Preserv Surg. 2014;1:82–95. https://doi.org/10.1093/jhps/hnu008.
13. Ganz R, Huff TW, Leunig M. Extended retinacular soft-tissue flap for intra-articular hip surgery: surgical technique, indications, and results of application. Instr Course Lect. 2009;58:241–55.
14. Siebenrock K-A, Ganz R. Osteochondroma of the femoral neck. Clin Orthop Relat Res. 2002;394:211–8. https://doi.org/10.1097/00003086-200201000-00025.
15. Ganz R, Aprato A, Mazziotta G, Pignatti G. Joint instability after anatomic reconstruction of severe, chronic slipped capital femoral epiphysis: a report

of 3 cases, with high femoral anteversion in 1 and adaptive acetabular roof deformation in 3. JBJS Case Connect. 2016;6:e50. https://doi.org/10.2106/JBJS.CC.15.00149.
16. Leunig M, Manner HM, Turchetto L, Ganz R. Femoral and acetabular re-alignment in slipped capital femoral epiphysis. J Child Orthop. 2017;11:131–7. https://doi.org/10.1302/1863-2548-11-170020.
17. Ganz R, Aprato A, Massè A. Femoral head reduction osteotomy. In: Tsiridis E, editor. The adult hip - master case series and techniques. Cham: Springer International Publishing; 2018. p. 3–47.

6 Femoro-Acetabular Impingement: Treatment Options—Arthroscopy

Ettore Sabetta and Michele Cappa

6.1 Introduction

Hip arthroscopy has become an alternative to open surgery after the femoro-acetabular impingement (FAI) has been described and treated with surgical dislocation by Ganz et al. [1, 2]. Possible advantages of arthroscopy compared with open surgery are reduced surgical invasiveness, shorter hospitalization, and easier recovery period [3–6]. The availability of dedicated arthroscopic instruments has resulted in constant improvement of the surgical techniques. Correct execution of hip arthroscopy, however, is not easy and time consuming even for experienced surgeons [7, 8]. While the learning curve for the technique is rather long, understanding of indication and contraindication is even more challenging. Very frequently, more than only one reason for impingement is present [9] and some may be extra-articular and not accessible with arthroscopy. Borderline acetabular dysplasia can be associated with cam deformity or retroversion, both eventually leading to impingement. Arthroscopy may treat the impinging deformity but may also increase the risk for joint destabilization [10]. Apparent general joint laxity, as nearly exclusively seen in female patients is a precondition to be very restrictive with any surgical attempt to treat a structural deformity. Very occasionally, advanced cartilage destruction may be an indication for arthroscopy, but the patient must be informed that the risk of pain persistence is high. Best evaluation for any joint preserving surgery of the hip is a careful and thorough clinical evaluation combined with plain radiographies and an arthro-MRI with radial sequences of the involved hip only, including cuts for acetabular and femoral version [11]. There is limited information at comprehensive complication rates of hip arthroscopy for impingement and labral repair. In a more recent multicenter study, the overall rate was 8.3%, the majority being grade 1 complications. Longer distraction time and arthroscopy in female patients were producing more complications. Compared with open surgery the overall complication rate was similar; however, severe complications were less [12]. To be kept in mind is that persistent structural disease is the most frequent cause of repeat hip preservation surgery [13].

E. Sabetta (✉) · M. Cappa
Orthopedics and Traumatology Complex Structure, Arcispedale Santa Maria Nuova, IRCCS Reggio Emilia Hospital Company, Reggio Emilia, Italy
e-mail: esabetta@tiscali.it

6.2 Instruments and Surgical Technique

We perform hip arthroscopy in supine position on a trauma table or a dedicated table allowing limb traction [14]. Joint diastasis is essential for the introduction of optical and surgical instruments between femoral epiphysis and acetabular cavity. Traction of the limb is applied trough the foot and

R. Ganz (ed.), *Modern Hip Preservation*, https://doi.org/10.1007/978-3-030-91967-2_6

ankle, after having positioned a counter-traction post on the perineal region. Foot, ankle, and the perineal zone are adequately padded in order to prevent skin or neurological injuries. An image intensifier must be available for preparation of the arthroscopic portals, for checking the amount of acetabular trimming, for anchor positioning and for femoral osteochondroplasty. Most commonly used portals are anterolateral and mid-anterior, they allow access to both the central joint and the periphery [15, 16]. The anterolateral portal is placed about 1 cm cranial and anterior to the apex of the greater trochanter. The antero-medial portal is placed about six centimeters caudal to the antero-superior iliac spine (ASIS), anteriorly on the thigh in the middle between the ASIS and the anterolateral portal (Fig. 6.1).

Accessory portals are used as needed, for example for optimal application of bony anchors and labral sutures (Fig. 6.2). The articulation is inspected and the antero-medial angle of the capsule is localized, this angle is defined by the inguinal portion of the acetabular labrum on the upper side and by the femoral epiphysis below. This is the location of the second portal from inside (Fig. 6.3). Once the two main arthroscopic portals are set up, the capsulotomy is executed while alternating the position of optics and surgical instruments. With this technique there is a risk of iatrogenic lesions of acetabular labrum and femoral head cartilage especially during preparation of the anterolateral portal [17, 18].

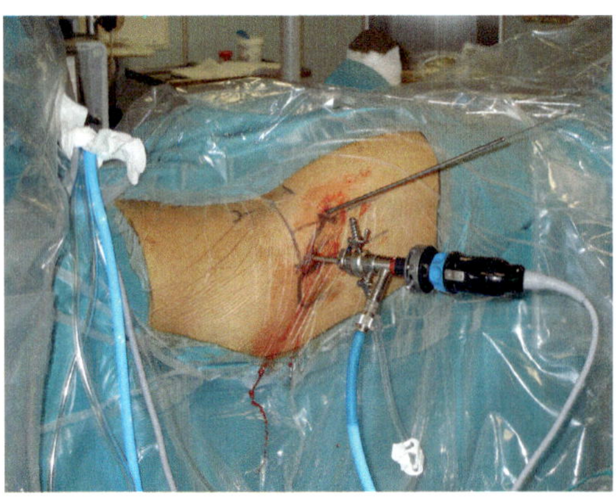

Fig. 6.1 Right hip. Anterolateral and mid-anterior portals. Optics in AL portal

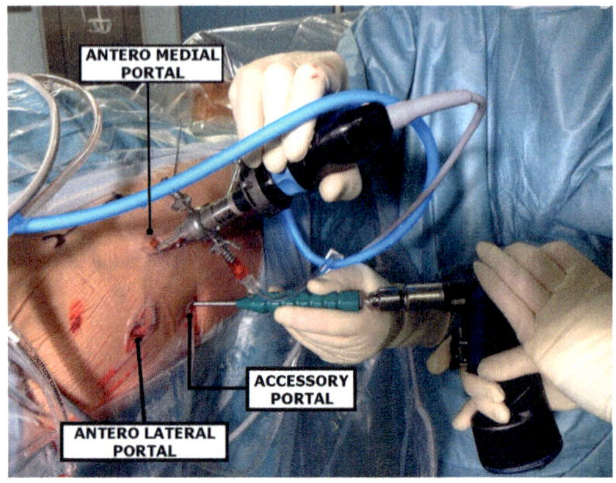

Fig. 6.2 Right hip. Accessory lateral-caudal portal used for the insertion of a suture anchor for refixation of the labrum. The optic is in the mid-anterior portal

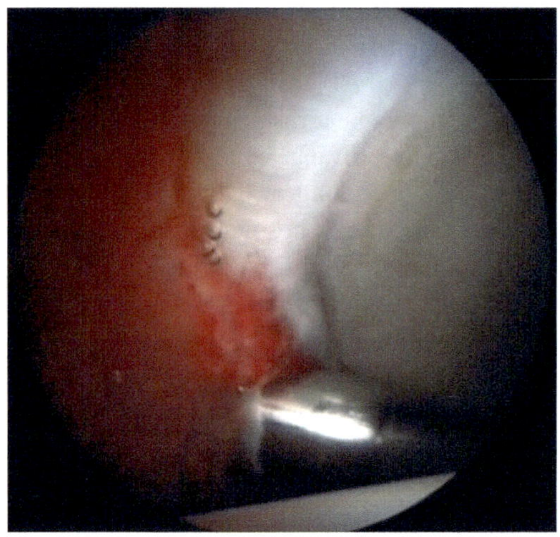

Fig. 6.3 Left hip. The optic is in the anterolateral portal. The mid-anterior portal is set under arthroscopic control by introducing the cannula in the antero-medial joint capsule, delimited by the inguinal portion of the acetabular labrum superiorly and by the femoral epiphysis inferiorly

While some authors access the peripheral compartment with the hip flexed at 40–45° [19, 20], we prefer the hip being extended, in abduction of about 10°, and internal rotation of 20–25°. Skin portals are the same. Capsular plane is reached by blunt dissection. The anterior capsule is isolated endoscopically, then capsulotomy is performed following the femoral neck axis (Fig. 6.4, line A). If necessary, the capsulotomy can be expanded to "L" or "T" in correspondence of the capsular insertion into the acetabulum (Fig. 6.4, B and C

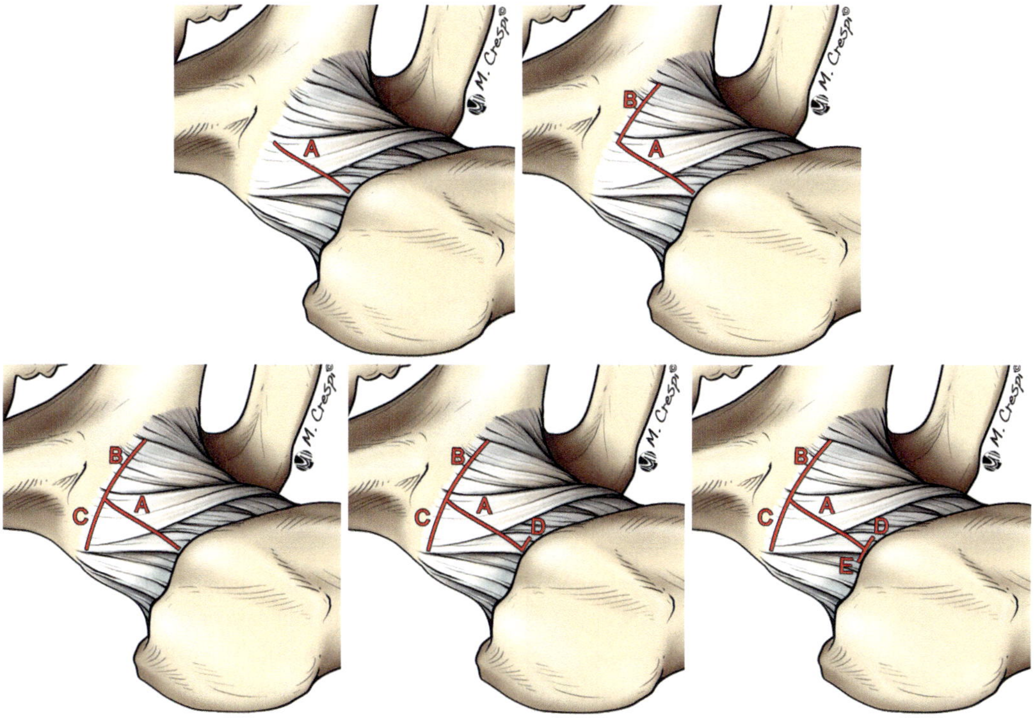

Fig. 6.4 Schematic drawing of the different capsulotomy steps. The first cut (*A*) is placed in the middle of and in line with the femoral neck. Close to the acetabular rim it can be expanded to an "L" (*B*) or a "T" (*C*). The extension to an "H" (*D* and *E*) near the base of the neck is rarely necessary

lines). Theoretically capsulotomy can be extended along lines D and E, but in our experience this has never been necessary. This type of capsular incision facilitates suturing at the end of surgery. Traction is applied only at the end of capsulotomy allowing for lower traction force and duration.

6.3 Treatment of Pincer Type Femoro-Acetabular Impingement (FAI)

Pincer impingement is primarily induced by acetabular over-coverage and can be aggravated by a low or negative femoral anteversion. It leads to a linear conflict between the femoral neck and the acetabular labrum even for physiological excursion angles [1, 21–26]. The labral tissue may become degenerated and shows intrasubstance ganglion formation and/or fissure lines. The adjacent acetabular cartilage may also become degenerated, but the extent of damage is much less deep than with cam impingement and outside-in cartilage disconnections are not seen [22]. The arthroscopic treatment of pincer FAI aims for correcting the acetabular deformity. Before doing so, the degenerated parts of the labrum are debrided and the intact part kept for later refixation. In case of larger areas of labrum degeneration, bucket handle like dissection of the labrum can make the execution easier. Trimming of the acetabular rim is undertaken with a 5.5 mm spherical burr after the surface of the bony rim is cleaned with radiofrequency tools or shavers. Extension and depth of bony removal has to be determined preoperatively and constantly controlled during surgery. For the planning an AP pelvis projection is used to measure Wiberg's angle (normally ranging from 25° to 35–40°) [27, 28]. By experience, 1 mm of trimming equals 1° of Wiberg's angle reduction. The trim depth can be estimated measuring the distance between the apex of the acetabular fossa and the rim. This distance should not be less than 25 mm (Fig. 6.5); in most cases the acetabular

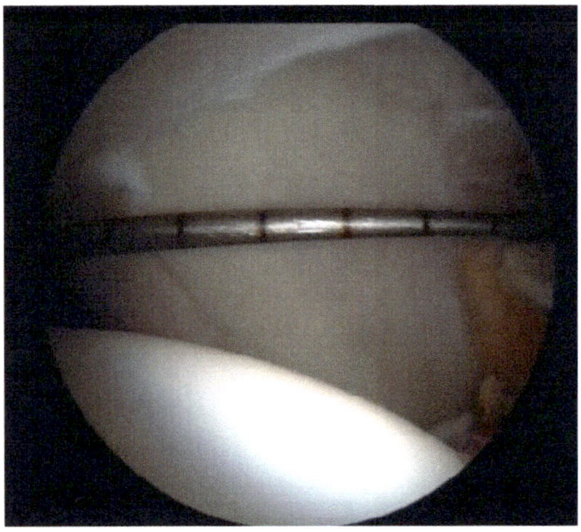

Fig. 6.5 Measuring the cartilage horseshoe depth with a calibrated nerve hook

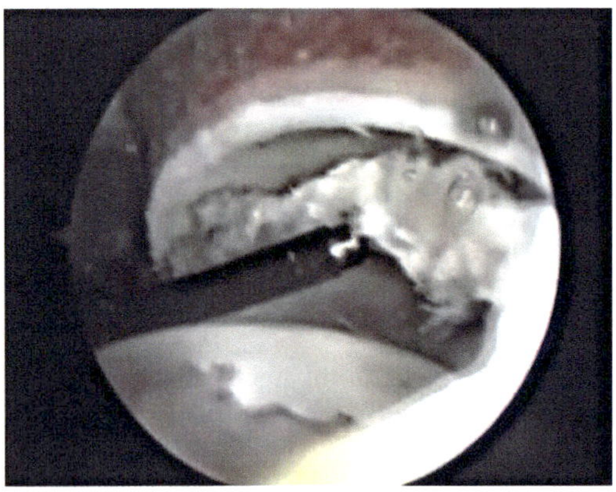

Fig. 6.6 After completion of the rim trimming, the detached and debrided portion of the labrum (backside visible) is ready for refixation

resection is less than 3 mm. The degeneration area is a further guide to determine the starting and end points of the area to be resected. The final resection plane should be leveed with smooth borders (Fig. 6.6). For greater extensions or depth of resection, the detached labrum should be sutured back to the bone at the end of the procedure.

6.4 Labral Suture

The labrum is a sealing device, keeping the fluid inside the articulating surfaces, it helps to avoid peak stresses along the joint and due to its innervation, it is a sensitive bumper. Therefore, it is very important to maintain or restore the function of the labrum [29, 30]. To ensure good fixation and stability we suggest using 2–3 mm suture anchors spaced not more than 7–8 mm one from each other. They should be placed within the subchondral bone avoiding any penetration into cartilage or even joint. If this goal cannot be reached and controlled through classical arthroscopic portals, accessory portals should be created more distal and lateral. Two portals are needed to re-suture the labrum. With one technique the suture embraces the labrum (Fig. 6.7), while with another technique the needle is passed through the labrum, allowing to avoid contact between suture and epiphyseal cartilage. The first technique is mechanically stronger while the second can be applied even when the remaining labrum is rather thin. The second technique is also more elegant because the suture material does not get in contact with the epiphyseal cartilage. With both suture techniques one must ensure that the re-fixed labrum levels the acetabular cartilage surface to create the desired gasket function.

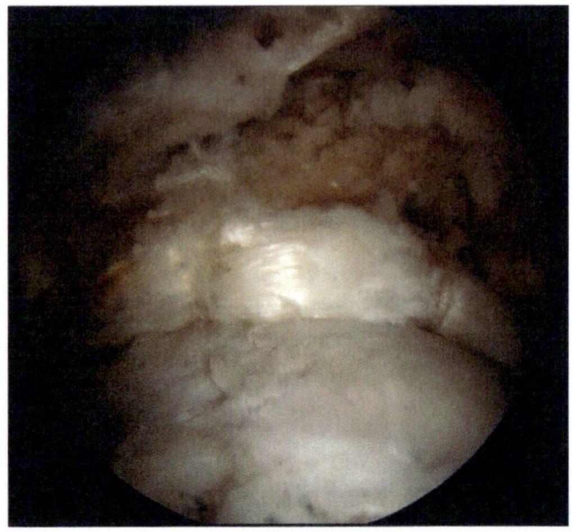

Fig. 6.7 Circumferential suture of the labrum

6.5 Cam Treatment

The cam type FAI is produced by a morphological abnormality of the anterolateral circumference of the head-neck junction. The reduced head-neck offset leads to an inclusion and jamming of a neck surface without cartilage cover into the joint. The repetition of this movement—mainly flection-internal rotation—leads to the acetabular cartilage abrasion. In high-speed movements, the jamming results in an outside-in avulsion of the cartilage, a phenomenon which is not seen in pincer type FAI. FAI is observed more frequently in men and, since the sensitive labrum is not primarily involved, pain becomes an issue rather late in the disease process [1, 22, 31]. Mild slipped capital femoral epiphysis, where the offset problem is produced by a retro tilt of the epiphysis, is a prototype of cam impingement. Arthroscopic removal of the "bump" (osteochondroplasty) by means of a circular motorized burr (diameter 5.5 mm) and recreation of a slightly waisted head/neck offset is the method of choice when the cam deformity is the unique deformity. The treatment will increase the range of internal rotation, mainly in flexion. To execute an osteochondroplasty, the limb is placed in neutral rotation, the hip joint is slightly abducted (about 10°) and flexed (about 45°) (Fig. 6.8). The caudal-cranial extension of the femoral osteochondroplasty goes from the anterior border of lateral retinaculum (where the branches of the medial femoral circumflex artery penetrate the femoral epiphysis [32]), to Weitbrecht's ligament, representing the medial retinaculum with the medial branch of the medial femoral circumflex artery. These two retinacular structures, which supply the femoral head, should not be injured. Medial-lateral extension and depth of the osteochondroplasty can be determined and controlled under fluoroscopy guidance and using dynamic maneuvers. These consist in flexion, adduction, and internal rotation of the hip (Fig. 6.9). If conflicting bone continues to exist, we proceed with a further bone removal (Fig. 6.10). Dynamic arthroscopic assessment is more reliable and more useful than radiologic assessment.

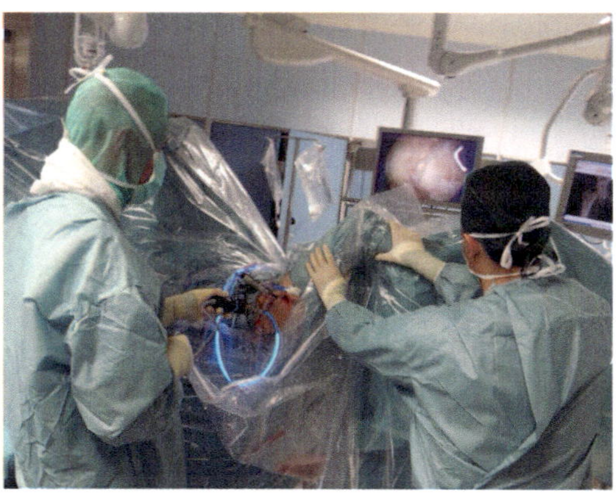

Fig. 6.8 The femoral osteochondral resection begins with the hip flexed to approximately 45°. Varying the angle of hip flexion allows the approach to the entire cam area

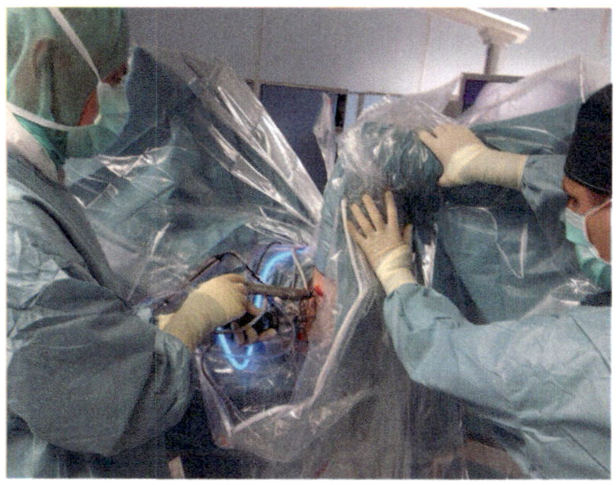

Fig. 6.9 The elimination of the conflict is confirmed by dynamic flexion-adduction and intrarotation under arthroscopic control

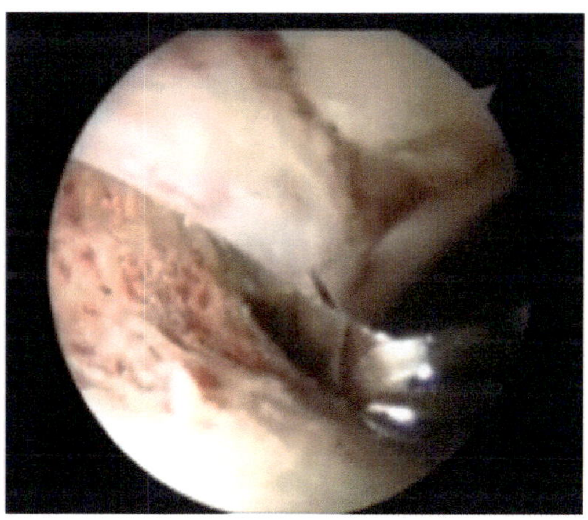

Fig. 6.10 If the dynamic maneuvers reveal the persistence of conflict areas, these are removed with a 5.5 mm burr

6.6 Capsular Suture

Suturing of the capsule after hip arthroscopy is a somewhat controversial subject. Some authors have documented iatrogenic instability after hip arthroscopy [33–36] and recommend capsular suture as the best prevention for post-surgical secondary instability [34, 37, 38]. In our opinion, a must for careful capsular suture after arthroscopic FAI treatment are the following conditions: borderline acetabular coverage before or after rim trimming; abnormal acetabular anteversion +/ combined with higher-than-normal femoral anteversion. Such morphological conditions may favor subluxation or even dislocation after arthroscopy. Ligamentous laxity but also sports and physical activities that need extensive articular excursions (gymnastics, dancing, etc.) are factors which can promote joint instability after arthroscopy.

To simplify the capsular suture, it is advisable to use a proximal accessory portal located at the midpoint between the anterolateral portal and the antero-superior iliac spine (Fig. 6.11). The optic is positioned in the anterolateral portal while the instruments for the suture are introduced through the two opposite portals, the mid-anterior and the proximal accessory one (Fig. 6.11). A semi-tubular probe is introduced through the proximal accessory portal to gain access to the superior capsular flap. A 30° angled bird-beak is introduced along the probe, carrying a suture wire (Vicryl 1) that will cross the superior capsular flap from outside to inside. The tip of this instrument and the loop of the transported suture are temporarily left against the femoral neck. A second semi-tubular probe is inserted through the mid-anterior portal until the lower capsular flap. Another bird-beak is introduced along this second probe to pierce the inferior capsular flap from outside to inside. The introduction will be stopped when the femoral neck is reached by the instrument. The suture loop is grabbed with the second bird-beak and one of the suture's ends is transported outside through the mid-anterior portal. At this point the two suture's ends protrude from the proximal accessory and from the mid-anterior portals (Fig. 6.11). The second end of the suture needs to be transported from the accessory portal to the mid-anterior portal. This maneuver can be difficult therefore we suggest mounting the suture that protrudes from the accessory portal on a knot pusher that will be inserted until the capsular flap is reached. The suture now can be grabbed with a ring clamp and transported out from the mid-anterior portal. The knot is executed with a standard technique. The entire operation can be repeated two or three times if necessary (Fig. 6.12). Usually, the suture is per-

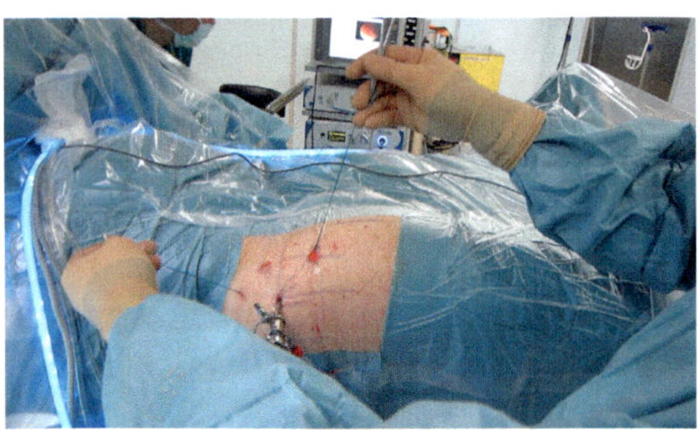

Fig. 6.11 Capsular suture: One suture end is inserted through the proximal accessory portal (*to the left*) to anchor the superior capsular flap from outside to inside and the inferior capsular flap from inside to outside. Exiting through the mid-anterior portal (*to the right*). Surgeon's hands are tensioning the suture. The left end of the suture will be grabbed through the mid-anterior portal (*to the right*) to tighten the knot

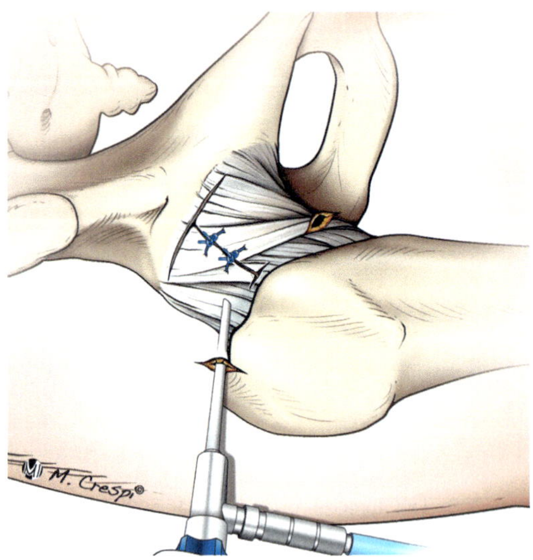

Fig. 6.12 In the majority of cases, the capsule is sufficiently stabilized with one or two stitches placed along the femoral neck axis

formed only along the femoral neck axis (line A in Fig. 6.4; Fig. 6.12).

The arthroscopic treatment of the global pincer FAI requires labral detachment and acetabular trimming for a broad sector of the acetabulum circumference. In such cases it is necessary to expand the capsulotomy for several centimeters, parallel to the edge of the cup (lines B and C, Fig. 6.4). A similar need arises in the case of labral reconstruction with autograft or allograft. In these cases, the suture of the single capsular gap parallel to the femoral neck (line A, Fig. 6.4) does not guarantee enough stability. The capsule must be stabilized on the supra-acetabular bone. For this purpose, an anchor is used (Fig. 6.13).

The sutures are tightened with sliding knots. The capsular suture restores the native stability of the joint. Care must be taken not to over-tighten the capsule to avoid joint stiffness. If the capsulotomy is performed with radiofrequencies, a portion of capsular tissue is lost due to tissue's vaporization. Often the capsular edges are regularized with the motorized shaver, destroying part of the capsular tissue. In such circumstances, capsular suturing inevitably involves reduction of the joint volume. The greater the sacrificed capsular tissue the looser the suture must be. The flap ends can only be approximated.

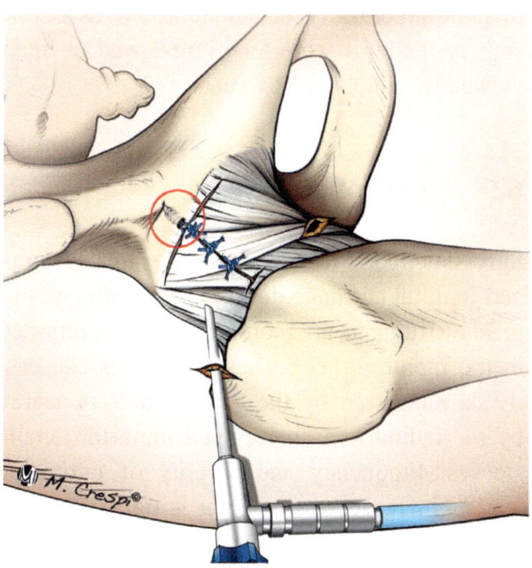

Fig. 6.13 When the capsulotomy is largely extended parallel to the acetabular margin (e.g., in cases with acetabular trimming), the capsule needs to be stabilized with a suture anchor placed above the acetabular border (*highlighted in red circle*)

6.7 Post-operative Treatment

The rehabilitation program following arthroscopic surgery for FAI must be designed according to the injuries, surgical procedures, and physiological healing time of the involved joint structures [39]. The rehabilitation program includes different sequential stages [40, 41]. In the immediate post-operative phase, joint mobilization is performed cautiously to prevent joint stiffness without the risk of adverse scaring and periarticular ossification. At the same time the joint capsule (sutured or not sutured) and the labrum (sutured or reconstructed) should be protected from pathological movements [42]. Sufficient pain and anti-inflammatory medication is another important aspect [43]. When properly managed, load and neuromuscular activation [44] do not interfere with the healing of capsule and labrum [45, 46]. Passive joint mobilization is an important aspect in the immediate post-operative period [47]. Flexion over 90° should be avoided in the first phase because it may overload the sutured labrum and stretch the capsule. Hyperextension tends to provoke an anterior subluxation, thus also overloading the labrum and the joint capsule. External rotation in extension has a subluxing effect too and should not be allowed in the first 2–3 weeks. Adduction is more painful than abduction in the early post-operative phases as it tends to reproduce the impingement mechanism. For circling motions, the physiotherapist flexes the hip to 20–30° and abduces it to about 10°. Rotational movement are gradually increased according to the patient's tolerance. The safest movements in the first post-operative phase are those executed along the femoral neck axis oriented against the acetabular opening plane and as such avoiding eccentric and subluxing forces. The combined flexion-abduction-rotation movement does not stretch the joint capsule; thus, it does not cause pain and it does not hinder tissue healing. This movement can be started from the very first day after surgery. Since introduction of this technique, we have observed quicker and less painful joint recovery.

6.8 Patient Group and Methods

From 2009 to 2015 we have performed 143 hip arthroscopies for FAI in 130 patients. All 11 bilateral arthroscopies were staged. Included are 2 revisions and 1 arthroscopy for extra-articular FAI due to ossifications after traumatic avulsion of the anterior inferior iliac spine. The 60 females and 70 males had an age distribution of 16–61 years.

In most cases the FAI was mixed, in few cases it was isolated cam or pincer. Absolute contraindications for surgery were a LCE Wiberg angle of less than 25°, a Tönnis angle >10°, or cases with poor joint congruency Arthro MRI of the hip was performed in all hips when pain lasted longer than 8–10 months, when the age was over 40 years in non-sportive individuals or when degenerative signs were seen in standard radiographs [48]. Arthro MRI was also indicated in those patients whose clinical and radiological examinations were in contrast with the described pain. Hips with MRI documented severe cartilage damage were excluded, with the exception of a 30-year-old judo instructor who insisted to have arthroscopy before THR. Of the two revisions in our case series, one had to be executed in the judo instructor's second side after he had benefited from the arthroscopy of the first side. The second revision was performed in a girl who had developed intra-articular adhesions. With arthroscopic removal the patient became pain free.

Prior to arthroscopy hip mobility was photographically documented. All patients had an orthograde AP pelvis radiography (sacro-coccyx in line with pubic symphysis) and axial view of the involved hip. When clinically in doubt a CT scan was performed to quantify the femoral version.

Evidence of acetabular cartilage lesions were found arthroscopically in 95% of our cases while femoral cartilage lesions were rare. Acetabular cartilage lesions ranged from cartilage dissociation from the subchondral bone, with the integrity of the labral junction (wave sign), to the complete absence of cartilage. In cam FAI, frequently outside-in detached cartilage flaps were seen. Labral lesions varied from intrasubstance degeneration to thinning, to complete absence, both mainly seen in pincer impingement. The most severe cartilage and labral lesion were always located at the peak area of impingement and the severity of lesions was proportional to the duration of symptoms. Treatment consisted in acetabular rim trimming when the local over-coverage was creating the impingement. It could be performed without further detachment of the labrum when the involved area was small. In larger impingement areas the labrum was detached to execute the necessary trimming and refixation using suture anchors of 2.3 mm. Exposed subchondral bone after debridement of disconnected cartilage was treated with micro-fracturing technique. In this series we did not use labrum reconstruction when it was absent or not anymore useful for refixation. All hips had post-operative radiographies as before surgery. All patients were first reviewed after 2 weeks. Four to six weeks after surgery we performed another clinical evaluation and control X-rays. A next clinical control was performed approximately 4 months after surgery to photographically document ROM as before surgery. Patients were finally reviewed or interviewed by telephone at 1 year.

6.9 Complications

Iatrogenic labral tears and damages to acetabular and femoral cartilage during introduction of surgical instruments are more frequent than reported in the literature [14]. These structures can easily be punctured by the needle guide or teared by the cylindrical dilators and the arthroscopic sleeves. Frequency and severity of iatrogenic lesions increase when a joint is tight. To avoid such damage when using traction of the limb, an articular diastasis of at least 10 mm must be reached. When traction is intense and prolonged beyond 60 min ischemic skin lesions on the dorsum of the foot or injuries of the pudendal nerve caused by the perineal post can be observed.

In this series, we observed 15 cases of perineal dysesthesia resolved within few days to several weeks. We also observed 2 cases of labrum perforation and several, mainly superficial lesions of the femoral cartilage during the anterolateral portal setup. More recently we began to use the traction-free technique for portal setup and capsulotomy reducing the overall traction time for surgery to about 30 min. Since this change has been adopted, we have not experienced traction-related complications anymore. Moreover, thanks to the application of the out-in capsulotomy technique the number of joint lesions dropped to zero.

6.10 Results

Our case series is very heterogeneous in terms of age, physical activity, duration of symptoms prior to intervention and comorbidities. Two patients were lost to follow-up. For this study, the evaluation of results is concentrating on two major aspects, namely patient's satisfaction and ROM improvement: Based on the mentioned parameters, the results were positive in most cases. Almost all patients reported improvement in amplitude and easiness of motion. All patients showed improved internal rotation in 90° flexion while external rotation did not clearly improve. Most patients reported significant improvement in pain, in 15% the symptoms disappeared completely. Residual discomfort was mainly evoked as groin pain with hip flexion more than 90°. All patients with bilateral surgery were evidently satisfied by the result of the first hip. The second side did not do well in a 46-year-old woman making THR necessary 2 years after, while the first side continued to be asymptomatic. The majority of patients had good to average benefit from the intervention and would repeat the surgery. Thirty percent reported that the result was below their expectations, although they are satisfied with the operation and they report an improvement. Ten percent, despite having reported improvements, would not repeat the surgery. A stable result has been achieved between 4 and 9 months in most cases. Some cases finally recovered about 1 year after surgery. In accordance with the literature, we observed that results are better in patient with a symptomatic period shorter than 1 year [49]. The results are better and are achieved more rapidly in patients below 30 years of age [50], especially in professional athletes [51, 52]. As already described, hips with advanced cartilage damage show rapid deterioration of results over time [53].

6.11 Conclusions

Arthroscopic treatment is ideal for isolated intra-articular FAI. Accurate diagnosis and careful patient selection are essential criteria for success. Nevertheless, in about 30% of the cases the results do not reflect the patient's expectations [54]. Therefore, the surgeon has to outline clearly the realistic possibilities of such treatment especially to young patients who often have unrealistic expectations, even when not being athletic.

References

1. Ganz R, Parvizi J, Beck M, et al. Femoroacetabular impingement: a cause for osteoarthritis of the hip. Clin Orthop Relat Res. 2003;(417):112–20. https://doi.org/10.1097/01.blo.0000096804.78689.c2.
2. Ganz R, Gill TJ, Gautier E, et al. Surgical dislocation of the adult hip. A technique with full access to the femoral head and acetabulum without the risk of avascular necrosis. J Bone Joint Surg Br. 2001;83:1119–24. https://doi.org/10.1302/0301-620x.83b8.11964.
3. Botser IB, Jackson TJ, Smith TW, et al. Open surgical dislocation versus arthroscopic treatment of femoroacetabular impingement. Am J Orthop Belle Mead NJ. 2014;43:209–14.
4. Domb BG, Stake CE, Botser IB, Jackson TJ. Surgical dislocation of the hip versus arthroscopic treatment of femoroacetabular impingement: a prospective matched-pair study with average 2-year follow-up. Arthroscopy. 2013;29:1506–13. https://doi.org/10.1016/j.arthro.2013.06.010.
5. Zingg PO, Ulbrich EJ, Buehler TC, et al. Surgical hip dislocation versus hip arthroscopy for femoroacetabular impingement: clinical and morphological short-term results. Arch Orthop Trauma Surg. 2013;133:69–79. https://doi.org/10.1007/s00402-012-1616-2.
6. Matsuda DK, Carlisle JC, Arthurs SC, et al. Comparative systematic review of the open dislocation, mini-open, and arthroscopic surgeries for femoroacetabular impingement. Arthroscopy. 2011;27:252–69. https://doi.org/10.1016/j.arthro.2010.09.011.

7. Fayad TE, Khan MA, Haddad FS. Femoroacetabular impingement: an arthroscopic solution. Bone Joint J. 2013;95-B:26–30. https://doi.org/10.1302/0301-620X.95B11.33016.
8. Kaplan KM, Shah MR, Youm T. Femoroacetabular impingement--diagnosis and treatment. Bull NYU Hosp Jt Dis. 2010;68:70–5.
9. Tibor LM, Liebert G, Sutter R, et al. Two or more impingement and/or instability deformities are often present in patients with hip pain. Clin Orthop. 2013;471:3762–73. https://doi.org/10.1007/s11999-013-2918-6.
10. Nepple JJ, Clohisy JC. The dysplastic and unstable hip: a responsible balance of arthroscopic and open approaches. Sports Med Arthrosc Rev. 2015;23:180–6. https://doi.org/10.1097/JSA.0000000000000096.
11. Locher S, Werlen S, Leunig M, Ganz R. MR-arthrography with radial sequences for visualization of early hip pathology not visible on plain radiographs. Z Orthop Ihre Grenzgeb. 2002;140:52–7. https://doi.org/10.1055/s-2002-22122.
12. Larson CM, Clohisy JC, Beaulé PE, et al. Intraoperative and early postoperative complications after hip arthroscopic surgery: a prospective multicenter trial utilizing a validated grading scheme. Am J Sports Med. 2016;44:2292–8. https://doi.org/10.1177/0363546516650885.
13. Clohisy JC, Nepple JJ, Larson CM, et al. Persistent structural disease is the most common cause of repeat hip preservation surgery. Clin Orthop. 2013;471:3788–94. https://doi.org/10.1007/s11999-013-3218-x.
14. Byrd JWT. Hip arthroscopy by the supine approach. Instr Course Lect. 2006;55:325–36.
15. Mannava S, Howse EA, Stone AV, Stubbs AJ. Basic hip arthroscopy: supine patient positioning and dynamic fluoroscopic evaluation. Arthrosc Tech. 2015;4:e391–6. https://doi.org/10.1016/j.eats.2015.05.005.
16. Byrd JW, Pappas JN, Pedley MJ. Hip arthroscopy: an anatomic study of portal placement and relationship to the extra-articular structures. Arthroscopy. 1995;11:418–23. https://doi.org/10.1016/0749-8063(95)90193-0.
17. Mlynarek RA, Cowan JB, Larson CM, et al. Arthroscopic approach to femoroacetabular impingement. J Arthroplast. 2015;30:1096–104. https://doi.org/10.1016/j.arth.2015.04.016.
18. Byrd JW. Avoiding the labrum in hip arthroscopy. Arthroscopy. 2000;16:770–3. https://doi.org/10.1053/jars.2000.7686.
19. Alwattar BJ, Bharam S. Hip arthroscopy portals. Oper Tech Sports Med. 2011;19:74–80. https://doi.org/10.1053/j.otsm.2010.12.003.
20. Dienst M, Seil R, Kohn DM. Safe arthroscopic access to the central compartment of the hip. Arthroscopy. 2005;21:1510–4. https://doi.org/10.1016/j.arthro.2005.09.014.
21. Clohisy JC, Carlisle JC, Beaulé PE, et al. A systematic approach to the plain radiographic evaluation of the young adult hip. J Bone Joint Surg Am. 2008;90(Suppl 4):47–66. https://doi.org/10.2106/JBJS.H.00756.
22. Beck M, Kalhor M, Leunig M, Ganz R. Hip morphology influences the pattern of damage to the acetabular cartilage. J Bone Joint Surg Br. 2005;87-B:1012–8. https://doi.org/10.1302/0301-620X.87B7.15203.
23. Kassarjian A, Brisson M, Palmer WE. Femoroacetabular impingement. Eur J Radiol. 2007;63:29–35. https://doi.org/10.1016/j.ejrad.2007.03.020.
24. Meyer DC, Beck M, Ellis T, et al. Comparison of six radiographic projections to assess femoral head/neck asphericity. Clin Orthop Relat Res. 2006;445:181–5. https://doi.org/10.1097/01.blo.0000201168.72388.24.
25. Eijer H, Myers SR, Ganz R. Anterior femoroacetabular impingement after femoral neck fractures. J Orthop Trauma. 2001;15:475–81. https://doi.org/10.1097/00005131-200109000-00003.
26. Barton C, Salineros MJ, Rakhra KS, Beaulé PE. Validity of the alpha angle measurement on plain radiographs in the evaluation of cam-type femoroacetabular impingement. Clin Orthop. 2011;469:464–9. https://doi.org/10.1007/s11999-010-1624-x.
27. Werner CML, Ramseier LE, Ruckstuhl T, et al. Normal values of Wiberg's lateral center-edge angle and Lequesne's acetabular index--a coxometric update. Skelet Radiol. 2012;41:1273–8. https://doi.org/10.1007/s00256-012-1420-7.
28. Zumstein M, Hahn F, Sukthankar A, et al. How accurately can the acetabular rim be trimmed in hip arthroscopy for pincer-type femoral acetabular impingement: a cadaveric investigation. Arthroscopy. 2009;25:164–8. https://doi.org/10.1016/j.arthro.2008.09.016.
29. Ferguson SJ, Bryant JT, Ganz R, Ito K. An in vitro investigation of the acetabular labral seal in hip joint mechanics. J Biomech. 2003;36:171–8. https://doi.org/10.1016/S0021-9290(02)00365-2.
30. Dwyer MK, Jones HL, Field RE, et al. Femoroacetabular impingement negates the acetabular labral seal during pivoting maneuvers but not gait. Clin Orthop. 2015;473:602–7. https://doi.org/10.1007/s11999-014-3760-1.
31. Ito K, Minka-II M-A, Leunig M, et al. Femoroacetabular impingement and the cam-effect. J Bone Joint Surg Br. 2001;83-B:171–6. https://doi.org/10.1302/0301-620X.83B2.0830171.
32. Gojda J, Bartoníček J. The retinacula of Weitbrecht in the adult hip. Surg Radiol Anat. 2012;34:31–8. https://doi.org/10.1007/s00276-011-0829-3.
33. Philippon MJ, Schenker ML, Briggs KK, et al. Revision hip arthroscopy. Am J Sports Med. 2007;35:1918–21. https://doi.org/10.1177/0363546507305097.
34. Ranawat AS, McClincy M, Sekiya JK. Anterior dislocation of the hip after arthroscopy in a patient with capsular laxity of the hip. A case report. J Bone Joint Surg Am. 2009;91:192–7. https://doi.org/10.2106/JBJS.G.01367.
35. Benali Y, Katthagen BD. Hip subluxation as a complication of arthroscopic debridement. Arthroscopy. 2009;25:405–7. https://doi.org/10.1016/j.arthro.2009.01.012.

36. Domb BG, Philippon MJ, Giordano BD. Arthroscopic capsulotomy, capsular repair, and capsular plication of the hip: relation to atraumatic instability. Arthroscopy. 2013;29:162–73. https://doi.org/10.1016/j.arthro.2012.04.057.
37. Abrams GD, Hart MA, Takami K, et al. Biomechanical evaluation of capsulotomy, Capsulectomy, and capsular repair on hip rotation. Arthroscopy. 2015;31:1511–7. https://doi.org/10.1016/j.arthro.2015.02.031.
38. Myers CA, Register BC, Lertwanich P, et al. Role of the acetabular labrum and the iliofemoral ligament in hip stability: an in vitro biplane fluoroscopy study. Am J Sports Med. 2011;39(Suppl):85S–91S. https://doi.org/10.1177/0363546511412161.
39. Garrison JC, Osler MT, Singleton SB. Rehabilitation after arthroscopy of an acetabular labral tear. North Am J Sports Phys Ther. 2007;2:241–50.
40. Spencer-Gardner L, Eischen JJ, Levy BA, et al. A comprehensive five-phase rehabilitation programme after hip arthroscopy for femoroacetabular impingement. Knee Surg Sports Traumatol Arthrosc. 2014;22:848–59. https://doi.org/10.1007/s00167-013-2664-z.
41. Cheatham SW, Kolber MJ. Rehabilitation after hip arthroscopy and labral repair in a high school football athlete. Int J Sports Phys Ther. 2012;7:173–84.
42. Stalzer S, Wahoff M, Scanlan M. Rehabilitation following hip arthroscopy. Clin Sports Med. 2006;25:337–57, x. https://doi.org/10.1016/j.csm.2005.12.008.
43. Wahoff M, Ryan M. Rehabilitation after hip femoroacetabular impingement arthroscopy. Clin Sports Med. 2011;30:463–82. https://doi.org/10.1016/j.csm.2011.01.001.
44. Philippon MJ, Decker MJ, Giphart JE, et al. Rehabilitation exercise progression for the gluteus medius muscle with consideration for iliopsoas tendinitis: an in vivo electromyography study. Am J Sports Med. 2011;39:1777–85. https://doi.org/10.1177/0363546511406848.
45. Edelstein J, Ranawat A, Enseki KR, et al. Postoperative guidelines following hip arthroscopy. Curr Rev Musculoskelet Med. 2012;5:15–23. https://doi.org/10.1007/s12178-011-9107-6.
46. Enseki KR, Martin R, Kelly BT. Rehabilitation after arthroscopic decompression for femoroacetabular impingement. Clin Sports Med. 2010;29:247–55, viii. https://doi.org/10.1016/j.csm.2009.12.007.
47. Enseki KR, Martin RL, Draovitch P, et al. The hip joint: arthroscopic procedures and postoperative rehabilitation. J Orthop Sports Phys Ther. 2006;36:516–25. https://doi.org/10.2519/jospt.2006.2138.
48. Yasunaga Y, Takahashi K, Ochi M, et al. Rotational acetabular osteotomy in patients forty-six years of age or older: comparison with younger patients. J Bone Joint Surg Am. 2003;85:266–72. https://doi.org/10.2106/00004623-200302000-00013.
49. Aprato A, Jayasekera N, Villar R. Timing in hip arthroscopy: does surgical timing change clinical results? Int Orthop. 2012;36:2231–4. https://doi.org/10.1007/s00264-012-1655-x.
50. Domb BG, Linder D, Finley Z, et al. Outcomes of hip arthroscopy in patients aged 50 years or older compared with a matched-pair control of patients aged 30 years or younger. Arthroscopy. 2015;31:231–8. https://doi.org/10.1016/j.arthro.2014.08.030.
51. Malviya A, Paliobeis CP, Villar RN. Do professional athletes perform better than recreational athletes after arthroscopy for femoroacetabular impingement? Clin Orthop Relat Res. 2013;471:2477–83. https://doi.org/10.1007/s11999-013-2787-z.
52. Philippon MJ, Weiss DR, Kuppersmith DA, et al. Arthroscopic labral repair and treatment of femoroacetabular impingement in professional hockey players. Am J Sports Med. 2010;38:99–104. https://doi.org/10.1177/0363546509346393.
53. Byrd JWT, Jones KS. Diagnostic accuracy of clinical assessment, magnetic resonance imaging, magnetic resonance arthrography, and intra-articular injection in hip arthroscopy patients. Am J Sports Med. 2004;32:1668–74. https://doi.org/10.1177/0363546504266480.
54. Kamath AF, Componovo R, Baldwin K, et al. Hip arthroscopy for labral tears: review of clinical outcomes with 4.8-year mean follow-up. Am J Sports Med. 2009;37:1721–7. https://doi.org/10.1177/0363546509333078.

Femoroacetabular Impingement: Treatment Options—Open Femoral Osteochondroplasty and Rim Trimming

7

Alessandro Aprato, Matteo Olivero, Alessandro Massè, and Reinhold Ganz

7.1 Introduction

The goal of femoroacetabular impingement (FAI) treatment is to restore the normal hip function removing pathomechanic femoral and/or acetabular deformities. The technique of safe surgical hip dislocation has been described more than 15 years ago [1] and it has been, for several years, the gold standard for the treatment of intra-articular hip pathology [2]. In the last decades hip arthroscopy became progressively more popular for FAI treatment and, in literature, it is reported an over 600% increase of hip arthroscopy between 2006 and 2010 [3]. However, this success was partially reduced with the increase of revision surgery, mainly required for insufficient resection or unrecognized co-deformities [4, 5].

Nowadays, open treatment is the method of choice when the deformity is complex, or more than one deformity are present. The main indications for the open treatment are global acetabular overcoverage as seen in coxa profunda, severe acetabular retroversion, impingement in combination with femoral retroversion and high riding greater trochanter. Severe femoral retro tilt as seen in SCFE, complex deformities of the head as in Perthes disease, and failure of arthroscopic treatment are also indications for open surgery. In any case, a comprehensive preoperative evaluation to identify the causes of impingement, often including MRI and CT, is essential.

A. Aprato (✉) · M. Olivero · A. Massè
University of Turin, Turin, Italy
e-mail: alessandro.masse@unito.it

R. Ganz
Faculty of Medicine, University of Bern, Bern, Switzerland

7.2 Surgical Dislocation of the Hip

General or spinal anesthesia can be used although general anesthesia is preferred for the possibility of muscle relaxation.

The patient is placed in lateral decubitus position with well-padded bolster. A single anterior squared pubic support is generally used during hip dislocation instead of the anterior support traditionally used for total hip arthroplasty (Fig. 7.1). Indeed, the latter may not allow a proper leg positioning when the hip is dislocated and the leg is placed in the bag on the anterior side of the table.

The trochanteric region is prepped and draped in standard sterile fashion and a sterile bag is hung on the edge of the table, anteriorly to the patient, to receive the foot during hip dislocation.

Kocher-Langenbeck or Gibson approach may be used to perform the surgical hip dislocation [6]. The Gibson approach is usually characterized by a better aesthetic results with less "saddleback deformation" of the subcutaneous tissues [7]. The skin is incised along the anterior third of the greater trochanter with the hip fully extended

R. Ganz (ed.), *Modern Hip Preservation*, https://doi.org/10.1007/978-3-030-91967-2_7

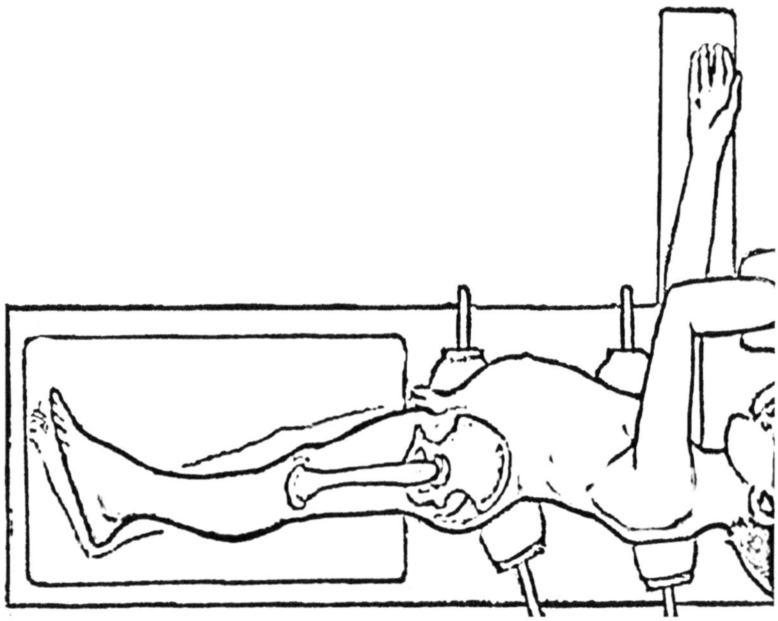

Fig. 7.1 Patient positioned in lateral decubitus with a single anterior support against the symphysis that allows better free leg positions

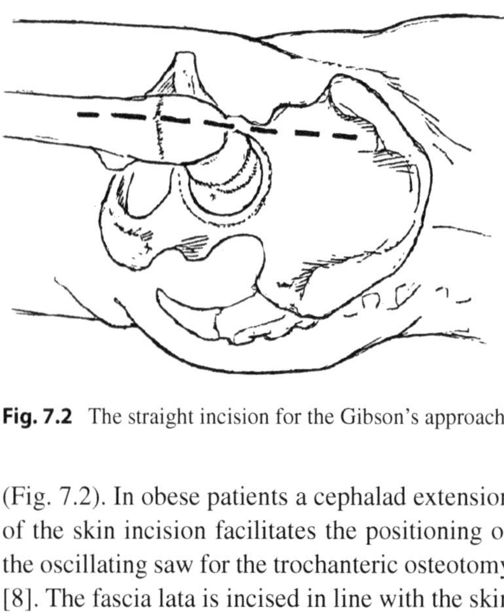

Fig. 7.2 The straight incision for the Gibson's approach

(Fig. 7.2). In obese patients a cephalad extension of the skin incision facilitates the positioning of the oscillating saw for the trochanteric osteotomy [8]. The fascia lata is incised in line with the skin incision. The gluteus maximus is retracted posteriorly, and not split, in order to avoid neurovascular damage to the anterior muscle's fibers [9].

The leg is then internally rotated to expose the posterior border of gluteus medius. No attempts should be made to mobilize the gluteus medius and to identify the tendon of piriformis [6].

After the incision of the trochanteric bursa, the trochanteric branch of the deep branch of the medial femoral circumflex artery (MFCA) can be identified. This branch serves as a landmark to identify the superior border of the quadratus femoris. In this area, the deep branch of the MFCA runs around the obturator externus tendon as a posterior sling [10]. This trochanteric branch can be cauterized at the level of the planned trochanteric osteotomy without compromising the vascular supply of the femoral head [8].

The trochanteric osteotomy should be performed with the leg internally rotated of 20–30°. The trochanteric fragment provides continuity between gluteus medius/minimus proximally and vastus lateralis distally. All the external rotators should remain on the stable part of the greater trochanter to protect and preserve the deep branch of MFCA, which becomes intracapsular at the level of the superior gemellus muscle [6].

A straight trochanteric osteotomy was reported in the original description of the surgical technique [6] (Fig. 7.3). The osteotomy line runs anterior to the posterior trochanteric crest with the proximal exit in the middle of the trochanteric tip. Usually some fibers of the gluteus medius insertion remain on the mobile fragment and have to be released during mobilization of the fragment [6, 7]. The osteotomy should not be

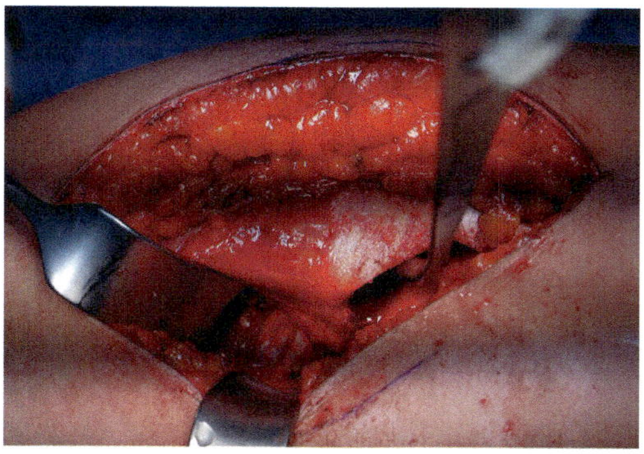

Fig. 7.3 The straight osteotomy of the greater trochanter as described in the original surgical technique. A straight line from the posterior edge of the greater trochanter to the posterior border of the ridge of vastus lateralis. The osteotomy is performed parallel to the long axis of the femoral shaft and should exit just anteriorly to the most posterior insertion of gluteus medius. Few fibers of the gluteus medius had to be left attached to the stable part of the femur and subsequently released

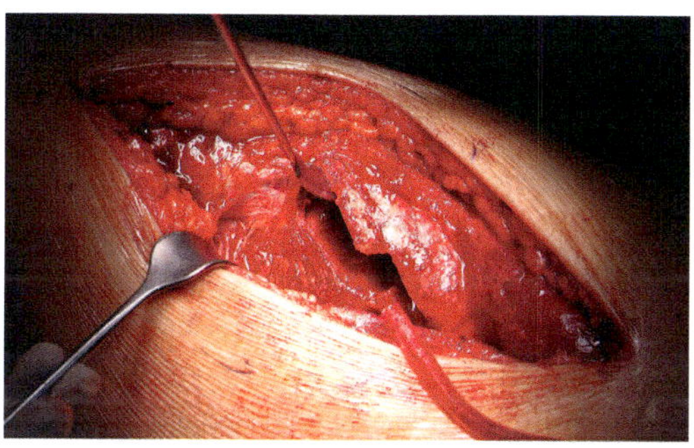

Fig. 7.4 "Z" osteotomy of the greater trochanter

completed with the oscillating saw but the anterior cortex of the trochanter can be broken by levering the fragment with an osteotome.

A trochanteric step osteotomy could be performed to achieve a more stable fixation of the fragment reducing the risk of trochanteric malunion and non-union [11]. The step between the two surfaces should be about 5 mm [8] (Fig. 7.4).

A straight osteotomy is indicated when distal advancement of the trochanter is necessary. In all the other cases, we prefer a step- or Z-osteotomy, although it is technically more demanding.

The osteotomized fragment can now be mobilized anteriorly with a Hohmann retractor. Strong fibrous connections at the anterosuperior circumference have to be released to obtain sufficient mobilization of the fragment. If a portion of the piriformis tendon remains attached to the mobile fragment, these fibers should be cut close to the trochanteric fragment. The fragment can now be tilted and completely mobilized anteriorly.

The limb is placed in slight flexion and external rotation to develop the safe interval between the piriformis tendon and gluteus minimus muscle. To find this interval, the dissection should start very close to the stable trochanter keeping in mind that all the vessels and anastomosis to the femoral head are distal to the piriformis tendon. The integrity of the tendon of piriformis ensures protection to the sciatic nerve and to the anastomosis between the inferior gluteal artery and the deep branch of the medial circumflex artery. This anastomosis runs along the lower margin of the piriformis tendon and it alone can guarantee sufficient vascularization to the femoral head also in cases of injury to the deep branch [10, 12]. The gluteus minimus muscle is dissected from the capsule and retracted cranially.

To obtain a complete exposure of the capsule, the leg is moved in different positions in flexion-extension and internal and external rotation. Usually a Z-capsulotomy is performed for the right hip and an inverse Z-capsulotomy for the left hip [6]. The first incision runs anterolaterally along the axis of the neck. Distally, the anterior branch of the capsulotomy starts close to the anterior femoral insertion of the capsule and is directed towards the anteroinferior border of the acetabulum. Proximally, the capsulotomy is extended posteriorly parallel to the acetabular rim until the retracted tendon of the piriformis (Fig. 7.5).

A Langenbeck retractor is used to keep the soft tissues back at the 12 o'clock position. The hip is now gently subluxed with traction, flexion, and external rotation while a bone hook is placed around the calcar to help the dislocation. The ligamentum teres is then cut and the hip is completely dislocated anteriorly with further flexion and external rotation.

The leg is than placed in the sterile bag anteriorly to the patient. In cases of scarring from previous surgery or trauma, sciatic nerve identification,

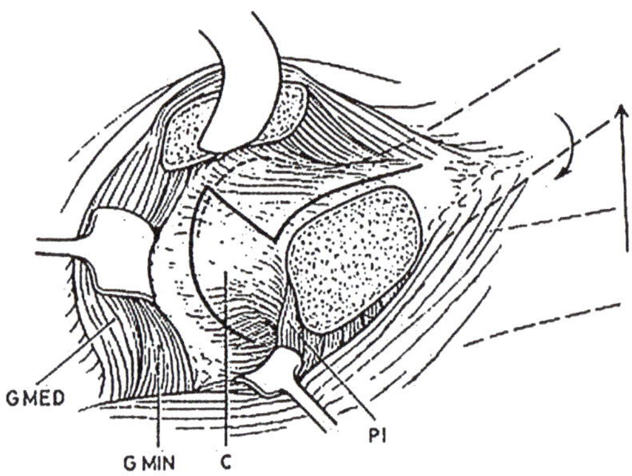

Fig. 7.5 Z-capsulotomy. The first incision runs anterolaterally along femoral neck; proximally is extended posteriorly parallel to the acetabular rim; distally is extended anteriorly towards the lesser trochanter

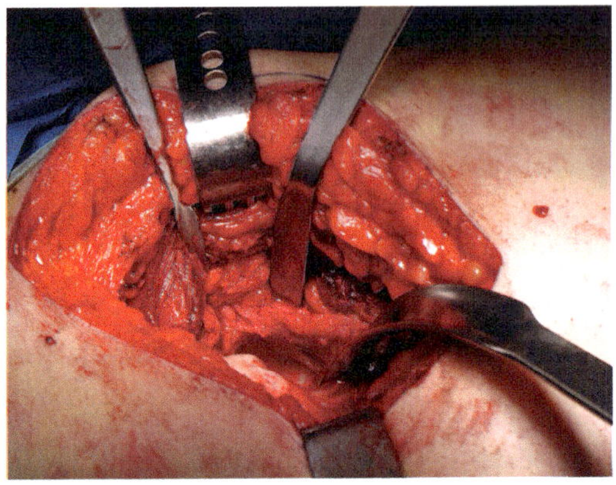

Fig. 7.6 Position of the retractors for acetabular exposure. One retractor at the 12 o'clock, one retractor anteriorly at the acetabular rim, and a large, narrow, curved Hohmann retractor posteriorly to the acetabular rim and against the femoral neck

inspection, and dissection had to be performed before complete dislocation of the hip to avoid injuries to the nerve [6].

After the complete dislocation, the hip is relocated to identify areas of impingement with the evaluation of a complete range of motion in flexion-extension and with combined movement of flexion-abduction-external rotation (FABER test) and flexion-adduction-internal rotation (FADIR test/impingement test). The posteroinferior rim area can be inspected with full extension and external rotation.

Complete 360° view and access to the acetabulum and nearly 360° to the proximal femur is now possible by manipulating the lower limb.

As soon as the hip is dislocated and the cartilage is fully exposed, it should be protected from drying out with frequent washes with saline solution [7, 8].

7.3 Acetabulum

Two additional retractors are used for the evaluation of the acetabulum: one anteriorly and the other inferiorly at the acetabular rim. Keeping the thigh parallel to the ground, the assistant pushes against the knee to obtain further exposure of the acetabulum. For the evaluation of the posterior rim area, the hip is extended to release the posterior muscle flap and the sciatic nerve. A small Hohmann placed posteriorly to the posterior rim pushes the neck away allowing inspection of the posteroinferior joint area (Fig. 7.6).

The pattern of damage to the acetabular cartilage and labrum depends on the morphology of the hip [13]. In pincer, or impacting impingement, the labrum is the first damaged structure. The typical damage patterns are ganglion formation within the labrum and degeneration of the adjacent cartilage. In retroverted hips the damaged area is anterosuperior, in deep sockets it can be circumferential [8, 13]. In advanced stages the labrum can be found torn. Bone apposition at the base of the labrum, induced by repetitive microtrauma, can worsen further the impingement [14]. If flexion is enforced, the increased pressure between the posteroinferior femoral head and the acetabulum can develop a contrecoup lesion both on femoral head and acetabular cartilage [8, 13].

In cam or inclusive impingement, the cartilage is usually damaged in the anterosuperior area of the acetabulum (1 o'clock position). Initially, the labrum is stable and uninjured while the cartilage is separated from the labrum towards the center of acetabulum. In later stages, the labrum becomes also part of the degeneration.

Isolated cam and pincer impingement are rare, the majority of patients have a combination of the two mechanism and, consequently, a mix of cartilage and labrum lesions [15]. In some patients, an

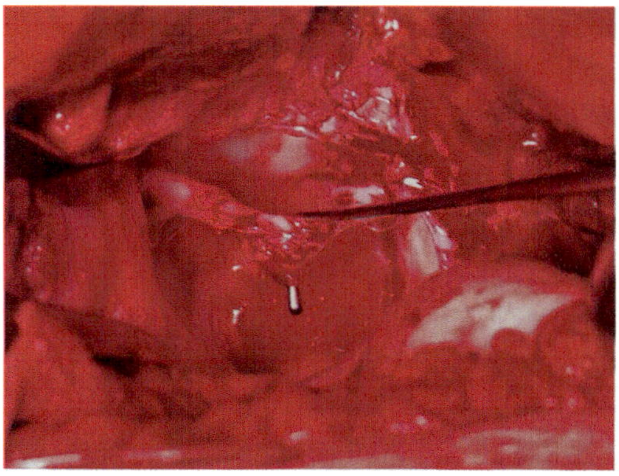

Fig. 7.7 Labrum detached from the acetabular rim by sharp dissection. Evaluation of the labrum with a small probe

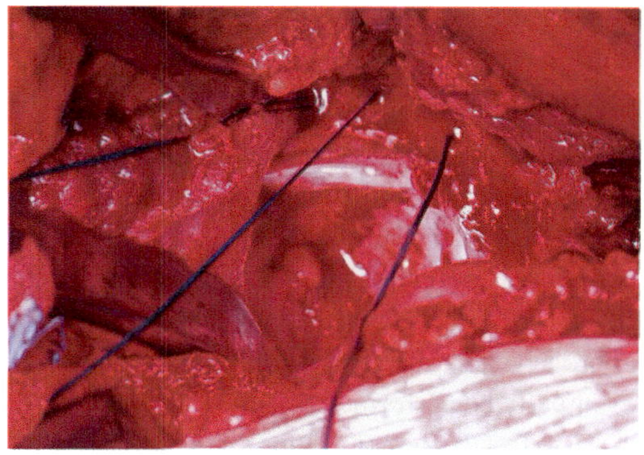

Fig. 7.8 Sutures are passed through the labral substance. The definitive suture tightening will be performed only after hip reduction to obtain a more anatomic alignment of the labrum and a perfect knots tension

extra-articular impingement between the greater or the lesser trochanter and the periacetabular bone is present. The extra-articular impingement sometimes becomes evident only after the removal of the intra-articular impingement [16].

A blunt probe can be used to evaluate the labrum for detachment or tears. If labral tears are irreparable, then part of the labrum may be debrided. Nowadays, results with labral reconstruction using autologous fascial tissue are encouraging [17].

In the area of maximum overcoverage, the labrum is detached from the acetabular rim by sharp dissection (Fig. 7.7). Then, the acetabular rim is resected with a curved osteotome or with a 5-mm high-speed burr. The amount of resection can be estimated pre-operatively on plain X-rays and CT scan based on the cross-over sign and on the lateral center-edge angle. The area of delaminated cartilage can be considered a good landmark for the magnitude of the rim resection and, as general rule, every 1 mm of lateral resection correspond to a reduction of 2° of acetabular coverage [8]. Intraoperatively, the rim excision is extended until no further impingement is present during repeatedly testing. Excessive resection can create hip instability and acetabular undercoverage similar to acetabular dysplasia.

If full-thickness chondral lesions are identified, microfractures can be performed.

Following rim resection, the labrum is debrided of fraying and unhealthy tissue leaving as much viable tissue as possible. Philippon et al. [18] recommend a minimum of 7 mm of width to repair and reattach the labrum without augmentation. The labrum had to be reattached on bleeding bone surfaces using absorbable suture anchors [18, 19]. In most cases, 3 to 4 suture anchors are used [20]. The anchors have to be placed 2–3 mm away from the cartilage surface and have to be directed away from the cartilage to avoid its penetration. The sutures are passed through the labrum in a piercing fashion (Fig. 7.8). Sutures can also be passed around the labrum in a loop fashion to avoid further tissue damages [18], a technique which has limited primary seal effect. Definitive tightening of the sutures has to be performed after hip reduction to provide a more homogeneous expansion of the labrum and tension on the knots [8]. The knots must be placed on the capsular side of the labrum to avoid contact with the articular surfaces [21, 22].

After an early phase of debridement of the labrum, labral re-attachment became the method of choice leading to better midterm results [7, 18, 21, 23, 24].

7.4 Femur

For an optimal exposure of the proximal femur, the leg remains in the sterile bag, the knee is lowered, and the hip adducted and externally rotated. Two blunt Hohmann retractors are placed around the femoral neck (Fig. 7.9). First of all the posterosuperior retinaculum with the vessels has to be identified and protected [10]. The retinacular area is about 2 cm large and can be visually identified. Femoral version can be easily evaluated on the dislocated hip. Impingement can be due to an excessive anteversion or to a retroversion of the femur. In these cases, caudal extension of the approach and a subtrochanteric osteotomy should eventually be performed.

Usually, the femoral bump is localized at the anterosuperior head-neck junction and can be identified by an inflammatory appearance. The cartilage can have pink appearance and sometimes cysts near the non-spherical area can be identified [8, 25]. Transparent plastic templates are helpful to better identify the amount and the extension of the non-spherical area and to control the amount of correction (Fig. 7.10).

The removal of the abnormal bone to restore a correct head-neck offset can be performed with a curved osteotome or with an high-speed burr [23]. Regular re-evaluation of the contouring with the templates is mandatory as well as testing of impingement free motion (Fig. 7.11).

During the osteochondroplasty, constant visual control of the retinacular integrity is

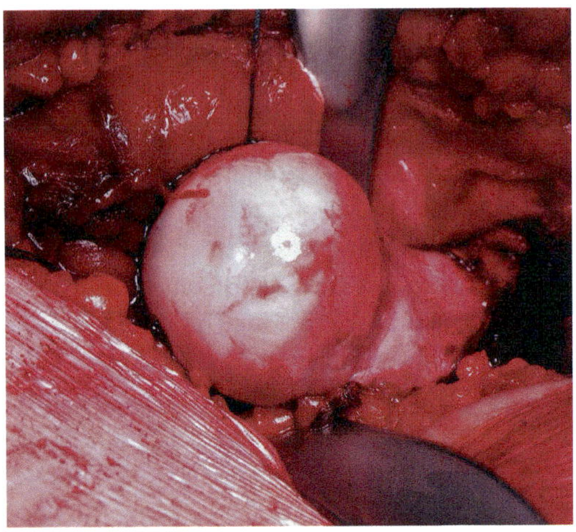

Fig. 7.9 Position of retractors for exposure of the femoral head and neck. The femoral head is further elevated with two blunt Hohmann retractors, placed around the neck

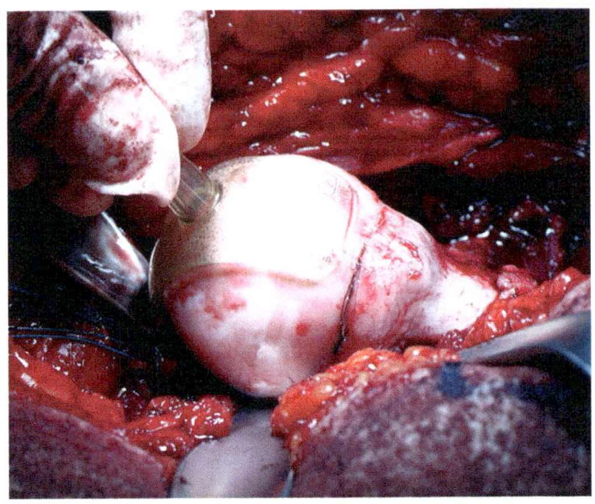

Fig. 7.10 Identification and evaluation of the femoral bump with sized transparent plastic template

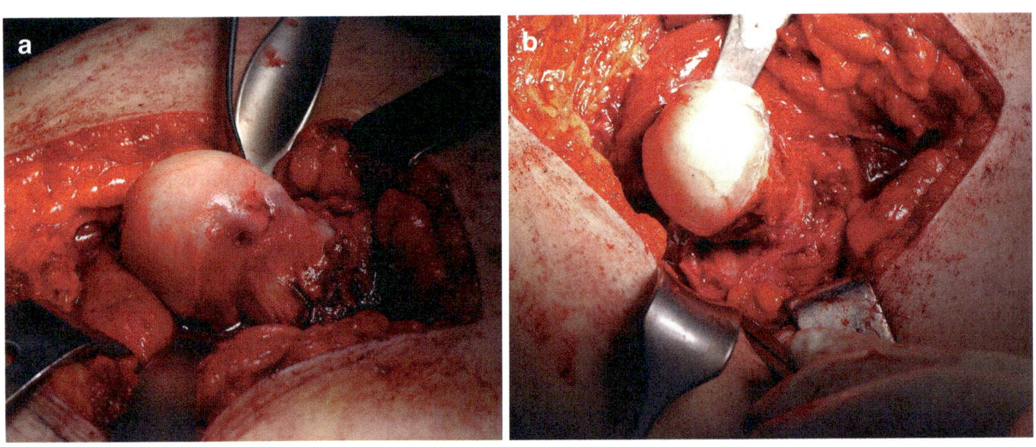

Fig. 7.11 (**a**) Bump at head-neck femoral junction before osteochondroplasty. (**b**) Head-neck junction after the osteochondroplasty

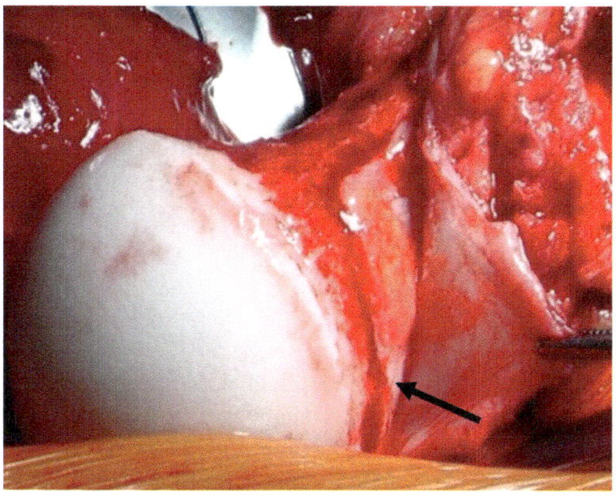

Fig. 7.12 Limited bone resection proximal to the retinacular flap. *Black arrow*: Posterosuperior periosteal flap

mandatory to preserve the vascularization of the femoral head. If a bump extends posteriorly over the retinaculum, resection has to respect not only the perforation area of the retinacular vessels (7) but also consider that the intraosseous course is rather superficially [26] (Fig. 7.12).

Over-resection of the neck increases the risk of neck fracture and compromises the seal effect of the labrum. Several authors reported that 30% of the diameter of the neck is the maximum amount of resection without an increased risk of fracture [27–29].

Before reduction of the hip, the stump of the ligamentum teres can be debrided and bone wax can be applied on the debrided bone surfaces to reduce the bleeding (Fig. 7.13).

During the dislocation, is reported a reduction of the perfusion of the femoral head circa by 10% [30]. Intraoperatively, the "bleeding sign" can confirm the adequate vascularization of the femoral head. This test consist in a 2.0 mm drill hole carried out on the non-weight bearing area of the femoral head and is considered positive for immediate appearance of active bleeding after drilling [6, 31]. This test has been validated as a reliable indicator of good femoral head prognosis after surgical dislocation [31]. Some authors reported the use of electronic devices to monitor the blood flow into the spongious bone [30, 32].

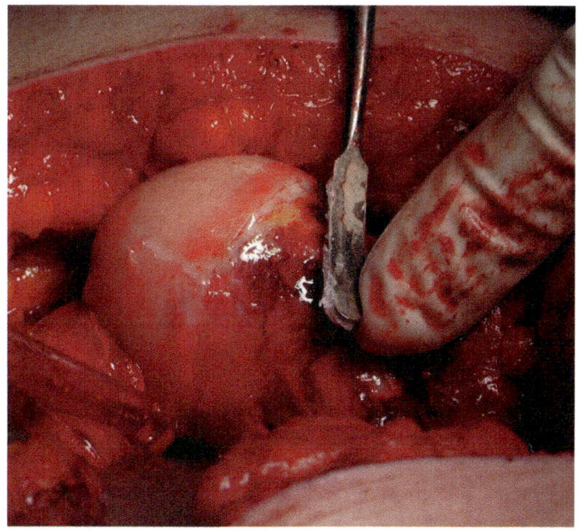

Fig. 7.13 Application of bone wax on the debrided bone surface

7.5 Reduction

Relocation of the femoral head is easily achieved with traction and controlled internal rotation with attention to not avulse labral sutures and to not invert the labrum.

Following hip reduction, the sutures of the labrum can be finally tightened and final assessment of the range of motion is performed to identify any residual impingement.

Only the vertical incision of the capsule is repaired with loose running absorbable suture. Excessive tension on the capsule should be avoided for the risk of stretching on the retinacular vessels and decrease the perfusion of femoral head [30, 31, 33, 34].

The trochanteric fragment is then reduced. If a Z-osteotomy was performed, the anatomical reduction is easily achieved [8]. In case of a straight osteotomy, the greater trochanter fragment can be reduced in an anatomic position or advanced distally to respect relative lengthening of the femoral neck and improve function of abductors muscles; overcorrection however should be avoided. Final fixation of the trochanteric fragment is performed with two or three 3.5-mm screws from the lateral aspect of the greater trochanter towards the medial calcar [19, 33] (Fig. 7.14).

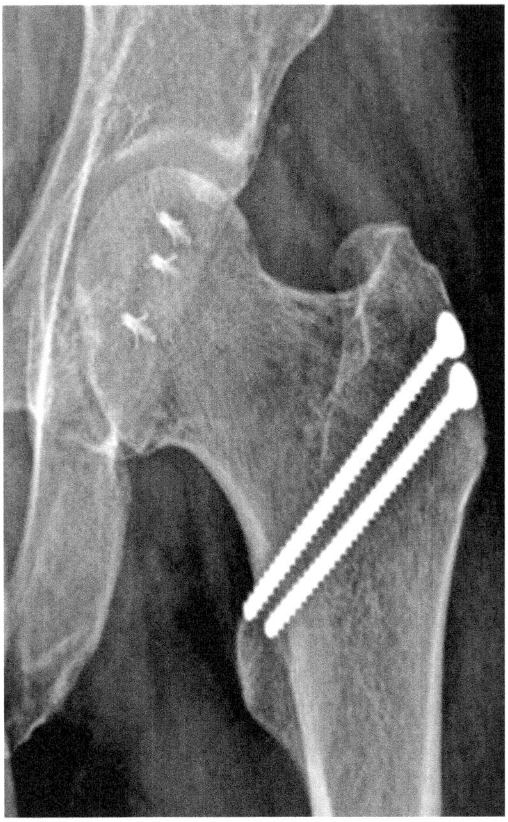

Fig. 7.14 Postoperative X-rays. Fixation of the trochanter with 3.5-mm screws

Fascia lata, subcutaneous tissue and skin are carefully sutured in a layered fashion.

7.6 Conclusions

Treatment of femoroacetabular impingement by open surgical dislocation is characterized by several advantages. First of all, the procedure is safe regarding the risk of avascular necrosis and the morbidity is low. Second, surgical dislocation provides a complete direct visualization of the entire acetabulum and proximal femur and consequently, major pathologic deformities can be identified and treated. Third, with a single surgical approach the surgeon can perform several surgical procedures on the acetabulum, the femur, and the soft tissues.

The efficacy of FAI treatment has been demonstrated for both arthroscopic and open surgery and both have specific indications. A careful evaluation of the deformity leading to impingement is essential.

References

1. Ganz R, Gill TJ, Gautier E, et al. Surgical dislocation of the adult hip. A technique with full access to the femoral head and acetabulum without the risk of avascular necrosis. J Bone Joint Surg Br. 2001;83:1119–24. https://doi.org/10.1302/0301-620x.83b8.11964.
2. Ryan MK, Youm T, Vigdorchik JM. Beyond the scope open treatment of femoroacetabular impingement. Bull Hosp Joint Dis. 2018;76:47–54.
3. Bozic KJ, Chan V, Valone FH, et al. Trends in hip arthroscopy utilization in the United States. J Arthroplast. 2013;28:140–3. https://doi.org/10.1016/j.arth.2013.02.039.
4. Philippon MJ, Schenker ML, Briggs KK, et al. Revision hip arthroscopy. Am J Sports Med. 2007;35:1918–21. https://doi.org/10.1177/0363546507305097.
5. Clohisy JC, Nepple JJ, Larson CM, et al. Persistent structural disease is the most common cause of repeat hip preservation surgery. Clin Orthop. 2013;471:3788–94. https://doi.org/10.1007/s11999-013-3218-x.
6. Ganz R, Gill TJ, Gautier E, et al. Surgical dislocation of the adult hip a technique with full access to the femoral head necrosis. J Bone Joint Surg Br. 2001;83(8):1119–24.
7. Beck M, Puloski S, Leunig M, et al. Surgical dislocation of the adult hip. A technique for the treatment of articular pathology of the hip. Semin Arthroplast. 2005;16:38–44.
8. Marín-peña Ó. Femoroacetabular Impingement. Berlin: Springer; 2012.
9. Gibson A. Posterior exposure of the hip joint: commentary. J Bone Jt Surg. 1950;32B:183–6. https://doi.org/10.1097/01.blo.0000150719.68914.a5.
10. Gautier E, Ganz K, Krugel N, et al. Anatomy of the medial femoral circumflex artery and its surgical implications. J Bone Joint Surg Br. 2018;83-B:149. https://doi.org/10.1302/0301-620x.83b1.0830149.
11. Schoeniger R, Lafrance AE, Oxland TR, et al. Does trochanteric step osteotomy provide greater stability than classic slide osteotomy? Clin Orthop. 2009;467:775–82. https://doi.org/10.1007/s11999-008-0668-7.
12. Kalhor M, Beck M, Huff TW, Ganz R. Capsular and pericapsular contributions to acetabular and femoral head perfusion. J Bone Joint Surg Am. 2009;91:409–18. https://doi.org/10.2106/JBJS.G.01679.
13. Beck M, Kalhor M, Leunig M, Ganz R. Hip morphology influences the pattern of damage to the acetabular

cartilage Femoroacetabular impingement as a cause of early osteoarthritis of the hip. J Bone Joint Surg Br. 2005;87:1012–8.
14. Corten K, Ganz R, Chosa E, Leunig M. Bone apposition of the acetabular rim in deep hips. J Bone Joint Surg Am. 2011;93:10–6. https://doi.org/10.2106/jbjs.j.01799.
15. Siebenrock KA, Steppacher SD, Haefeli PC, et al. Valgus hip with high antetorsion causes pain through posterior extraarticular FAI. Clin Orthop. 2013;471:3774–80. https://doi.org/10.1007/s11999-013-2895-9.
16. Ganz R, Slongo T, Turchetto L, et al. The lesser trochanter as a cause of hip impingement: pathophysiology and treatment options. Hip Int. 2013;23:S35. https://doi.org/10.5301/hipint.5000063.
17. Domb BG, Hartigan DE, Perets I. Decision making for labral treatment in the hip: repair versus débridement versus reconstruction. J Am Acad Orthop Surg. 2017;25:e53–62. https://doi.org/10.5435/JAAOS-D-16-00144.
18. Philippon MJ, Briggs KK, Fagrelius T, Patterson D. Labral refixation: current techniques and indications. HSS J. 2012;8(3):240–4. https://doi.org/10.1007/s11420-012-9290-z.
19. Graves ML, Mast JW. Femoroacetabular impingement: do outcomes reliably improve with surgical dislocations? Clin Orthop. 2009;467:717–23. https://doi.org/10.1007/s11999-008-0648-y.
20. Slikker W, Van Thiel GS, Chahal J, Nho S. The use of double-loaded suture anchors for labral repair and capsular repair during hip arthroscopy. Arthrosc Tech. 2012;1:e213–7. https://doi.org/10.1016/j.eats.2012.08.002.
21. Espinosa N, Beck M, Rothenfluh DA, et al. Treatment of femoro-acetabular impingement: preliminary results of labral refixation. J Bone Joint Surg Am. 2007;89-A:36–53.
22. Aprato A, Jayasekera N, Villar RN. Revision hip arthroscopic surgery: outcome at three years. Knee Surg Sports Traumatol Arthrosc. 2013;22(4):932–7.
23. Peters CL, Erickson JA. Treatment of femoroacetabular impingement with surgical dislocation and débridement in young adults. J Bone Joint Surg Am. 2006;88:1735–41. https://doi.org/10.2106/JBJS.E.00514.
24. Philippon MJ, Briggs KK, Yen Y-M, Kuppersmith DA. Outcomes following hip arthroscopy for femoroacetabular impingement with associated chondrolabral dysfunction. J Bone Joint Surg Br. 2008;91-B:16–23. https://doi.org/10.1302/0301-620x.91b1.21329.
25. Wilson AS. Current concepts in management of femoroacetabular impingement. World J Orthop. 2013;3:204. https://doi.org/10.5312/wjo.v3.i12.204.
26. Rego P, Mascarenhas V, Collado D, et al. Arterial topographic anatomy near the femoral head-neck perforation with surgical relevance. J Bone Joint Surg Am. 2017;99:1213–21. https://doi.org/10.2106/JBJS.16.01386.
27. Rothenfluh E, Zingg P, Dora C, et al. Influence of resection geometry on fracture risk in the treatment of femoroacetabular impingement: a finite element study. Am J Sports Med. 2012;40:2002–8. https://doi.org/10.1177/0363546512456011.
28. Mardones RM, Gonzalez C, Chen Q, et al. Surgical treatment of femoroacetabular impingement: evaluation of the effect of the size of the resection. J Bone Joint Surg Am. 2005;87:273–9. https://doi.org/10.2106/JBJS.D.01793.
29. Loh BW, Stokes CM, Miller BG, Page RS. Femoroacetabular impingement osteoplasty. Bone Joint J. 2015;97-B:1214–9. https://doi.org/10.1302/0301-620x.97b9.35263.
30. Nötzli HP, Siebenrock KA, Hempfing A, et al. Perfusion of the femoral head during surgical dislocation of the hip: monitoring by laser doppler flowmetry. J Bone Joint Surg Br. 2003;84:300–4. https://doi.org/10.1302/0301-620x.84b2.12146.
31. Aprato A, Bonani A, Giachino M, et al. Can we predict femoral head vitality during surgical hip dislocation? J Hip Preserv Surg. 2014;1:77–81. https://doi.org/10.1093/jhps/hnu010.
32. Madhuri V, Dutt V, Samuel K, Gahukamble AD. Intra-operative femoral head vascularity assessment: an innovative and simple technique. Indian J Orthop. 2012;45:231–5. https://doi.org/10.4103/0019-5413.91649.
33. Masse A, Aprato A, Rollero L, et al. Surgical dislocation technique for the treatment of acetabular fractures. Clin Orthop Relat Res. 2013;471:4056–64. https://doi.org/10.1007/s11999-013-3228-8.
34. Massè A, Aprato A, Alluto C, et al. Surgical hip dislocation is a reliable approach for treatment of femoral head fractures. Clin Orthop Relat Res. 2015;473:3744–51. https://doi.org/10.1007/s11999-015-4352-4.

Acetabular Reorientation Procedure

8

Luigino Turchetto, Stefano Saggin, and Reinhold Ganz

8.1 Introduction

There is a clear correlation between osteoarthritis of the hip and acetabular dysplasia [1, 2] subsequent to global or local growth retardation, mainly of the acetabulum [3]. Growth retardation [4, 5] may persist over time with the result that at the end of acetabular growth the femoral head remains within the acetabulum but coverage of the head is insufficient, the proximal femur frequently shows also some minor deformity.

The major deformity is represented by a shallow acetabulum; requiring thus a correction on the acetabular side increasing the load transmission area.

Correction of acetabular dysplasia in the skeletally mature patient has shown to improve symptoms and longevity of the hip [6–8], In this paper, we describe the technique of periacetabular osteotomy that was first described and popularized by Reinhold Ganz [9].

The main advantage of this osteotomy over the triple pelvic osteotomies is the preservation of part of the posterior column of the hemipelvis. It increases the overall stability, it helps to protect the sciatic nerve, and it guarantees an undisturbed birth canal.

L. Turchetto (✉) · S. Saggin
Orthopedics and Traumatology Unit of Portogruaro Hospital, Portogruaro, Italy
e-mail: lturchetto@tin.it

R. Ganz
Faculty of Medicine, University of Bern, Bern, Switzerland

8.2 Pathophysiology of Hip Dysplasia

The pathomorphology of residual acetabular dysplasia in adults is commonly understood as excessive anteversion from the sagittal plane and the insufficiency of coverage is anterolateral [10]. More recent studies, [11, 12] however, have shown that 17–34% of classic acetabular dysplasias are retroverted; approximately 10% show a pure anterior and less than 5% an exclusively lateral deficiency.

Recognition of such variants of version is important to understand that some hips may suffer from impingement rather than from dysplasia [13] and such parameters must be considered during corrective surgery [14].

8.3 Association of Hip Dysplasia with Osteoarthritis

It is common understanding that residual acetabular dysplasia is a mechanical abnormality frequently leading to osteoarthritis (OA) of the hip [2, 15]. As a consequence of pathological loading of a reduced area of force transmission [16], it is reported that by the age of 50 years 25–50% of the patients may suffer from secondary joint degeneration [17]. Murphy et al. [18] found that with a smaller load transmission area, represented by a Wiberg LCE angle of 16°, all hips would undergo end-stage OA. When combined

R. Ganz (ed.), *Modern Hip Preservation*, https://doi.org/10.1007/978-3-030-91967-2_8

iliac muscle during the entire operation. The exposure is continued by detaching the origin of the iliac muscle along the interspinous crest.

The floor of TFL muscle is incised longitudinally and the lateral border of the rectus femoris with the reflect tendon is visualized.

In the distal part of the fascia incision, the ascending branch of the lateral femoral circumflex artery that is an important source of vascularization of the tensor fasciae latae muscle is exposed and mobilized distally (Fig. 8.3).

The direct head of the rectus femuris muscle is detached from di Anterior Inferior Iliac Spine (AIIS) and the reflected ramus is divided.

The rectus muscle is reflected distally and medially and the lateral border of the iliocapsularis muscle is identified (Fig. 8.4) and detached from the capsule by lateral to medial dissection until the iliopectineal bursa is opened and psoas tendon becomes visible. A pointed Hohmann retractor is inserted into the pubic ramus 1 cm medial to the iliopectineal eminence (Fig. 8.5) [49].

The iliocapsularis muscle is completely detached exposing the anteroinferior part of the capsule around the calcar. A curved scissor is advanced along the anteroinferior capsule and the space between the capsule and the obturator externus muscle is opened by spreading the scissors (Fig. 8.6).

It is safe to maintain the instrument in close contact with the anteroinferior capsule in a posterior direction because the medial femoral circumflex artery that supplies the femoral head runs distal to the obturator externus muscle belly.

With the tip of the scissors, we can palpate the posterior and inferior border of acetabulum called infracotyloid groove and the ischium width is evaluated by gliding the scissors medially into the obturator foramen for understanding the position of medial ischial border and lamina quadrilatera orientation without any risk of injuring the obturator vessel which lie more superior. The lateral border of ischial ramus is formed by the tendinous origin of the ischiocrural muscles which

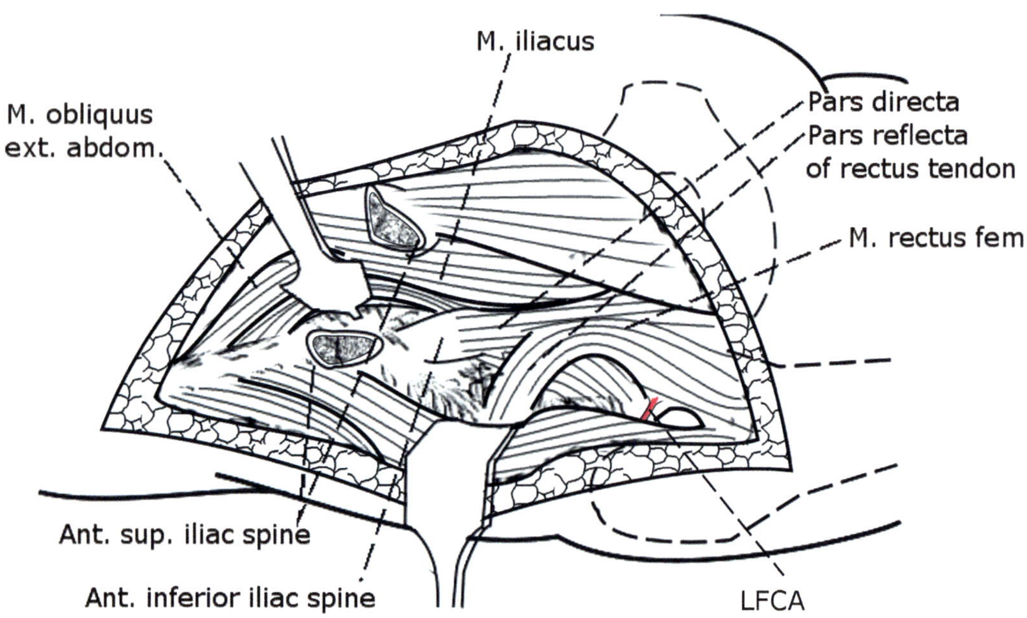

Fig. 8.3 (Modified from Weber and Ganz [49]) The *Anterior Superior Iliac spine* is detached through a V-Shaped osteotomy from lateral over a distance of ca 1.5 cm and a depth of ca. 1 cm. The origins of tensor fascia latae muscle, *M. Obliquus abdominis externus*, inguinal and sartorius ligament are reflected medially. The origin of the *external obliquus muscle* is lifted and its distal half is detached subperiosteally. The ascending branch of the lateral femoral circumflex artery (*LCFA*) is exposed and mobilized distally

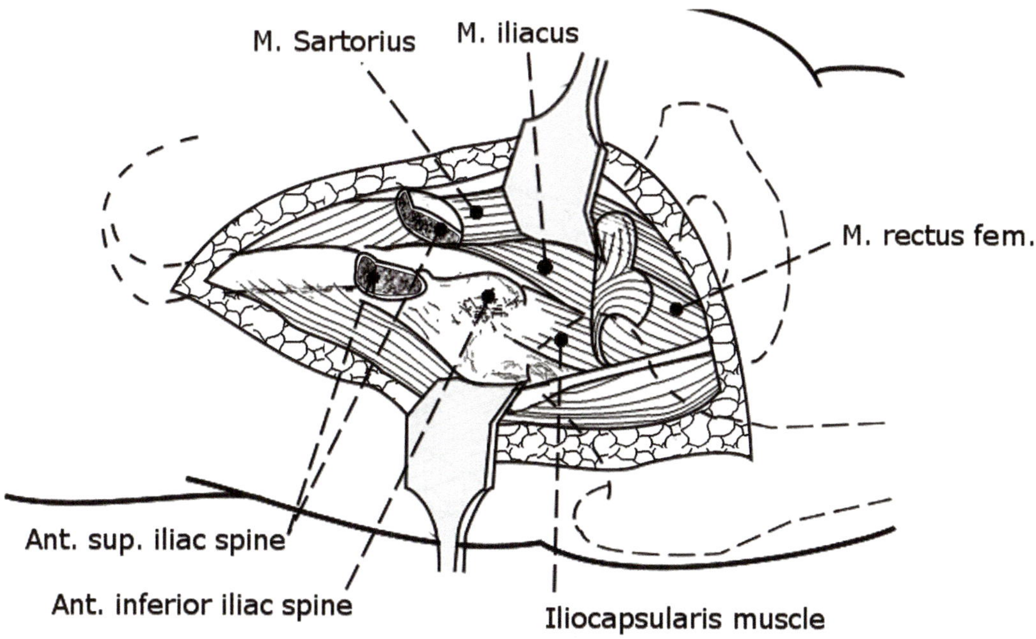

Fig. 8.4 (Modified from Weber and Ganz [49]) *M. Rectus femuris* is retracted medially. The *Iliocapsularis muscles* can be seen over the anterior joint capsule originating mainly from the *anterior inferior iliac spine*

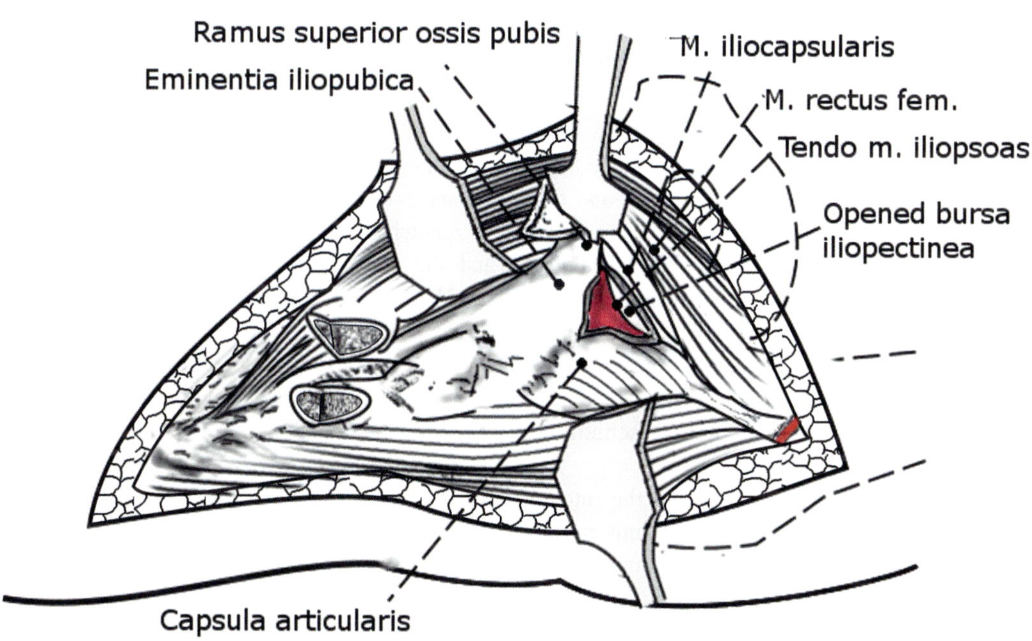

Fig. 8.5 (Modified from Weber and Ganz [49]) The *Iliocapsularis muscle* is detached from the capsule, the *iliopectineal bursa* is opened, and the *psoas tendon* becomes visible. The *psoas tendon* is undermined and retracted medially with an Homann retractor pointed in the pubic ramus 1.5–2 mm medially to the iliopectineal eminence. The *psoas tendon* protects the femoral nerves and vessels from overstretching

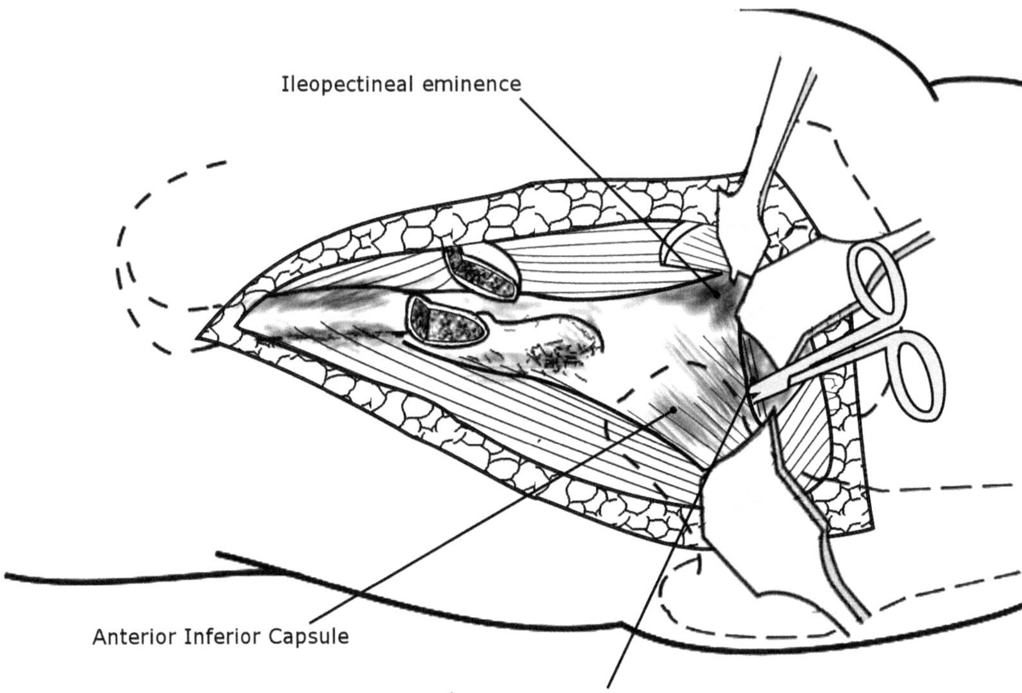

Fig. 8.6 (Modified from Weber and Ganz [49]) A large curved pair of scissors with rounded ends is inserted along the *anteroinferior capsule* and the space between the capsule and the *obturator externus muscle* is opened by spreading the scissors

exceed the lateral border of the ischium while flexing the hip. They offer a soft resistance to the instruments avoiding a lateral slipping and thus injury to the sciatic nerve (Fig. 8.7).

The periacetabular osteotomy can be divided into five steps and their sequence must be followed and done with the hip in 45° of flexion.

The first, incomplete, osteotomy of the ischium is done when the transverse diameter and the topography of the infracotyloid ischium are well known and memorized.

A Cobb elevator is inserted into the interval between capsule and obturator externus muscle which is mobilized distally for assisting the introduction of a 15 mm curved pelvic osteotomy chisel onto the anterior aspect of the ischium (Fig. 8.7). The axilla of the ischium and the posteroinferior acetabular rim are palpated with the chisel. The handle of curved osteotome is pointed in a slight posteroinferior direction and it is oriented towards the opposite shoulder (Figs. 8.8 and 8.9). If the surgeon feels unsecure regarding the first step, he may control position and advancement of the osteotome with fluoroscopy.

A notch is made in the central part of the ischium and the chisel is driven slowly to a depth of 20–25 mm while changing gradually its direction so that at the end of the insertion the handle points posterosuperiorly. With wiggling motion, the surgeon can feel if the medial and lateral cortical border is still intact and the chisel is drawn back till the blade remains in contact with the entry point. The osteotome is moved onto the remaining bone bridge. The medial cortex should be cut completely (Fig. 8.10), whereas the lateral cortex should only be notched because of the narrowing of the posterior column and the proximity of the sciatic nerve.

At the end the posterior column is not osteotomized completely, but a sufficiently deep cut is important to allow an easy fracture completion into the last osteotomy from the inside of the pelvis at the end of all five osteotomies.

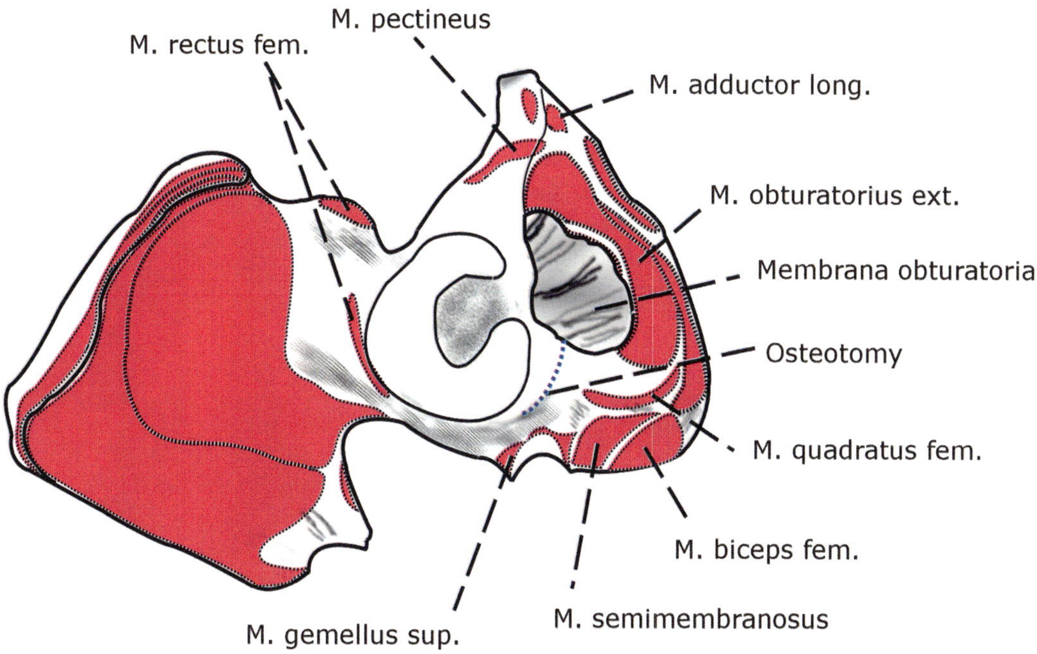

Fig. 8.7 *Blue dotted line* indicating the path of the ischial osteotomy onto the anterior aspect of the ischium

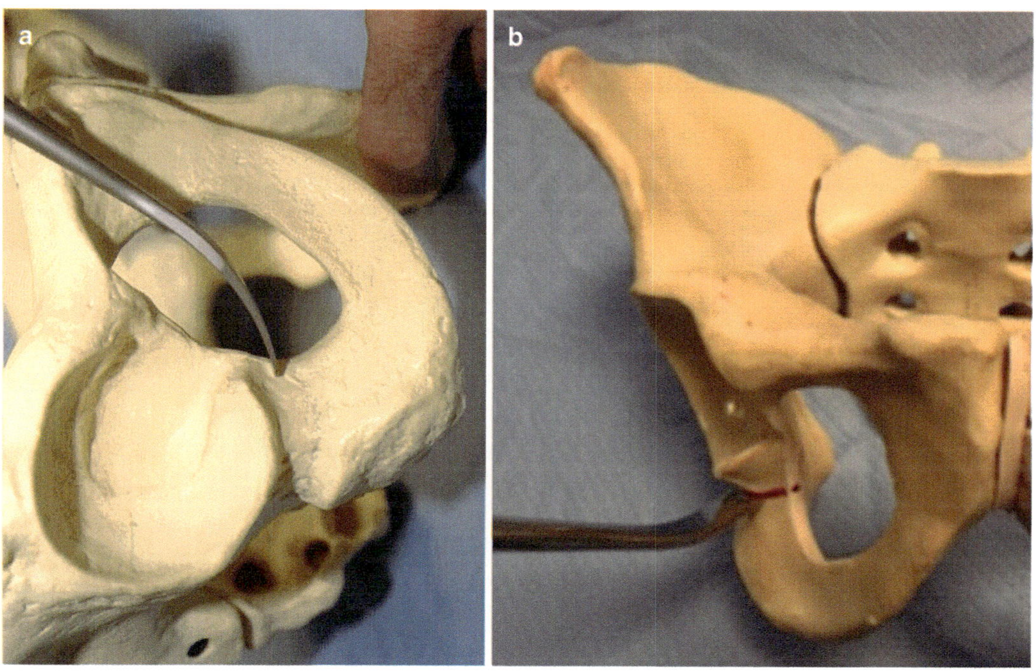

Fig. 8.8 (**a**) Lateral view of the pelvis from the right, indicating the position and orientation of the curved pelvic osteotomy chisel. (**b**) Frontal view of the same action. The handle of curved osteotome is pointed in a slight posteroinferior direction and it is oriented toward the opposite shoulder and a notch is made in the central part of the ischium

During this last ischial cut, the flexed hip must be abducted and externally rotated to relax and protect the sciatic nerve.

The osteotomy of the superior pubic ramus is made just medial to the iliopectineal eminence (Fig. 8.11). The flexed hip is adducted, the pointed Hohmann is placed 1 cm. medial to the iliopectineal eminence, and the superior pubic ramus is exposed subperiosteally with a small elevator. Two blunt curved retractors are placed subperiosteally around it to protect the obturator nerve and vessels.

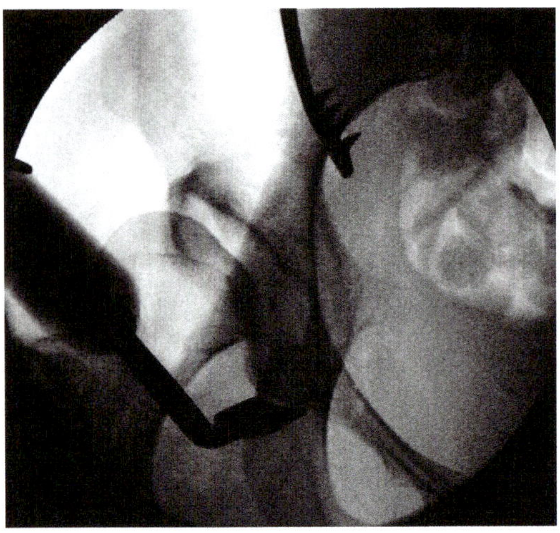

Fig. 8.9 Intra-op fluoroscopy to check correct position and advancement of the chisel that is driven slowly to a depth of 20–25 mm while changing gradually its direction so that at the end of the insertion the handle points postero-superiorly

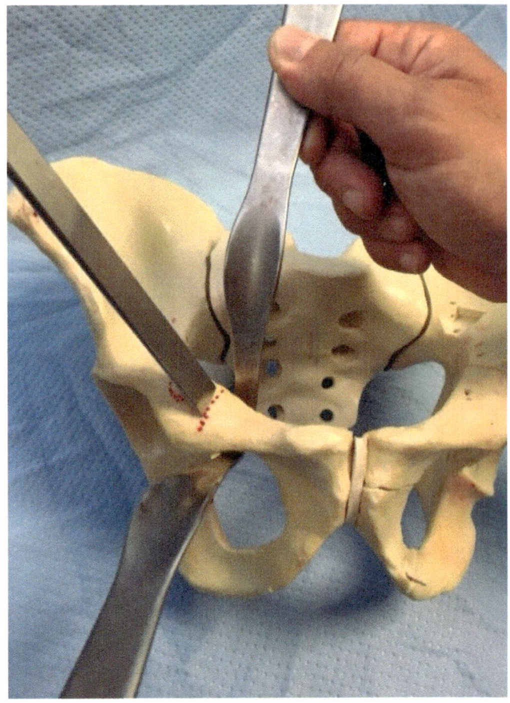

Fig. 8.11 Osteotomy of the superior pubic ramus: The osteotomy is performed subperiosteally and it is perpendicular to the longitudinal axis of the pubic ramus; the 15 mm Lexer osteotome is maintained at 45° with respect to the bony surface

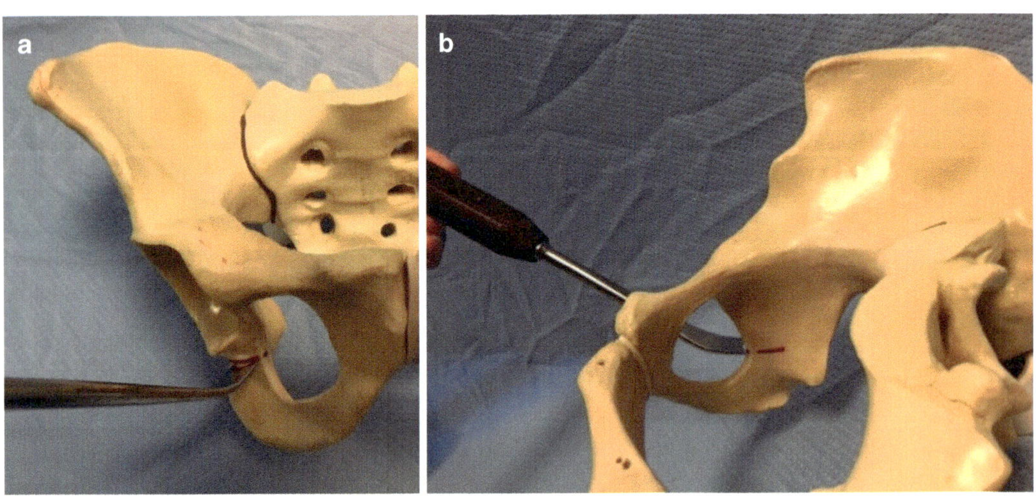

Fig. 8.10 (**a**) Cut of the medial ischial cortex. (**b**) Notching of the lateral cortex of the ischium. The narrowing of the posterior column and the proximity of the sciatic nerve (not represented) are shown

The osteotomy is made with a 15 mm Lexer osteotome, medial to the eminence, angled away from the joint and pointed caudally at an angle of 45°. Mobility between the two fragments is confirmed by wiggling the osteotome to ensure completion of the osteotomy. At the end one of the blunt retractors is placed into the osteotomy of the superior pubic ramus.

The ilium and the quadrilateral surface are prepared for the remaining three osteotomies, the periosteum along the anterior wall is incised and detached medially and inferiorly along the quadrilateral surface with the use of a curved periosteal elevator.

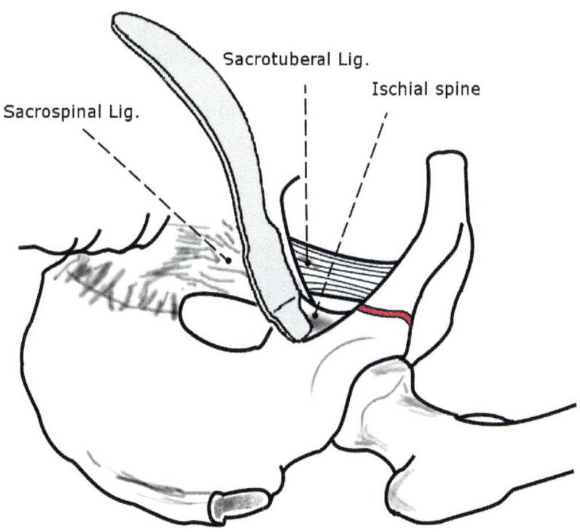

Fig. 8.12 (Modified from Weber and Ganz [49]) Preparation for the supra- and retro-acetabular osteotomies: placement of a reversed Homann with its tip near the *ischial spine*

A reversed Hohmann is placed with its tip near the ischial spine (Fig. 8.12) and a limited subperiosteal tunnel is created at the outer wall of the ilium to insert a reverse blunt Hohmann retractor toward the greater sciatic notch (Fig. 8.13) to protect the muscles and the sciatic nerve during the following osteotomies.

The supra- and retro-acetabular cuts are performed in two parts. The osteotomy line is marked with a straight 10 mm osteotome starting at the distal border of the osteotomized SIAS and continues perpendicularly to a point 1 cm lateral to the pelvic brim line (Fig. 8.14a). The mark continues at an angle of 110–120° in the direction of the ischial spine (Fig. 8.14b). It is important that the retro-acetabular cut be made at the distance of about 1.5 cm away from the sciatic notch (Fig. 8.15a).

The supra-acetabular cut is performed with an oscillating saw and the remaining distance to the pelvic brim is osteotomized with a curved osteotome at an angle of 110–120° to the first cut (Fig. 8.15b).

Only the first 30 mm of the quadrilateral plate is cut with a straight osteotome at the distance

Fig. 8.13 (Modified from Weber and Ganz [49]) Preparation of the supra- and retro-acetabular osteotomies: a limited subperiosteal tunnel is created at the outer wall of the ilium to insert a reverse blunt Hohmann retractor toward the greater sciatic foramen (*Foramen isch. maj.*) to protect the muscles and the sciatic nerve during the following osteotomies

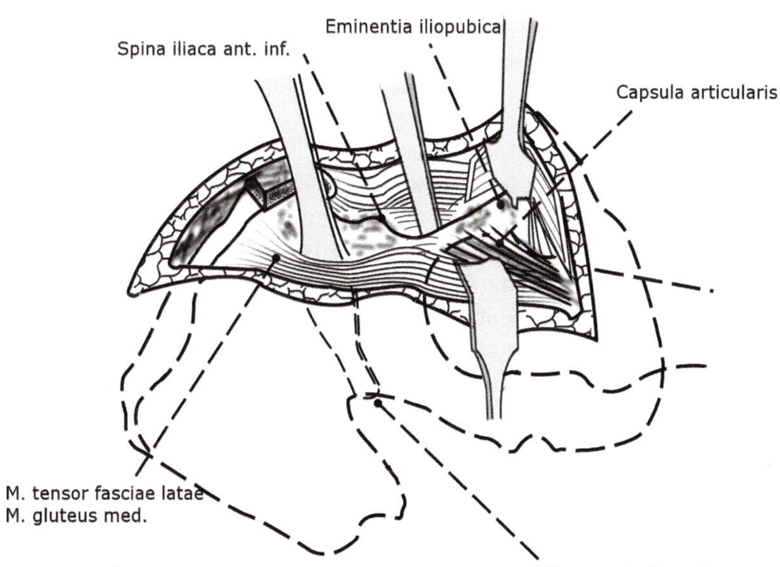

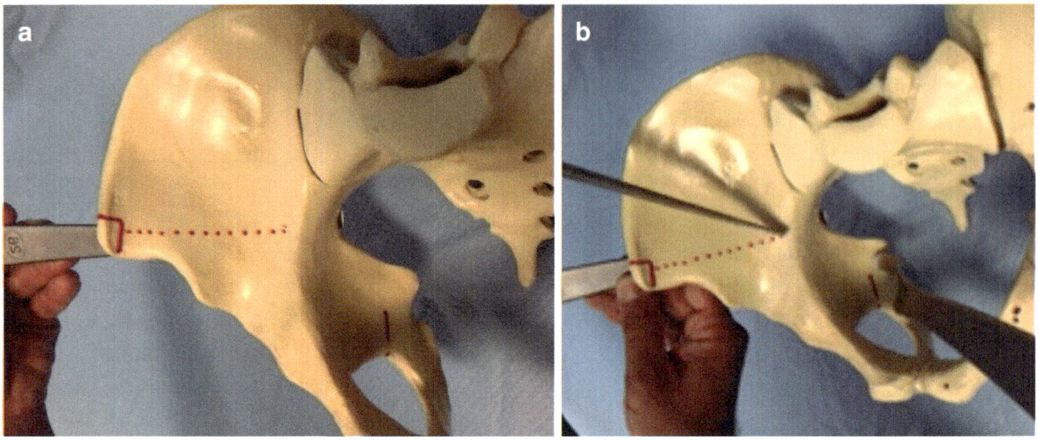

Fig. 8.14 (**a**) Supra-acetabular cut starting point: The osteotomy line is marked with a straight 10 mm osteotome starting at the distal border of the osteotomized ASIS. (**b**) Supra-acetabular cut end point: The osteotomy line continues perpendicularly from ASIS to a point 1 cm lateral to the pelvic brim line

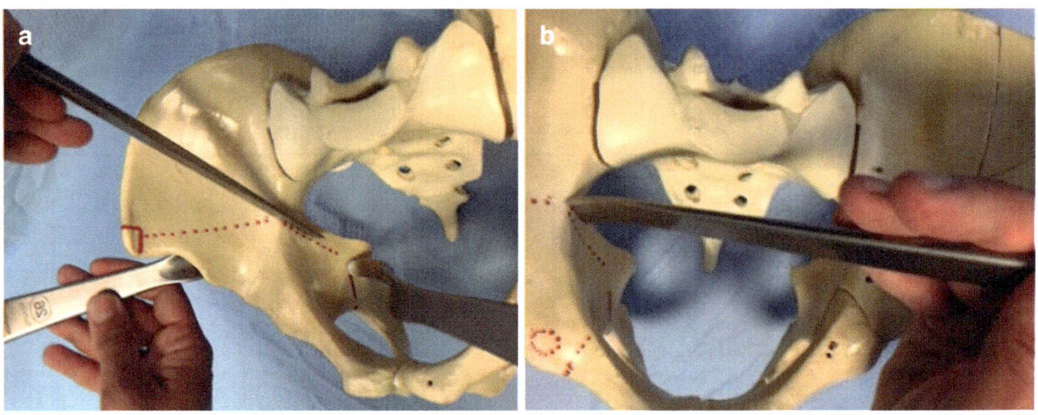

Fig. 8.15 (**a**) Retro-acetabular cut path: the retro-acetabular cut is performed generally at 110°–120° from the supra-acetabular cut, maintaining a distance of about 1.5 cm away from the greater sciatic foramen. (**b**) A curved osteotome is used to initiate the retro-acetabular cut

mentioned, to the greater sciatic notch (Fig. 8.16a) and the lateral cortex of the supra-acetabular area is notched with a curved osteotome (Fig. 8.16b). A 15 mm Lexer osteotome is inserted into the posterior part of the osteotomy and by pulling the handle a lever movement is created against the acetabulum until the bone bridge breaks toward the sciatic spine in a controlled fashion.

A Schantz screw is placed into the acetabular fragment in the supra-acetabular region and with a large spreader the remaining bone bridge between the ischial and supra-acetabular osteotomy is put under tension (Fig. 8.18).

The final cut is performed 4 cm below the pelvic brim with a 20 mm wide curved special chisel to bone posterior to the quadrilateral plate which remains between the first ischial and the supra-retro-acetabular osteotomy (Figs. 8.17 and 8.18). During this maneuver we recommend extending and abducting the hip slightly to move the sciatic nerve out of the way as much as possible.

When the iliac osteotomy is completed, with a combined maneuver the Schantz screw is rotated medially, whereas the spreader is rotated externally (Fig. 8.18). In this way the last part of the posteroinferior bone bridge is fractured and the

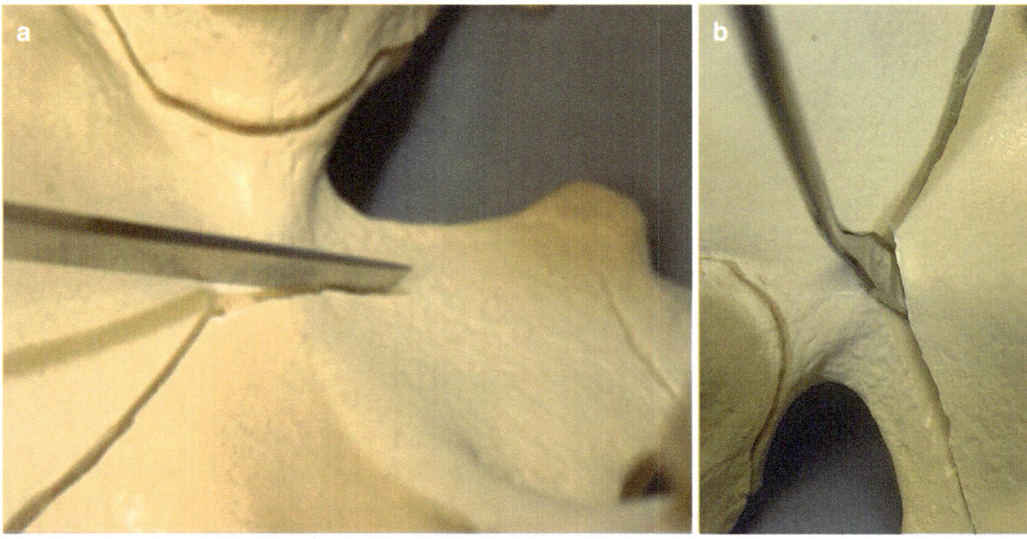

Fig. 8.16 (**a**) The first 30 mm of the quadrilateral plate is cut with a straight osteotome maintaining a distance of 1.5 cm from the greater sciatic notch. (**b**) Inner view of the pelvis: the lateral cortex of the supra-acetabular area is notched with a curved osteotome

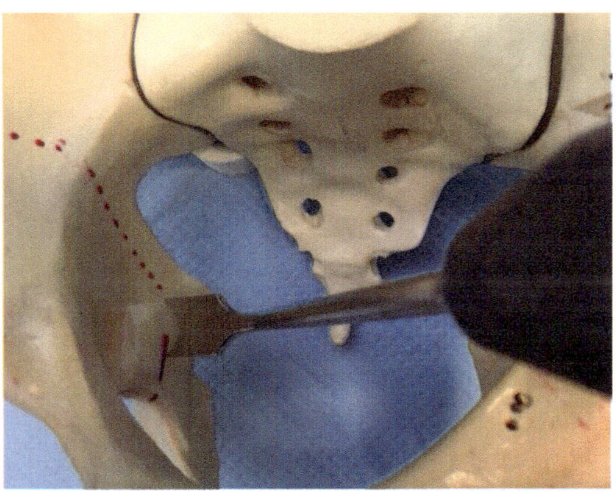

Fig. 8.17 The final cut is performed 4 cm below the pelvic brim with a 20 mm curved special chisel posterior to the quadrilateral plate which remains between the first ischial and the supra-retro-acetabular osteotomy

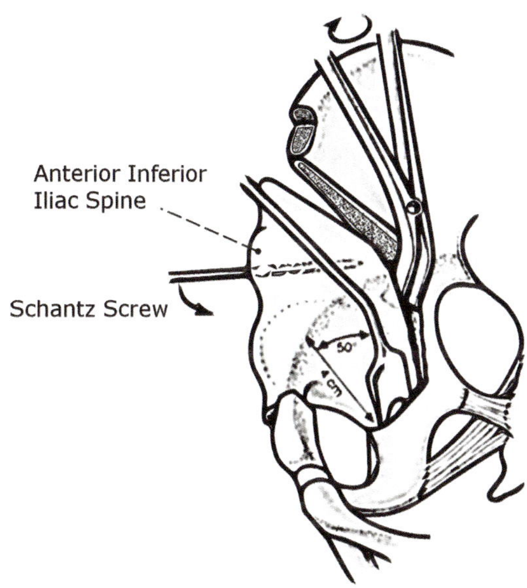

Fig. 8.18 (Modified from Weber and Ganz [49]) Lateral manipulation of the bony fragment: a *Schantz screw* is inserted parallelly to the inner wall through the *Anterior Inferior Iliac Spine* into the supra-acetabular bony bridge. A spreader is inserted into the posterior part of the supra-acetabular osteotomy. With a combined maneuver the *Schantz screw* is rotated medially whereas the spreader is rotated externally provoking a controlled fracture of last part of the posteroinferior bone bridge. The acetabular fragment becomes movable

acetabular fragment is now movable. This allows for free rotation around the center of the femoral head (Fig. 8.19b). A correct and sufficient rotation of the acetabular fragment over the head is only possible in presence of completely movable fragment. A supra-acetabular cleft appearing during correction is due to an incomplete postero-caudal mobilization (Fig. 8.19a).

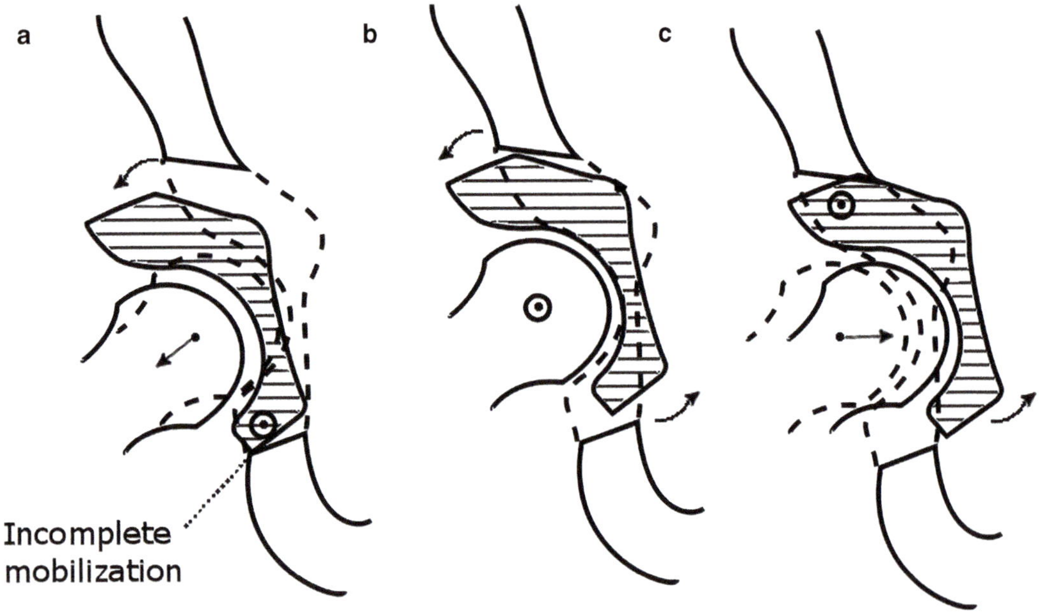

Fig. 8.19 (Modified from Weber and Ganz [49]) (**a**) a supra-acetabular cleft appearing during correction is always associated with an incomplete postero-caudal mobilization and/or a persisting bony bridge. (**b**) If the joint is in correct position, the correction is achieved through a rotation of the acetabular fragment around the femoral head center. (**c**) To contrast the tendency of dysplastic hips toward a lateralization of the center of rotation, the fragment must be medialized correspondingly

The correction depends on the area of deficient coverage. As the anterolateral deficit is most frequent, the correction maneuver is an anterior rotation, which also results in improvement of the lateral coverage. Care is taken to maintain or correct anteversion of the acetabular fragment by respective rotation of the acetabulum. If the correction maneuver produces a gap between acetabular fragment and stable ilium, the fragment is not completely free and the cuts have to be controlled again. The correction is stabilized preliminary with 2.5 mm Kirschner wires (Fig. 8.20) and controlled with an orthograde anteroposterior radiograph of the entire pelvis centered over the pubic symphysis. This is necessary to control neutral tilt and rotation of the pelvis, both contributing to the projection of the acetabular version.

The joint is opened with an anterior "T" shaped incision, the labrum is inspected and if necessary debrided if a free flap or an intra-labial ganglion is present. The anterolateral head neck junction is inspected and eventually shaped to recreate a normal waisting and avoid potential impingement.

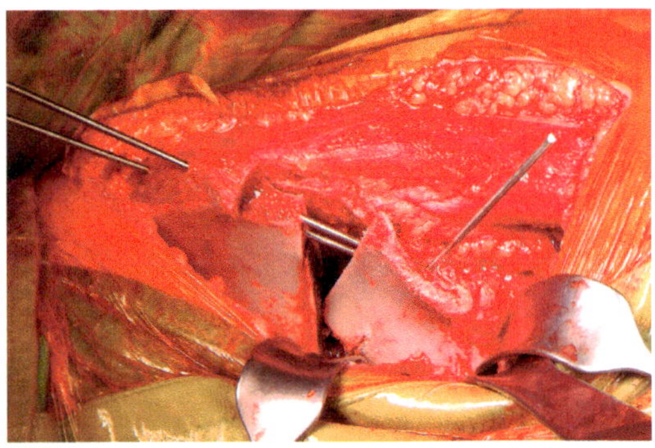

Fig. 8.20 Intra-op picture of provisional stabilization of the bony fragment with 2.5 mm Kirschner wires

As a standard role 90° of passive hip flexion and 30° of internal rotation at 90° of flexion are required.

The final fixation is achieved with two 3.5 mm cortical screws introduced from the iliac crest to the acetabular fragment. An additional screw is inserted from the AIIS through the fragment

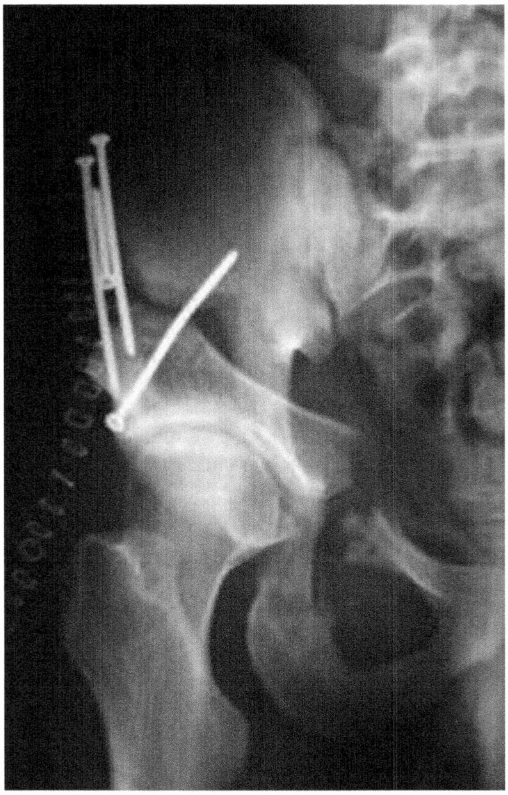

Fig. 8.21 Post-op X-ray showing the final fixation achieved by two 3.5 mm cortical screws introduced from the iliac crest to the acetabular fragment and a third screw inserted from the AIIS (Anterior Inferior Iliac Spine) through the fragment toward the sacroiliac joint

toward the sacroiliac joint (Fig. 8.21). The prominent anterior spike of the acetabular fragment is removed with an oscillating saw and is used to fill the gap with the stable ilium. The capsule is closed and the direct and reflect heads of the rectus are re-inserted with transosseous non-resorbable sutures. The osteotomized ASIS is fixed with a 1 mm cortical screw. Normally, no suction drains are necessary. The superficial wound is closed in a routine fashion.

8.7 Conclusions

Osteotomies around the hip, especially the periacetabular osteotomy have made a tremendous impact on modern hip joint surgery.

Several authors in their 20 years' follow-up study, concluded that periacetabular osteotomies provide better coverage of the femoral head with hyaline cartilage and mean clinical hip scores at intermediate- to long-term follow-up seem superior to published studies for other osteotomies techniques around the acetabulum [40, 47, 51, 55].

References

1. Aronson J. Osteoarthritis of the young adult hip: etiology and treatment. Instr Course Lect. 1986;35:119–28.
2. Harris WH. Etiology of osteoarthritis of the hip. Clin Orthop Relat Res. 1986;(213):20–33.
3. Strayer LM. Embryology of he human hip joint. Clin Orthop Relat Res. 1971;74:221–40.
4. Clohisy JC, Schutz AL, St John L, et al. Periacetabular osteotomy: a systematic literature review. Clin Orthop Relat Res. 2009;467:2041–52. https://doi.org/10.1007/s11999-009-0842-6.
5. Wynne-Davies R. Acetabular dysplasia and familial joint laxity: two etiological factors in congenital dislocation of the hip. A review of 589 patients and their families. J Bone Joint Surg Br. 1970;52:704–16.
6. Nakamura S, Ninomiya S, Takatori Y, et al. Long-term outcome of rotational acetabular osteotomy: 145 hips followed for 10-23 years. Acta Orthop Scand. 1998;69:259–65. https://doi.org/10.3109/17453679809000926.
7. Siebenrock KA, Leunig M, Ganz R. Periacetabular osteotomy: the Bernese experience. Instr Course Lect. 2001;50:239–45.
8. Clohisy JC, Nepple JJ, Ross JR, et al. Does surgical hip dislocation and periacetabular osteotomy improve pain in patients with Perthes-like deformities and acetabular dysplasia? Clin Orthop. 2015;473:1370–7. https://doi.org/10.1007/s11999-014-4115-7.
9. Ganz R, Klaue K, Vinh TS, Mast JW. A new periacetabular osteotomy for the treatment of hip dysplasias. Technique and preliminary results. Clin Orthop Relat Res. 1988;(232):26–36.
10. Salter RB. Innominate osteotomy in the treatment of congenital dislocation and subluxation of the hip. J Bone Joint Surg Br. 1961;43:518–39.
11. Li PLS, Ganz R. Morphologic features of congenital acetabular dysplasia: one in six is retroverted. Clin Orthop Relat Res. 2003;(416):245–53. https://doi.org/10.1097/01.blo.0000081934.75404.36.
12. Mast JW, Brunner RL, Zebrack J. Recognizing acetabular version in the radiographic presentation of hip dysplasia. Clin Orthop Relat Res. 2004;(418):48–53. https://doi.org/10.1097/00003086-200401000-00009.
13. Ganz R, Parvizi J, Beck M, et al. Femoroacetabular impingement: a cause for osteoarthritis of the hip. Clin Orthop Relat Res. 2003;(417):112–20. https://doi.org/10.1097/01.blo.0000096804.78689.c2.

14. Tannast M, Hanke MS, Zheng G, et al. What are the radiographic reference values for acetabular under- and overcoverage? Clin Orthop Relat Res. 2015;473:1234–46. https://doi.org/10.1007/s11999-014-4038-3.
15. Hadley NA, Brown TD, Weinstein SL. The effects of contact pressure elevations and aseptic necrosis on the long-term outcome of congenital hip dislocation. J Orthop Res. 1990;8:504–13. https://doi.org/10.1002/jor.1100080406.
16. Kummer B. Biomechanical aspects of hip dislocation. Orthopade. 1988;17:452–62.
17. Cooperman DR, Wallensten R, Stulberg SD. Acetabular dysplasia in the adult. Clin Orthop Relat Res. 1983;(175):79–85.
18. Murphy SB, Ganz R, Müller ME. The prognosis in untreated dysplasia of the hip. A study of radiographic factors that predict the outcome. J Bone Joint Surg Am. 1995;77:985–9. https://doi.org/10.2106/00004623-199507000-00002.
19. Wedge JH, Wasylenko MJ. The natural history of congenital dislocation of the hip: a critical review. Clin Orthop Relat Res. 1978;(137):154–62.
20. Hartofilakidis G, Karachalios T, Stamos KG. Epidemiology, demographics, and natural history of congenital hip disease in adults. Orthopedics. 2000;23:823–7.
21. Werlen S, Leunig M, Ganz R. Magnetic resonance arthrography of the hip in femoroacetabular impingement: technique and findings. Oper Tech Orthop. 2005;15:191–203. https://doi.org/10.1053/j.oto.2005.07.007.
22. Locher S, Werlen S, Leunig M, Ganz R. MR-arthrography with radial sequences for visualization of early hip pathology not visible on plain radiographs. Z Orthop Ihre Grenzgeb. 2002;140:52–7. https://doi.org/10.1055/s-2002-22122.
23. Leunig M, Werlen S, Ungersböck A, et al. Evaluation of the acetabular labrum by MR arthrography. J Bone Joint Surg Br. 1997;79:230–4. https://doi.org/10.1302/0301-620x.79b2.7288.
24. Beaulé PE, Zaragoza E, Copelan N. Magnetic resonance imaging with gadolinium arthrography to assess acetabular cartilage delamination. A report of four cases. J Bone Joint Surg Am. 2004;86:2294–8. https://doi.org/10.2106/00004623-200410000-00025.
25. Schmid MR, Nötzli HP, Zanetti M, et al. Cartilage lesions in the hip: diagnostic effectiveness of MR arthrography. Radiology. 2003;226:382–6. https://doi.org/10.1148/radiol.2262020019.
26. Zilkens C, Miese F, Kim Y-J, et al. Three-dimensional delayed gadolinium-enhanced magnetic resonance imaging of hip joint cartilage at 3T: a prospective controlled study. Eur J Radiol. 2012;81:3420–5. https://doi.org/10.1016/j.ejrad.2012.04.008.
27. Ferguson SJ, Bryant JT, Ganz R, Ito K. The acetabular labrum seal: a poroelastic finite element model. Clin Biomech. 2000;15:463–8. https://doi.org/10.1016/S0268-0033(99)00099-6.
28. Parvizi J, Bican O, Bender B, et al. Arthroscopy for labral tears in patients with developmental dysplasia of the hip: a cautionary note. J Arthroplast. 2009;24:110–3. https://doi.org/10.1016/j.arth.2009.05.021.
29. Klaue K, Durnin CW, Ganz R. The acetabular rim syndrome. A clinical presentation of dysplasia of the hip. J Bone Joint Surg Br. 1991;73:423–9.
30. Tönnis D. The prearthrotic deformity as origin of coxarthrosis. Radiographic measurements and their value in the prognosis. Z Orthop Ihre Grenzgeb. 1978;116:444–6.
31. Wiberg G. Studies on dysplastic acetabula and congenital subluxation of the hip joint with special reference to the complication of osteoarthritis. Exp., Norstedt; 1939.
32. Lequesne M, de Seze. False profile of the pelvis. A new radiographic incidence for the study of the hip. Its use in dysplasias and different coxopathies. Rev Rhum Mal Osteoartic. 1961;28:643–52.
33. Tönnis D. Congenital dysplasia and dislocation of the hip in children and adults. Berlin: Springer-Verlag; 1987.
34. Albers C, Steppacher S, Ganz R, et al. Optimal acetabular reorientation and offset correction improve the long term results after periacetabular osteotomy. Orthop Proc. 2012;94-B:585. https://doi.org/10.1302/1358-992X.94BSUPP_XXXVII.EFORT2011-585.
35. Beck M, Kalhor M, Leunig M, Ganz R. Hip morphology influences the pattern of damage to the acetabular cartilage: femoroacetabular impingement as a cause of early osteoarthritis of the hip. J Bone Joint Surg Br. 2005;87:1012–8. https://doi.org/10.1302/0301-620X.87B7.15203.
36. Steel HH. Triple osteotomy of the innominate bone. J Bone Joint Surg Am. 1973;55:343–50.
37. Wagner H. Osteotomies for congenital hip dislocation. In: The hip: proceedings of the fourth meeting of the hip society. CV Mosby Co; 1976. p. 45–66.
38. Ninomiya S, Tagawa H. Rotational acetabular osteotomy for the dysplastic hip. J Bone Joint Surg Am. 1984;66:430–6.
39. Flückiger G, Eggli S, Kosina J, Ganz R. Birth after peri-acetabular osteotomy. Orthopade. 2000;29:63–7. https://doi.org/10.1007/s001320050009.
40. Steppacher SD, Tannast M, Ganz R, Siebenrock KA. Mean 20-year followup of Bernese periacetabular osteotomy. Clin Orthop. 2008;466:1633–44. https://doi.org/10.1007/s11999-008-0242-3.
41. Yasunaga Y, Takahashi K, Ochi M, et al. Rotational acetabular osteotomy in patients forty-six years of age or older: comparison with younger patients. J Bone Joint Surg Am. 2003;85:266–72. https://doi.org/10.2106/00004623-200302000-00013.
42. Millis MB, Kain M, Sierra R, et al. Periacetabular osteotomy for acetabular dysplasia in patients older than 40 years: a preliminary study. Clin Orthop. 2009;467:2228–34. https://doi.org/10.1007/s11999-009-0824-8.

43. Cunningham T, Jessel R, Zurakowski D, et al. Delayed gadolinium-enhanced magnetic resonance imaging of cartilage to predict early failure of Bernese periacetabular osteotomy for hip dysplasia. J Bone Joint Surg Am. 2006;88:1540–8. https://doi.org/10.2106/JBJS.E.00572.
44. Troelsen A, Elmengaard B, Søballe K. Medium-term outcome of periacetabular osteotomy and predictors of conversion to total hip replacement. J Bone Joint Surg Am. 2009;91:2169–79. https://doi.org/10.2106/JBJS.H.00994.
45. Davey JP, Santore RF. Complications of periacetabular osteotomy. Clin Orthop Relat Res. 1999;(363):33–7.
46. Schramm M, Hohmann D, Radespiel-Troger M, Pitto RP. Treatment of the dysplastic acetabulum with Wagner spherical osteotomy. A study of patients followed for a minimum of twenty years. J Bone Joint Surg Am. 2003;85:808–14. https://doi.org/10.2106/00004623-200305000-00006.
47. Takatori Y, Ninomiya S, Nakamura S, et al. Long-term results of rotational acetabular osteotomy in patients with slight narrowing of the joint space on preoperative radiographic findings. J Orthop Sci. 2001;6:137–40. https://doi.org/10.1007/s007760100061.
48. Sharifi E, Sharifi H, Morshed S, et al. Cost-effectiveness analysis of periacetabular osteotomy. J Bone Joint Surg Am. 2008;90:1447–56. https://doi.org/10.2106/JBJS.G.00730.
49. Weber M, Ganz R. The Bernese periacetabular osteotomy. Orthop Traumatol. 2002;10:93–112.
50. Clohisy JC, Barrett SE, Gordon JE, et al. Periacetabular osteotomy for the treatment of severe acetabular dysplasia. J Bone Joint Surg Am. 2005;87:254–9.
51. Matheney T, Kim Y-J, Zurakowski D, et al. Intermediate to long-term results following the Bernese periacetabular osteotomy and predictors of clinical outcome. J Bone Joint Surg Am. 2009;91:2113–23.
52. Leunig M, Siebenrock KA, Mahomed MN, Ganz R. Bernese periacetabular osteotomy: technical aspects and clinical results. Hip Int. 1999;9:119–26.
53. Turchetto L, Masse A, Aprato A, et al. Developmental dysplasia of hip: joint preserving surgery in the adolescent and young adult. Minerva Ortopedica e Traumatologica. 2013;64:41–52.
54. Leunig M, Siebenrock KA, Ganz R. Rationale of periacetabular osteotomy and background work. J Bone Joint Surg Am. 2001;83:438–48.
55. Ito H, Tanino H, Yamanaka Y, et al. The Chiari pelvic osteotomy for patients with dysplastic hips and poor joint congruency: long-term follow-up. J Bone Joint Surg Br. 2011;93:726–31.

9 How to Reduce the Risk of Nerve Injury During Bernese PAO?

Morteza Kalhor

9.1 Introduction

Bernese PAO is the widely accepted surgical procedure for treatment of adolescent and adult dysplastic hip [1–12]. The modified Smith-Petersen approach as described in original technique is used by the majority of orthopedic surgeons [1, 13], but other types of approaches are sometimes used [14–19]. Depending on the experience of surgeon and the type of used approach, varying rates of nerve injury have been reported [1, 3, 7, 9, 12, 15, 20–24]. For lateral femoral cutaneous nerve this was 30% after iliofemoral and 100% after ilioinguinal approach [15, 23]. The reported rate of major nerve damages like femoral and sciatic was up to 15% [24]. The etiology of neurological injury during PAO has not been specifically studied so far. Intraoperative nerve monitoring was effective as a diagnostic tool but ineffective as preventive measure [22]. The purpose of this chapter is to demonstrate topographic anatomy of the nerves located in vicinity of the periacetabular bone and to evaluate the potential risk of nerve injury during various steps of operation. All findings and illustrations are based on a cadaveric study performed in a realistic surgical environment and previously published [25, 26].

M. Kalhor (✉)
Department of Orthopedic Surgery, Firoozgar Medical Center, Iran University of Medical Sciences, Tehran, Iran

9.2 Methods

Modified Smith-Petersen approach was used in 20 fresh cadaver hips in order to study the risk of femoral, obturator, sciatic, and lateral femoral cutaneous nerve during execution of Bernese periacetabular osteotomy. In 10 hips all stages of operation from beginning to the end that is, approach, osteotomy steps, mobilization and stabilization of the acetabulum were performed as described in original technique. The corresponding nerves were exposed after completion of the operation by extension of the original wound or addition of new incisions.

In the remaining 10 hips, the corresponding nearby nerve was exposed during each osteotomy step in order to evaluate the risk of injury under direct vision. For sciatic nerve evaluation, the specimens turned to lateral position and the nerve exposed through Kocher-Langenbeck approach. After repositioning of the acetabular fragment, the position of nerves was checked in different correction severities.

9.3 Results

9.3.1 LCNT: Lateral Cutaneous Nerve of the Thigh

This is the most superficial nerve located in operation field. It is vulnerable to injury during dissection and exposure. LCNT exits from the

R. Ganz (ed.), *Modern Hip Preservation*, https://doi.org/10.1007/978-3-030-91967-2_9

pelvis usually in close proximity to the medial aspect of ASIS, passing usually under the inguinal ligament and over the tendon of sartorius muscle (Fig. 9.1). Distal to the inguinal ligament and in anterior aspect of the proximal thigh the nerve runs superficially between sartorius and tensor muscle and is prone to damage if this plane is taken for access to deep structures. Incising the fascia over the tensor muscle and intra-facial lateral retraction of the muscle can keep the nerve in femoral part of the approach (Fig. 9.2). In inguinal area, the nerve is more susceptible to damage during iliofemoral and even more often during ilioinguinal approach. Osteotomy of the ASIS pedicled by sartorius and inguinal ligament, when in continuous with subperiosteal exposure of iliac fossa, can protect the nerve in iliac part of the iliofemoral approach (Figs. 9.3 and 9.4). Without osteotomy of the ASIS the nerve remains unprotected in this area and prone to compression or stretching by the soft tissue retractors (Fig. 9.5).

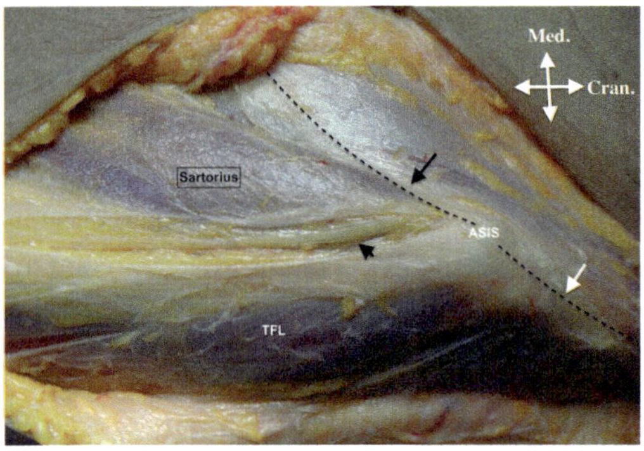

Fig. 9.1 Anterior aspect of left hip after superficial exposure to show the topography of the *LFCN* after exit from pelvis. The *dotted line* shows the inguinal ligament (*black arrow*) and the iliac crest (*white arrow*). *ASIS* = anterior superior iliac spine. *Arrowhead* shows the LFCN. *TFL* = tensor fasciae latae (*Cran.* = cranial; *Med.* = medial)

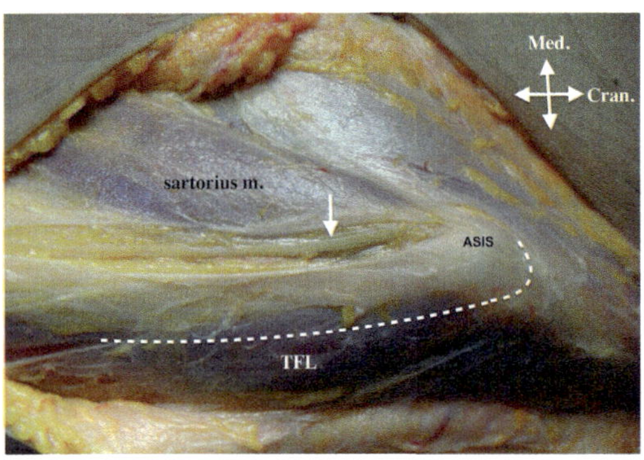

Fig. 9.2 The same as Fig. 9.1 to show the line of incision on tensor fascia for access to the deep layers in order to avoid cutaneous nerve damage. *ASIS* = anterior superior iliac spine. *TFL* = tensor fasciae latae. *Arrow* shows the lateral femoral cutaneous nerve (*Cran.* = cranial; *Med.* = medial)

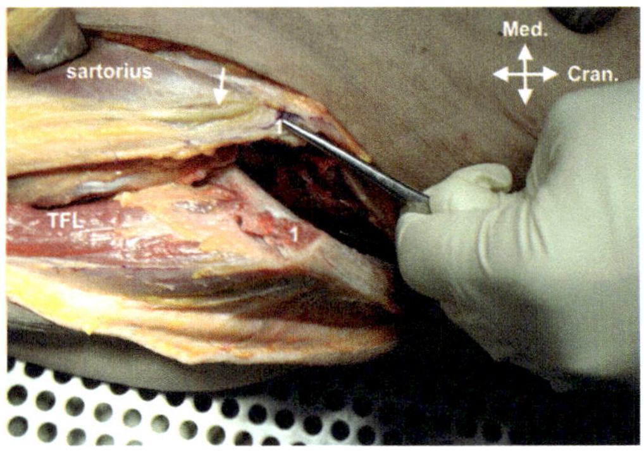

Fig. 9.3 Osteotomy of ASIS with sartorius tendon attached to it in iliofemoral approach in order to protect the LFCN. *White arrow* shows the LFCN. *TFL* = tensor fasciae latae. *1*: Osteotomized ASIS (*Cran.* = cranial; *Med.* = medial)

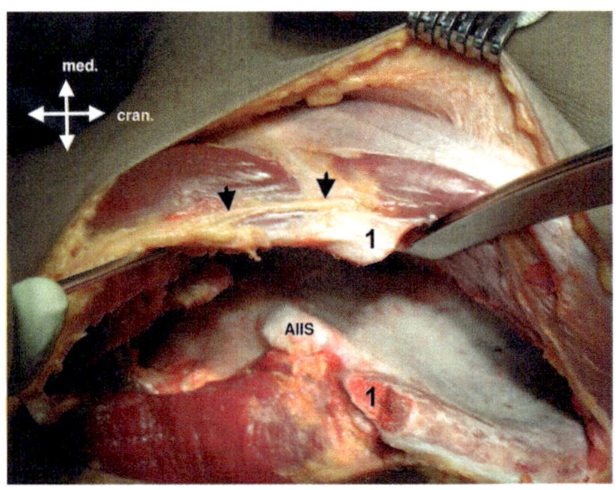

Fig. 9.4 Exposure of internal surface of left ilium in iliofemoral approach after osteotomy of ASIS, to show its effect in protection of the LFCN. *Black arrows* show the cutaneous nerve. *AIIS* = anterior inferior iliac spine. *1*: anterior superior iliac spine osteotomized (*Cran.* = cranial; *Med.* = medial)

9.3.2 ON: Obturator Nerve

When passing through obturator foramen the obturator nerve is located under the superior ramus of the pubis and close to the acetabulum where the pubic osteotomy is usually done. Direct injury of the nerve is possible by the osteotome blade if far cortex penetration is more than five millimeters (Fig. 9.6). Proper development of periosteal sleeve around the pubic bone and subperiosteal placement of blunt Hohmann retractors can protect the nerve from direct injury by osteotome (Fig. 9.7). Inclining the tip of the osteotome 45 degree medially and or performing the osteotomy at least 2 cm. medial to the most

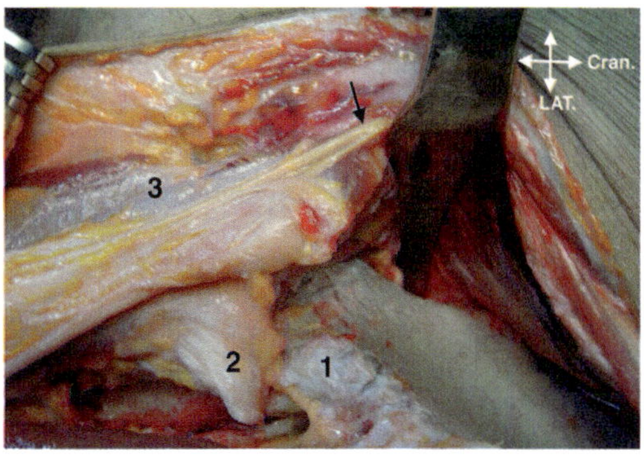

Fig. 9.5 The same as Fig. 9.4 but without osteotomy of ASIS to show the likelihood of LFCN injury. *Arrow* shows the LFCN (*1*: Anterior inferior iliac spine; *2*: Rectus tendon detached from AIIS; *3*: Sartorius; *Cran.* = cranial; *Med.* = medial). Reproduced with permission from [25]

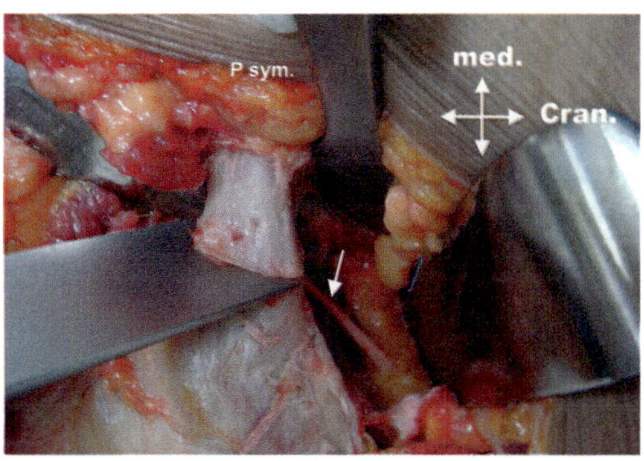

Fig. 9.6 Exposure of superior ramus of left pubis during osteotomy to demonstrate the likelihood of obturator nerve injury during unprotected osteotomy. *Arrow* shows the obturator nerve. *P sym.* = pubic symphysis (*Cran.* = cranial; *Med.* = medial)

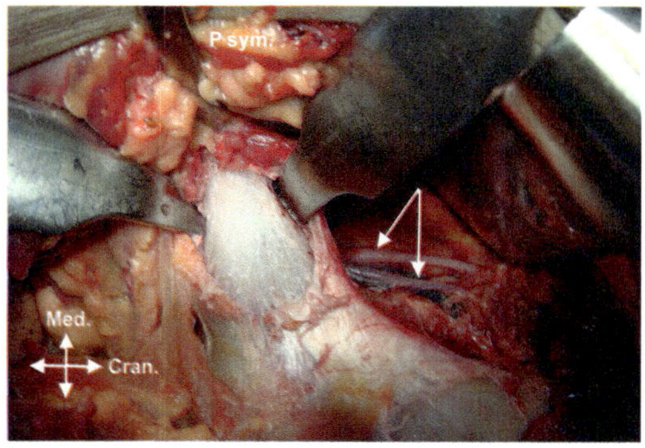

Fig. 9.7 The photograph shows exposure of left pubis for osteotomy. Proper development of periosteal sleeve around pubic ramus and subperiosteal placement of blunt retractors helps to reduce the risk of obturator nerve injury during osteotomy. *Arrows* show the obturator nerve and vessels (*Cran.* = cranial; *Med.* = medial)

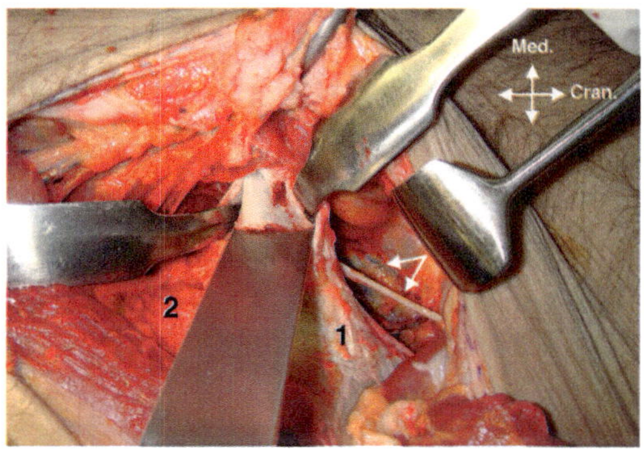

Fig. 9.8 Oblique osteotomy of the pubis helps to avoid obturator nerve injury. *Arrows* indicate to the obturator nerve and vessels (*1*: Iliopectineal eminence; *2*: Anteromedial aspect of hip capsule; *Cran.* = cranial; *Med.* = medial). Reproduced with permission from [25]

prominent part of the iliopectineal eminence are the other practical ways to reduce the risk of nerve damage (Fig. 9.8).

9.3.3 FN: Femoral Nerve

Outside the pelvis the femoral nerve is located on anterior surface of the iliopsoas muscle, overlying by the rectus and sartorius muscles. Proximal to the inguinal ligament the nerve is protected by iliopsoas and abdominal muscles. For primary osteotomy of ischium and pubis, the nerve must be retracted medially along with the medial soft tissue flap comprising of sartorius, rectus, and iliopsoas muscle.

The deep part of the flap that is the iliopsoas muscle is the principal protector of the nerve and prevents the nerve from being in direct contact with the soft tissue retractors. When iliopsoas is missing or atrophied, the risk of femoral nerve damage is higher [27, 28]. Entrapment or engagement of the nerve in pubic osteotomy gap is likely after large corrections (Fig. 9.9).

Flexion of the hip during pubic osteotomy can lower the tension on the nerve. Also finger control of the pubic osteotomy gap after repositioning of the acetabulum is necessary to prevent nerve entrapment. After extreme medialization of acetabulum specially when the iliopsoas is atrophied or damaged the nerve may be stretched over the iliac part of the osteotomy inside the pelvis (Fig. 9.10a, b). Anterior displacement and lateral rotation of the acetabulum also put the femoral nerve in more tension because of anterior transposition. Combination of anterior displacement and lateral rotation may further increase the tension on the nerve.

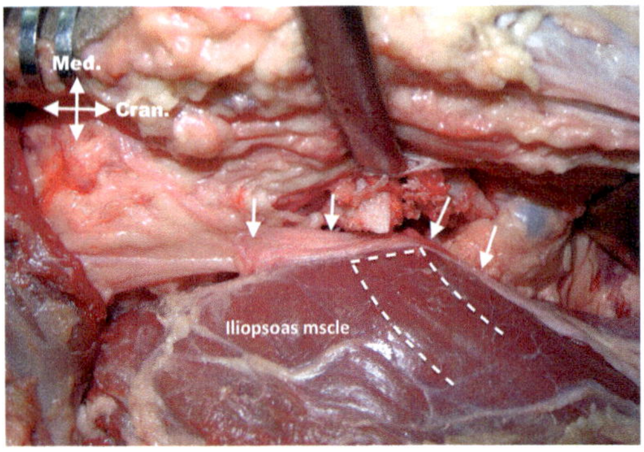

Fig. 9.9 Anterior aspect of left hip after repositioning of the acetabulum to show the entrapment of the femoral nerve in the pubic osteotomy gap. Broken line shows the position of the lateral segment of the pubis after osteotomy that is covered by the iliopsoas muscle. Arrows show the femoral nerve course (*Cran.* = cranial, *Med.* = medial). Reproduced with permission from [25]

9.3.4 SN: Sciatic Nerve

Sciatic nerve injury is likely during the first and last osteotomy steps in Bernese PAO. In first step the ischium is cut incompletely from anterior aspect of hip joint without direct vision. Sciatic nerve is located very close to the lateral cortex of ischial tuberosity and only intervened by the short external rotators. Penetrating the lateral cortex of the ischium beyond the thickness of the short external rotators may put the sciatic nerve in danger (Fig. 9.11). To avoid penetration of ischial lateral cortex the blade of special osteotome must be oriented toward the contralateral shoulder during first osteotomy step. In last osteotomy step from inside of the pelvis the iliac and ischial cuts are connected at ilio-ischial junction

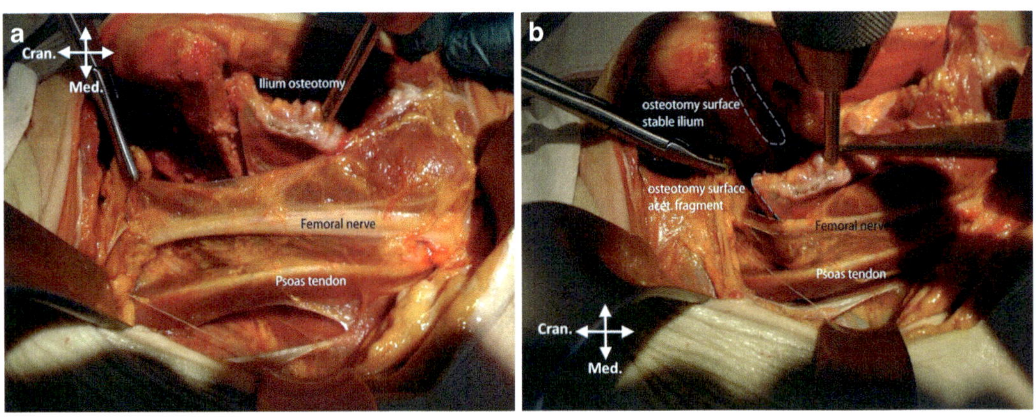

Fig. 9.10 (**a**) Anterior aspect of left hip after PAO and before repositioning the acetabular fragment to demonstrate the internal aspect of ilium and position of the femoral nerve (*Cran.* = cranial, *Med.* = medial). (**b**) The same picture as figure **a** after excessive medial displacement of the acetabular fragment to show the likelihood of femoral nerve stretching by the edge of the acetabular fragment (*Cran.* = Cranial, *Med.* = medial). Reproduced with permission from [25]

in order to free the acetabulum. Advancement of the osteotome should stop when it penetrates the lateral cortex. This can be recognized by the sound change during osteotomy. Short external rotator muscles protect the sciatic nerve from direct injury by the osteotome. But again, excessive penetration of lateral iliac cortex beyond the thickness of short external rotators can irritate or damage the sciatic nerve (Fig. 9.12).

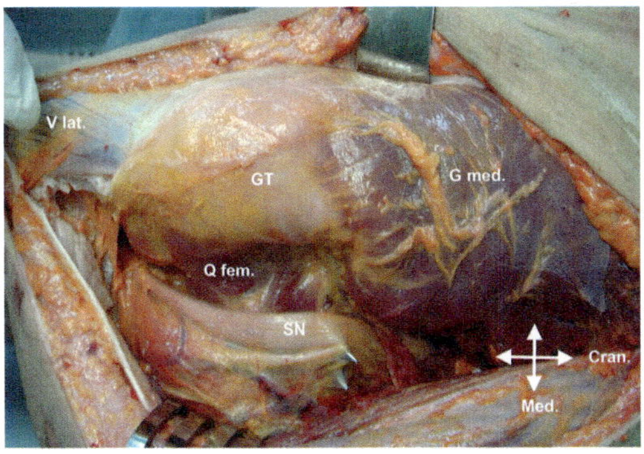

Fig. 9.11 Posterior aspect of left hip exposing the sciatic nerve during the first stage of ischial osteotomy from anterior approach. If the osteotome is driven too far and in wrong direction, sciatic nerve damage is likely (*V lat.* = Vastus lateralis; *GT* = Greater trochanter; *G med.* = Gluteus medius; *Q fem.* = Quadratus femoris; *SN* = Sciatic nerve; *Cran.* = cranial; *Med.* = medial). Reproduced with permission from [25]

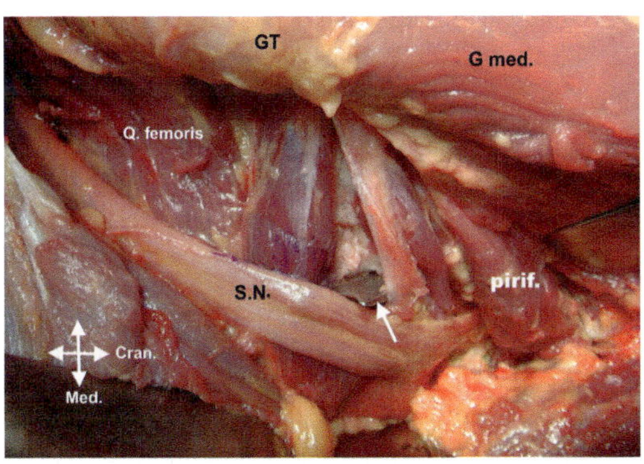

Fig. 9.12 Posterior aspect of left hip to demonstrate the likelihood of sciatic nerve damage during osteotomy of posterior column if the osteotome penetrates the posterior cortex beyond the thickness of the short hip external rotators. *Arrow* shows the tip of the bifid osteotome (*GT* = greater trochanter, *G med.* = gluteus medius, *Q. femoris* = quadratus femoris, *Pirif.* = piriformis, *S.N.* = sciatic nerve, *Cran.* = cranial, *Med.* = medial). Reproduced with permission from [25]

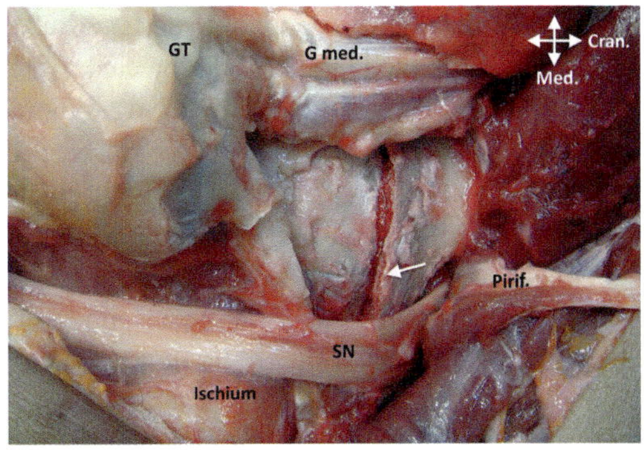

Fig. 9.13 Posterior aspect of left hip after medial displacement of the distal fragment showing compression of the sciatic nerve by the edge of the stable fragment if the acetabular fragment is excessively shifted medially. *Arrow* indicates the edge of stable fragment (*GT* = greater trochanter, *G med.* = gluteus medius, *Pirif.* = piriformis, *SN* = sciatic nerve, *Cran.* = cranial, *Med.* = medial). Reproduced with permission from [25]

Abduction and extension of the hip during primary and secondary ischial osteotomy can help to reduce the rate of nerve injury by decreasing the sciatic nerve tension.

The nerve is unlikely to be damaged after repositioning of the acetabulum except in excessive medialization of the joint that may bring the sciatic nerve into contact with the stable part of the posterior column (Fig. 9.13).

9.4 Discussion

Neurological complications following PAO, although not common in experienced hands, can be discouraging. In previous studies, the incidence of nerve injury has been reported but the etiology has not been investigated specifically [24]. In this cadaveric study, we tried to show the critical occasions during which the periacetabular nerves (LFCN, femoral, obturator, and sciatic nerve) are more likely to be damaged.

The incidence of LFCN injury depends on the approach used for performing PAO. Temporary or permanent dysfunction of this nerve was 100% in ilioinguinal approach as reported by Murphy et al. [15]. Following modified Smith-Petersen approach as described in original technique the rate of injury was 30% [23].

In ilioinguinal approach, the nerve usually remains unprotected or poorly protected when crossing the inguinal area, but in iliofemoral approach the nerve can efficiently be protected by osteotomy of the ASIS pedicled by its attachments (sartorius tendon and inguinal ligament).

For primary osteotomy of ischium and pubic superior ramus, the femoral nerve must be retracted medially along with the iliopsoas muscle. Sierra et al. [24] attributed femoral nerve injuries to traction during exposure for the primary ischial and pubic osteotomies. However, the nerve is usually well protected by the iliopsoas muscle. Overstretching of the nerve is likely especially in patients with atrophied, damaged, or transferred iliopsoas muscle. Flexion and adduction of hip decrease the nerve tension during primary ischial and pubic osteotomy.

The incidence of obturator nerve injury following PAO has not been specifically reported. This lack of information is partly because subjective and objective signs of obturator nerve damage are not prominent enough to be detected early after PAO. For this reason, obturator nerve injury is more likely to remain unnoticed postoperatively in comparison to the sciatic and femoral nerve. Subperiosteal placement of retractors around pubic bone if associated with using right osteotomy technique can substantially reduce the risk of obturator nerve injury.

Sciatic nerve may be damaged during first and last osteotomy steps. During primary ischial osteotomy, orientation of osteotome is the determining factor. If the blade of bifid osteotome is faced laterally and penetrates the lateral cortex of the ischium more than five millimeters, sciatic nerve damage is likely. To avoid nerve damage the osteotome should be positioned toward the contralateral shoulder. During the last osteotomy step from inside of the pelvis in order to connect the iliac and ischial cuts, the sciatic nerve may be damaged if the lateral cortex of ilium and ilio-ischial junction is penetrated 10 mm or more. The short external rotators as the only intervening soft tissues can help to protect the nerve from direct injury, provided the penetration of the external iliac cortex is less than 10 mm.

In conclusion, neurological damage in Bernese periacetabular osteotomy may occur during approach, osteotomy steps, or even after repositioning of the acetabulum. Precise knowledge of topographic anatomy, observing the details of surgical technique, appropriate positioning, and correct orientation of osteotome associated with experience of the surgeon are the main factors effective to reduce the incidence of neurological damage in Bernese PAO.

References

1. Ganz R, Klaue K, Vinh TS, Mast JW. A new periacetabular osteotomy for the treatment of hip dysplasias. Technique and preliminary results. Clin Orthop Relat Res. 1988;(232):26–36.
2. Siebenrock KA, Schöll E, Lottenbach M, Ganz R. Bernese periacetabular osteotomy. Clin Orthop Relat Res. 1999;363:9–20.
3. Crockarell JJ, Trousdale RT, Cabanela ME, Berry DJ. Early experience and results with the periacetabular osteotomy: the Mayo Clinic experience. Clin Orthop Relat Res. 1999;363:45–53.
4. Siebenrock KA, Leunig M, Ganz R. Periacetabular osteotomy: the Bernese experience. Instr Course Lect. 2001;50:239–45.
5. Leunig M, Siebenrock KA, Ganz R. Rationale of periacetabular osteotomy and background work. J Bone Joint Surg Am. 2001;83:438.
6. Trousdale R, Cabanela M. Lessons learned after more than 250 periacetabular osteotomies. Acta Orthop Scand. 2003;74:119–26. https://doi.org/10.1080/00016470310013824.
7. Clohisy JC, Barrett SE, Gordon JE, et al. Periacetabular osteotomy for the treatment of severe acetabular dysplasia. J Bone Joint Surg Am. 2005;87:254–9.
8. Peters CL, Erickson JA, Hines JL. Early results of the Bernese periacetabular osteotomy: the learning curve at an academic medical center. J Bone Joint Surg Am. 2006;88:1920–6.
9. Clohisy JC, Nunley RM, Curry MC, Schoenecker PL. Periacetabular osteotomy for the treatment of acetabular dysplasia associated with major aspherical femoral head deformities. J Bone Jt Surg Am. 2007;89:1417–23. https://doi.org/10.2106/JBJS.F.00493.
10. Garras DN, Crowder TT, Olson SA. Medium-term results of the Bernese periacetabular osteotomy in the treatment of symptomatic developmental dysplasia of the hip. J Bone Joint Surg Br. 2007;89-B:721–4. https://doi.org/10.1302/0301-620X.89B6.18805.
11. Steppacher SD, Tannast M, Ganz R, Siebenrock KA. Mean 20-year followup of Bernese periace-

tabular osteotomy. Clin Orthop. 2008;466:1633–44. https://doi.org/10.1007/s11999-008-0242-3.
12. Clohisy JC, Schutz AL, St John L, et al. Periacetabular osteotomy: a systematic literature review. Clin Orthop. 2009;467:2041–52. https://doi.org/10.1007/s11999-009-0842-6.
13. Sierra RJ, Leunig M, Ganz R. Bernese periacetabular osteotomy. Eur Surg Orthop Traumatol. 2014;2343–2364.
14. Matta JM, Stover MD, Siebenrock K. Periacetabular osteotomy through the Smith-Petersen approach. Clin Orthop Relat Res. 1999;(363):21–32.
15. Murphy SB, Millis MB. Periacetabular osteotomy without abductor dissection using direct anterior exposure. Clin Orthop Relat Res. 1999;(364):92–8. https://doi.org/10.1097/00003086-199907000-00013.
16. Ko J-Y, Wang C-J, Lin C-FJ, Shih C-H. Periacetabular osteotomy through a modified Ollier transtrochanteric approach for treatment of painful dysplastic hips. J Bone Joint Surg Am. 2002;84:1594.
17. Mayman DJ, Rudan J, Yach J, Ellis R. The Kingston periacetabular osteotomy utilizing computer enhancement: a new technique. Comput Aided Surg. 2002;7:179–86. https://doi.org/10.3109/10929080209146028.
18. Pogliacomi F, Stark A, Vaienti E, Wallensten R. Periacetabular osteotomy of the hip: the ilioinguinal approach. Acta Biomed. 2003;74:38–46.
19. Bernstein P, Thielemann F, Günther K-P. A modification of periacetabular osteotomy using a two-incision approach. Open Orthop J. 2007;1:13–8. https://doi.org/10.2174/1874325000701010013.
20. Thawrani D, Sucato DJ, Podeszwa DA, DeLaRocha A. Complications associated with the Bernese periacetabular osteotomy for hip dysplasia in adolescents. J Bone Joint Surg Am. 2010;92:1707–14. https://doi.org/10.2106/JBJS.I.00829.
21. Davey JP, Santore RF. Complications of periacetabular osteotomy. Clin Orthop Relat Res. 1999;(363):33–37.
22. Pring ME, Trousdale RT, Cabanela ME, Harper CM. Intraoperative electromyographic monitoring during periacetabular osteotomy. Clin Orthop Relat Res. 2002;400:158–64.
23. Hussell JG, Rodriguez JA, Ganz R. Technical complications of the Bernese periacetabular osteotomy. Clin Orthop Relat Res. 1999;363:81–92.
24. Sierra RJ, Beaule P, Zaltz I, et al. Prevention of nerve injury after periacetabular osteotomy. Clin Orthop. 2012;470:2209–19. https://doi.org/10.1007/s11999-012-2409-1.
25. Kalhor M, Gharehdaghi J, Schoeniger R, Ganz R. Reducing the risk of nerve injury during Bernese periacetabular osteotomy: a cadaveric study. Bone Joint J. 2015;97:636–41.
26. Kalhor M, Collado D, Leunig M, Rego P, Ganz R. Recommendations to reduce risk of nerve injury during Bernese periacetabular osteotomy (PAO). JBJS Essent Surg Tech. 2017;7(4):e34.
27. Stillwell A, Menelaus MB. Walking ability after transplantation of the iliopsoas. A long-term follow-up. J Bone Joint Surg Br. 1984;66:656–9.
28. Sierra RJ, Schoeniger SR, Millis M, Ganz R. Periacetabular osteotomy for containment of the nonarthritic dysplastic hip secondary to poliomyelitis. J Bone Joint Surg Am. 2010;92:2917–23.

10 Surgical Hip Dislocation for Anatomic Reorientation of Slipped Capital Femoral Epiphysis

Alessandro Aprato, Chiara Arrigoni, and Alessandro Massè

10.1 Introduction

Slipped capital femoral epiphysis (SCFE) is a common hip disorder in children and adolescents and it consists by a postero-inferior migration of the epiphysis in metaphysis through the physis in proximal femur. The current incidence of SCFE ranges from 0.33/100,000 to 24.58/100,000 children 8 to 15 years of age, depending upon gender and ethnicity. There is significant variability within racial groups and the relative frequency, relative to Caucasians at 1.0, is 5.6 for Polynesians, 3.9 for Blacks, and 2.5 for Hispanics. The average age is 12.0 years for boys and 11.2 years for girls; obese children present earlier than light weighted children [1]. Regarding gender males are more affected than females (13.35 vs 8.07 cases/100.000) [2].

Nowadays SCFE etiology remains unknown but it seems that both mechanical factors and metabolic causes are involved [3].

Mechanical factors include a greater retroversion of the femoral neck or a "coxa profunda" [3] related to major weakness of the growth plate during the period of rapid growth [4].

Gebhart et al. examine the differences in 2 common anatomic measurements: pelvic incidence (PI) and acetabular retroversion and their associations with post-SCFE deformity. They explain that, when a subject has a small PI, the pelvis will often tilt forward to maintain normal lumbar lordosis and balance sagittal alignment of the spine. This anterior pelvic tilt would load the anterior aspect of the hip joint and propagate the stresses across the physis of the proximal femur that are experienced in SCFE. This increased stress, combined with other insults experienced as a result of obesity, physeal sloping angle, femoral retroversion and size of the epiphyseal tubercle, could potentially result in the development of an SCFE.

In their study, made in a large cohort of osteological specimens, they report that decreased PI wasn't associated with SCFE but they didn't find significant difference between acetabular version of specimens with and without SCFE deformity. Moreover, the contralateral or unaffected acetabulum of SCFE specimens was not more retroverted than the affected side [5].

Furthermore, from a histological point of view, physeal cellular columnar height and organization are significantly altered in SCFE. Because the perichondrial ring is thinned, the large surface area of the undulating, interlocking mammillary processes provide the greatest internal support of the normal physis. In contrast, SCFE is characterized by physeal widening up to 12 mm (normal range: 2–6 mm), a widened hypertrophic zone comprising 60–80% of the physeal height, enlargement of chondrocytes, cellular columnar disorganization, higher proteoglycan and extracellular matrix concentrations throughout the physis, and a general disruption

A. Aprato (✉) · C. Arrigoni · A. Massè
School of Medicine, University of Turin, Turin, Italy

R. Ganz (ed.), *Modern Hip Preservation*, https://doi.org/10.1007/978-3-030-91967-2_10

in orderly chondrocyte differentiation and endochondral ossification [6]. Radiographic physeal widening implies a mechanically weakened physis susceptible to unlocking of the mammillary processes and further destabilization. The epiphyseal tubercle is also an anatomic feature that needs increased attention. It is a prominence consistently located among the mammillary processes of the posterosuperior quadrant of the epiphysis [6]. The tubercle averages 4 mm in height, it is always below the foramina for the lateral epiphyseal vessels and it is postulated to confer mechanical strength to the physeal plate. It is considered a possible keystone for physeal stability, but it decreases in size and surface area during childhood and adolescence as peripheral physeal cupping increases. Liu and colleagues [7] postulate that the epiphysis internally rotates on the epiphyseal tubercle and that a widened physis could contribute to epiphyseal dislodgement. Because the lateral epiphyseal arteries are immediately adjacent to and above the epiphyseal tubercle, this could explain the low rate of osteonecrosis in chronic, stable slips (i.e., minimal displacement of the lateral epiphyseal vessels).

Metabolic causes implicated in SCFE are obesity [8] and some endocrinological diseases such as hypothyroidism, kidney failure and the treatment with growth hormone [3].

As already said, the onset of SCFE usually occurs during the period of maximum growth but, because of recently observed tendency to an earlier growth, the age of onset is continuously changing [9].

Most series report bilateral involvement in as many as 63% of patients [2].

Kohno et al. in their study found that approximately 70% of contralateral hips in unilateral SCFE patients had subclinical posterior inclination of the capital femoral epiphysis, indicating the possibility of bilateral involvement. The contralateral posterior sloping angle (PSA) was a reliable predictor of a contralateral slip and a PSA of 19° was the cut-off value for developing SCFE [10].

10.2 Classification and Clinical Presentation

Several classifications of SCFE have been described in orthopedic literature [4]. The traditional classification subdivides SCFE into acute, chronic, and acute-on-chronic slips [11]. Another useful classification is based on Southwick's method to assess the magnitude of the sliding, measuring the angle between the head and femoral diaphysis on X-ray antero-posterior and axial projection [12]. The angle is then compared with the non-affected side, in case of one side lesion, or with normal values (145° in antero-posterior projection and 18° in axial projection).

The sliding is defined slight when the angle differs less than 30°, mild if the angle is between 30° and 60°, and severe if it exceeds 60° [3].

The most frequently employed classification divides SCFE into "stable" or "unstable" cases and is based on the ability of the patient to walk [4].

From a clinical point of view, patient with stable SCFE is an obese teen, with a brief history of hip, thigh, and knee pain. The patient may present a slight or mild limp, a gait with external rotation of the foot, a limitation of internal rotation of the hip or with a fixed position in external rotation and flexion of the hip.

A patient with an unstable SCFE, however, often has a severe hip pain that does not allow him to walk.

Medical history is often positive for hip, thigh, and knee pain and a previous trauma (of a minor entity that does not justify the fracture).

During the clinical exam the patient, lying on the couch, has an attitude in external rotation of the side affected and counteracting any passive movement of the hip.

10.3 Treatment

Most investigators agree that once SCFE is diagnosed surgical treatment is indicated, but significant controversies exist regarding the best treatment [13].

The goals of treatment are to correct the deformity, to prevent further slippage, to promote the closure of the growth plate, and to avoid osteonecrosis and chondrolysis.

Classical treatment of SCFE consists in percutaneous fixation with cannulated screw. Other treatments used are "compensatory" trochanteric osteotomies and direct correction of the deformity at the head-neck junction [14]. Percutaneous fixation and compensatory osteotomies are not intended to achieve an anatomically aligned epiphysis and correction at the site of deformity is reported to risk the blood supply to the epiphysis and therefore has not found wide acceptance [15].

In a study on "pinning in situ," Castañeda [16] reported a high incidence of unsatisfactory results because of technique difficulties to achieve an anatomic reduction; Boyer, in his work, emphasized that in long-term follow-up 12% of the patients had to undergo further surgery and reported a prevalence of early arthritis in 15% of cases [17].

On the basis of these data it can be said that pinning in situ, in mild or severe cases, does not reach the main goal that's early arthritis prevention [3]. Furthermore, osteonecrosis rate varies between 10% and 40% with this technique [13].

In regard to the compensatory osteotomies, the most commonly used are intertrochanteric osteotomies and cuneiform osteotomies at the base of the neck.

The intertrochanteric osteotomies limits are the distance between the osteotomy and the joint, the inability to treat the impingement that is created by the sliding of the head and the inability to restore a correct anatomy of the hip.

Furthermore, intertrochanteric osteotomies create an unwanted deformity that may complicate further hip joint prosthesis; many authors showed poor results: Kartenbender [18] reported 23% of poor clinical results and 33% of poor radiographic results in a 13.7 years of follow-up.

Cuneiform osteotomies also reached poor results: Velasco [19] has shown at 16 years of follow-up osteonecrosis rates of 11%, chondrolysis rates of 12% and 40% of early arthritis.

Nowadays better understanding of femoroacetabular impingement [20], a pathomechanical process of which SCFE can be an initiator [21], has renewed interest in direct correction of the deformity following SCFE.

Ganz, while recognizing the role of screw fixation in slight cases, proposed as a method of open reduction an alignment using surgical hip dislocation [22]. This technique (Figs. 10.1 and 10.2) allows an anatomic reorientation of the epiphysis protecting retinacular vessels and epiphyseal vascularization [23, 24].

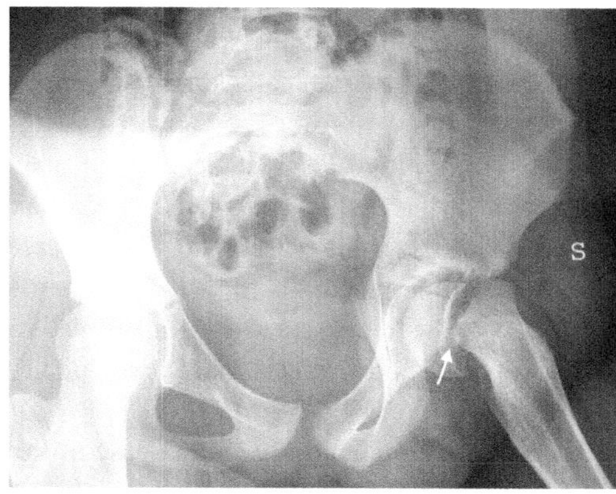

Fig. 10.1 Unstable slip in a 12-year-old female. Slight callus formation at the postero-medial neck (arrow), indicating that the slipping process was active more than only few days

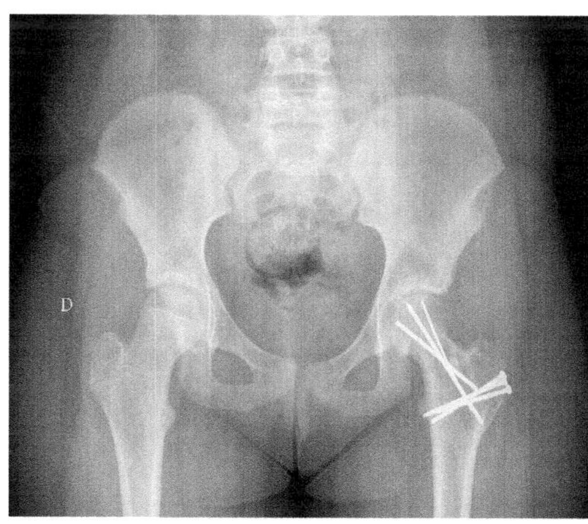

Fig. 10.2 Result 3 years after surgery: Preliminary fixation in situ followed by surgical hip dislocation, preparation of lateral and medial retinacular flap, callus resection at the posterior neck, and subcapital reorientation of the epiphysis. Fixation was achieved with 3 fully threaded pins (the one through the fovea was inserted in a retrograde fashion). Refixation of the trochanteric fragment was performed with 3.2 mm screws

Also, in non-recent onset SCFE you can possibly associate the treatment of acetabular labrum lesions and/or make a relative elongation of the femoral neck by retraction of the greater trochanter. This surgical technique is described below [15].

10.4 Surgical Technique

The authors perform this technique in lateral decubitus position through a straight lateral incision and the length of the incision itself depends on the thickness of the subcutaneous tissue [22].

The fasciotomy must be performed in line with the perforating vessels indicating the anterior border of the gluteus maximus muscle. The entire gluteus maximus muscle must be released from caudad to cephalad and retracted posteriorly together with the thin fascia of the gluteus medius containing the blood vessels and nerves of this muscle.

To obtain a sufficient proximal release of this muscle, the skin incision must be undermined, allowing the full exposure of the posterior margin of gluteus medius, the posterosuperior tip of the greater trochanter and the insertion of gluteus maximus. Now a digastric trochanteric osteotomy must be performed using an oscillating saw; the fragment must not be thicker than 1.5 cm.

Further dissection is needed to expose the joint capsule between the piriformis tendon and the gluteus minimus muscle; this is a very important interval for the preservation of the blood supply to the femoral head. The trochanteric fragment is then flipped anterosuperiorly, facilitated by releasing residual fibers of the gluteus medius and posterior insertion of the vastus lateralis down to the mid-level of the gluteus maximus tendon. The gradual mobilization of the posterior, superior, and anterior parts of gluteus minimus expose the capsule to beyond the acetabular rim. All external rotators initially remain attached to the stable trochanter. A Z-shaped capsulotomy follows, whereby the component axial to the femoral neck begins close to the anterosuperior edge of the stable trochanter. The inside-out direction of the capsulotomy along the femoral neck helps to avoid injury to retinaculum, cartilage, and labrum, and it's followed by the anterior capsular cut directed toward the anteroinferior acetabular rim and the posterior branch of the capsulotomy along the acetabular rim. Thereafter, the stability of the epi-metaphyseal connection is observed as well as the amount of slip. With gentle flexion and internal rotation, the presence and the range of impingement are assessed. If the epiphysis is disconnected, it must be immediately stabilized in situ, without any attempt of correcting the position, using two 2-mm Kirschner wires. Now the femoral head must be subluxed, moving the leg into external rotation, adduction, and flexion and placing the lower part of the leg into a sterile bag on the opposite side of the table.

To obtain the entire dislocation the round ligament has to be cut; now a 360° exposure of the acetabulum can be achieved. In this way it can be demonstrated any cam impingement at the metaphysis, along with any damage to the acetabular cartilage and labrum. If necessary, at this point, any labral refixation with suture anchors can be performed.

To create the retinacular flap the head is put back into the socket. The posterolateral portion of this flap contains the main vessels to the epiphysis and extends from the head-neck junction down to the lesser trochanter, and creation of the flap allows exposure of the posterolateral surface of the neck.

To allow retinacular flap preparation without damaging the vessels, the bone of the stable trochanter proximal to the physis is subperiosteally taken down to the level of the femoral neck using a "piece-meal" technique.

Thereafter, the subperiosteal release of the retinaculum is gradually continued from the lateral and posterior femoral neck using a scalpel and periosteal elevator. The same subperiosteal preparation is applied to the medial flap containing the branch of the medial circumflex femoral artery to the inferior portion of the epiphysis [25].

This step is easier to perform with the hip dislocated. The final result of the subperiosteal dissection is a soft tissue tube around the neck containing the vessels to the epiphysis and a circumferentially accessible bony neck.

Any tension applied to it is distributed over a long distance reducing the risk of adverse tension or rupture of the vessels. A curved chisel is then driven into the growth plate to slowly separate the epiphysis from the metaphysis. Before and after this step, the perfusion of the epiphysis must be tested with a 2 mm drill hole.

Careful external rotation of the leg allows further exposure of the metaphyseal stump, while spontaneous reduction of the epiphysis into the acetabulum is avoided with a cotton swab placed in the socket. With the epiphysis out of the socket, adverse movements are less likely to produce harmful tension in the retinaculum compared with the situation when the head is reduced.

There is always some callus formation at the posterior aspect of the metaphysis, even in acute slips, and if it can't be seen it can be palpated. This callus is removed using a straight osteotome. Shortening of the neck should not be performed, as it may be dangerous because it may create a relatively longer retinaculum that can be followed by compression of the retinacular vessels. The next step is the curettage of the remainder of the growth plate from the epiphysis, best performed with its manual stabilization. Thereafter, the epiphysis can be reduced onto the neck stump without abnormal tension in the retinacular flap, but care must be taken that the flap is not folded during the reduction. A 3.0 mm fully threaded wire is then drilled through the fovea capitis in a retrograde direction and, after retraction of this wire below the articular surface, the head is carefully repositioned into the acetabulum. Normal alignment of the retinacular flap is assessed and perfusion is tested again. Precise spatial alignment of the epiphysis is important and intraoperative fluoroscopic control is recommended after preliminary fixation. When the head position is correct, one or two more fully threaded wires are inserted in an anterograde direction to secure the position of the head. After final repositioning a further check that the retinaculum is falling back in place without a fold has to be made. Positioning sutures are applied to the retinaculum and capsule avoiding any tension. Finally, the trochanteric fragment is refixed about 5 mm more distally with 2 screws. Care is taken that the trochanter does not compress the soft tissue of capsule and retinaculum.

10.5 Results, Pros and Contras of This Technique

The most used SCFE treatment is pinning in situ with single or multiple screws with the goal of preventing further slip progression. However, even mild slips may lead to early acetabular labrum and cartilage damage and the metaphyseal bump, limiting internal rotation, leads to femoroacetabular impingement [21, 26]. For this reason, in case of mild or severe slips osteotomies have been recommended.

Several correction osteotomies have been proposed for those patients. Intertrochanteric osteotomy [27] and anterior cuneiform wedge osteotomy of the base of the neck [28] have been the most popular ones. Simulation of different corrections for different slip angles can show how limited these osteotomies are in terms of impingement, although an antero-posterior radiograph may show a satisfactory alignment.

Dunn [29] introduced a posterolateral dissection of the retinaculum to allow some trimming of the callus formation at the posterior neck, adding a trochanteric osteotomy to facilitate the procedure. The created space reaching from the head-neck junction to the axilla with the greater trochanter is rather narrow for perfect control of the retinacular tension during callus removal, and this may explain why necrosis of the epiphysis could not sufficiently be eliminated with this procedure [29, 30]. With current and detailed knowledge of the vascular supply of the femoral head and its topography [25], surgical hip dislocation is a safe procedure and has become a well-accepted technique for the treatment of SCFE [31]. This technique allows the creation of an extended retinacular flap [32] that is 3 times longer than the retinacular release made in Dunn's procedure.

The extended flap permits to distribute the tension over a larger distance that decreases the risk of negative effect on epiphysis perfusion. A crescent number of articles appears in literature about the treatment of SCFE with surgical dislocation [2, 3, 15, 22, 33–35]. Leunig et al. [22] provided one of the first reports using this technique for the reduction of SCFE. The approach is derived from the concern that slip displacement in patients with SCFE regularly produces acetabular cartilage damage and early clinical symptoms. Spencer et al. [33] presented a comparison between surgical dislocation with femoral head-neck osteoplasty only and the same procedure associated with intertrochanteric osteotomy. They affirmed that this technique is effective, particularly in patients of the second group (osteoplasty and osteotomy) who showed better clinical and radiographic findings. None showed avascular necrosis of the femoral head and all the trochanteric osteotomies healed.

Ziebarth et al. [34] have combined two case series from two institutions. Rebello et al. [35] compared surgical dislocation in different hip deformities. Patients with SCFE seem to have a greater benefit from the technique than patients with Perthes or osteonecrosis. They have justified this result to the underlying cartilage damage and to the inability to restore the normal anatomy in the last two conditions. In addition, at the time of surgery, patients with SCFE were younger than the others.

In a recent multicenter report by Sankar et al. [36], the authors reviewed the outcomes of 27 hips (27 patients) that had been treated with this technique for unstable SCFE. At a mean follow-up of 22.3 months, 4 patients (15%) had broken implants at 3–18 weeks after surgery and required revision fixation. A total of 7 patients (26%) developed osteonecrosis at a mean of 21.4 weeks and each surgeon in the series had at least 1 case of AVN. The authors also reported that patients who did not develop AVN had a significantly lower pain score, higher level of post-operative satisfaction, and higher University of California Los Angeles activity score.

Ganz and the GICCA group reviewed the patients they operated with surgical dislocation in the period between January 2007 and October 2009. All patients presenting to one of the author's clinics with stable or unstable SCFE in that period were included in a retrospective study [15].

Criteria for exclusion were hips with established necrosis before the procedure, those with chronic SCFE of 30° or less (for which trimming of the metaphyseal overhang and pinning was performed), and hips with advanced ankylosis.

All patients were treated with surgical dislocation and preservation of an extended retinacular flap, allowing an anatomic subcapital realignment. In four cases, the epiphysis was disconnected from the metaphysis or the connection was very weak. Non-weight bearing on the affected limb with crutches was recommended for 6–8 weeks after surgery, and active abduction and passive adduction were restricted for 4–6 weeks. Unrestricted function was allowed after 12 weeks.

Patients were clinically examined by monitoring pain, stiffness and function. Moreover, radiological follow-up examinations were carried out at the time of the most recent post-operative control and compared with the pre-operative series. On pre-operative and post-operative AP and L images were measured Southwick [37] and alpha angles [38] (this one only in post-operative images).

They try to compare their case series with other published series regarding age, follow-up, pre- and post-operative Southwick angles, alpha angles, post-operative pain and function and a statistical analysis was performed showing that there was no significant difference between their study and the other papers.

Doing the procedure carefully and following exactly the correct steps, the pioneers of this approach reported no cases of avascular necrosis [22, 34] and the GICCA group too, demonstrating clinical and radiological follow-up results comparable with those of others using the same technique. The disadvantages are that it's a technically demanding approach, there is however the risks of avascular necrosis in case of technique not correctly followed, has a long learning curve and uses an important skin access.

In recent literature, only few studies compared the modified Dunn procedure with pinning in situ.

In one of them, Souder et al. reported a 20% rate of osteonecrosis after the modified Dunn procedure for stable SCFE; however, the severity of their cases was not reported [39].

In a study of Novais et al. [40] were compared children with severe stable SCFE treated with the modified Dunn procedure or in situ pinning in terms of proximal femoral radiographic deformity, Heyman and Herndon clinical outcome, complication rate, and number of reoperations performed after the initial procedure. In a total of 30 hip treated for severe stable slip (15 with the modified Dunn procedure and 15 with pinning in situ, statistically comparable regarding age at surgery, sex, affected side, and duration of follow-up), they found that the modified Dunn subcapital realignment procedure using a surgical hip dislocation approach allows for better radiographic correction of the femoral head and neck deformity, better clinical Heyman and Herndon outcome classification, and lower reoperation rate when compared with in situ pinning for treatment of severe stable SCFE at an average of 2 years of follow-up.

They affirmed that despite historically better long-term outcomes after in situ pinning compared with reorientation procedures for mild and moderate SCFE, the residual deformity in severe SCFE is recognized to negatively affect its prognosis. They agreed with the authors of this chapter that the modified Dunn subcapital realignment procedure using a surgical hip dislocation approach has been reported to provide restoration of the femoral head-neck anatomy with low rates of osteonecrosis for treatment of stable SCFE even if it may have a higher risk than pinning in situ.

In their study, they concluded that because of the learning curve associated with the technically demanding modified Dunn procedure, the decision between its use versus in situ pinning often is based on surgeon experience rather than available evidence; their data suggest that the modified Dunn procedure is to be considered a safer treatment in terms of definitive treatment.

In agreement with recent studies published in the literature the author of this chapter may affirm that the modified Dunn procedure is safe, efficient, and reproducible, but it has a long learning curve and it should be learned in a specialized center before using it in clinical practice.

References

1. Loder RT, Skopelja EN. The epidemiology and demographics of slipped capital femoral epiphysis. ISRN Orthop. 2011;2011:486512. https://doi.org/10.5402/2011/486512.
2. Lehmann CL, Arons RR, Loder RT, Vitale MG. The epidemiology of slipped capital femoral epiphysis: an update. J Pediatr Orthop. 2006;26:286–90. https://doi.org/10.1097/01.bpo.0000217718.10728.70.
3. Massè A, Aprato A, Favuto M, et al. Epifisiolisi. Lo Scalpello-OTODI Educ. 2010;24:177–83.
4. Iwinski HJJ. Slipped capital femoral epiphysis. Curr Opin Orthop. 2006;17:511–6. https://doi.org/10.1097/01.bco.0000247364.51879.16.
5. Gebhart JJ, Bohl MS, Weinberg DS, et al. Pelvic incidence and acetabular version in slipped capital femoral epiphysis. J Pediatr Orthop. 2015;35:565–70. https://doi.org/10.1097/BPO.0000000000000342.
6. Georgiadis AG, Zaltz I. Slipped capital femoral epiphysis: how to evaluate with a review and update of treatment. Pediatr Clin N Am. 2014;61:1119–35. https://doi.org/10.1016/j.pcl.2014.08.001.
7. Liu RW, Armstrong DG, Levine AD, et al. An anatomic study of the epiphyseal tubercle and its importance in the pathogenesis of slipped capital femoral epiphysis. J Bone Joint Surg Am. 2013;95:e341–8. https://doi.org/10.2106/JBJS.L.00474.
8. Bhatia NN, Pirpiris M, Otsuka NY. Body mass index in patients with slipped capital femoral epiphysis. J Pediatr Orthop. 2006;26:197–9. https://doi.org/10.1097/01.bpo.0000218526.36362.3f.
9. Loder RT, Starnes T, Dikos G. The narrow window of bone age in children with slipped capital femoral epiphysis: a reassessment one decade later. J Pediatr Orthop. 2006;26:300–6. https://doi.org/10.1097/01.bpo.0000214919.77490.36.
10. Kohno Y, Nakashima Y, Kitano T, et al. Subclinical bilateral involvement of the hip in patients with slipped capital femoral epiphysis: a multicentre study. Int Orthop. 2014;38:477–82. https://doi.org/10.1007/s00264-013-2131-y.
11. Fahey JJ, O'Brien ET. Acute slipped capital femoral epiphysis: review of the literature and report of ten cases. J Bone Joint Surg Am. 1965;47:1105–22.
12. Southwick WO. Osteotomy through the lesser trochanter for slipped capital femoral epiphysis. J Bone Joint Surg Am. 1967;49:807–35.
13. Loder RT. Unstable slipped capital femoral epiphysis. J Pediatr Orthop. 2001;21:694–9.
14. Gholve PA, Cameron DB, Millis MB. Slipped capital femoral epiphysis update. Curr Opin Pediatr. 2009;21:39–45. https://doi.org/10.1097/MOP.0b013e328320acea.
15. Massè A, Aprato A, Grappiolo G, et al. Surgical hip dislocation for anatomic reorientation of slipped capital femoral epiphysis: preliminary results. Hip Int. 2012;22:137–44. https://doi.org/10.5301/HIP.2012.9208.

16. Castañeda P, Macías C, Rocha A, et al. Functional outcome of stable grade III slipped capital femoral epiphysis treated with in situ pinning. J Pediatr Orthop. 2009;29:454–8. https://doi.org/10.1097/BPO.0b013e3181aab7c3.
17. Boyer DW, Mickelson MR, Ponseti IV. Slipped capital femoral epiphysis. Long-term follow-up study of one hundred and twenty-one patients. J Bone Joint Surg Am. 1981;63:85–95.
18. Kartenbender K, Cordier W, Katthagen BD. Long-term follow-up study after corrective Imhäuser osteotomy for severe slipped capital femoral epiphysis. J Pediatr Orthop. 2000;20:749–56. https://doi.org/10.1097/00004694-200011000-00010.
19. Velasco R, Schai PA, Exner GU. Slipped capital femoral epiphysis: a long-term follow-up study after open reduction of the femoral head combined with sub capital wedge resection. J Pediatr Orthop B. 1998;7:43–52.
20. Ganz R, Parvizi J, Beck M, et al. Femoroacetabular impingement: a cause for osteoarthritis of the hip. Clin Orthop Relat Res. 2003;417:112–20. https://doi.org/10.1097/01.blo.0000096804.78689.c2.
21. Leunig M, Casillas MM, Hamlet M, et al. Slipped capital femoral epiphysis: early mechanical damage to the acetabular cartilage by a prominent femoral metaphysis. Acta Orthop Scand. 2000;71:370–5. https://doi.org/10.1080/000164700317393367.
22. Leunig M, Slongo T, Kleinschmidt M, Ganz R. Subcapital correction osteotomy in slipped capital femoral epiphysis by means of surgical hip dislocation. Oper Orthop Traumatol. 2007;19:389–410. https://doi.org/10.1007/s00064-007-1213-7.
23. Sucato DJ, De La Rocha A. High-grade SCFE: the role of surgical hip dislocation and reduction. J Pediatr Orthop. 2014;34(Suppl 1):S18–24. https://doi.org/10.1097/BPO.0000000000000297.
24. Ricciardi BF, Sink EL. Surgical hip dislocation: techniques for success. J Pediatr Orthop. 2014;34(Suppl 1):S25–31. https://doi.org/10.1097/BPO.0000000000000296.
25. Kalhor M, Beck M, Huff TW, Ganz R. Capsular and pericapsular contributions to acetabular and femoral head perfusion. J Bone Joint Surg Am. 2009;91:409–18. https://doi.org/10.2106/JBJS.G.01679.
26. Rab GT. The geometry of slipped capital femoral epiphysis: implications for movement, impingement, and corrective osteotomy. J Pediatr Orthop. 1999;19:419–24.
27. Schai PA, Exner GU. Corrective Imhäuser intertrochanteric osteotomy. Oper Orthop Traumatol. 2007;19:368–88. https://doi.org/10.1007/s00064-007-1212-8.
28. Kramer WG, Craig WA, Noel S. Compensating osteotomy at the base of the femoral neck for slipped capital femoral epiphysis. J Bone Joint Surg Am. 1976;58:796–800.
29. Dunn DM. The treatment of adolescent slipping of the upper femoral epiphysis. J Bone Joint Surg Br. 1964;46:621–9.
30. Fron D, Forgues D, Mayrargue E, et al. Follow-up study of severe slipped capital femoral epiphysis treated with Dunn's osteotomy. J Pediatr Orthop. 2000;20:320–5.
31. Ganz R, Gill TJ, Gautier E, et al. Surgical dislocation of the adult hip. A technique with full access to the femoral head and acetabulum without the risk of avascular necrosis. J Bone Joint Surg Br. 2001;83:1119–24. https://doi.org/10.1302/0301-620x.83b8.11964.
32. Ganz R, Huff TW, Leunig M. Extended retinacular soft-tissue flap for intra-articular hip surgery: surgical technique, indications, and results of application. Instr Course Lect. 2009;58:241–55.
33. Spencer S, Millis MB, Kim Y-J. Early results of treatment of hip impingement syndrome in slipped capital femoral epiphysis and pistol grip deformity of the femoral head-neck junction using the surgical dislocation technique. J Pediatr Orthop. 2006;26:281–5. https://doi.org/10.1097/01.bpo.0000217726.16417.74.
34. Ziebarth K, Zilkens C, Spencer S, et al. Capital realignment for moderate and severe SCFE using a modified Dunn procedure. Clin Orthop. 2009;467:704–16. https://doi.org/10.1007/s11999-008-0687-4.
35. Rebello G, Spencer S, Millis MB, Kim Y-J. Surgical dislocation in the management of pediatric and adolescent hip deformity. Clin Orthop. 2009;467:724–31. https://doi.org/10.1007/s11999-008-0591-y.
36. Sankar WN, Vanderhave KL, Matheney T, et al. The modified Dunn procedure for unstable slipped capital femoral epiphysis: a multicenter perspective. J Bone Joint Surg Am. 2013;95:585–91. https://doi.org/10.2106/JBJS.L.00203.
37. Southwick WO. Slipped capital femoral epiphysis. J Bone Joint Surg Am. 1984;66:1151–2.
38. Tannast M, Siebenrock KA, Anderson SE. Femoroacetabular impingement: radiographic diagnosis--what the radiologist should know. AJR Am J Roentgenol. 2007;188:1540–52. https://doi.org/10.2214/AJR.06.0921.
39. Souder CD, Bomar JD, Wenger DR. The role of capital realignment versus in situ stabilization for the treatment of slipped capital femoral epiphysis. J Pediatr Orthop. 2014;34:791–8. https://doi.org/10.1097/BPO.0000000000000193.
40. Novais EN, Hill MK, Carry PM, et al. Modified Dunn procedure is superior to in situ pinning for short-term clinical and radiographic improvement in severe stable SCFE. Clin Orthop. 2015;473:2108–17. https://doi.org/10.1007/s11999-014-4100-1.

11 Relative Lengthening of the Femoral Neck

Luigino Turchetto, Stefano Saggin, and Reinhold Ganz

11.1 Introduction

Extra-articular femoroacetabular impingement (FAI) is defined as a premature pathological, extracapsular contact of the proximal femur and the pelvis [1, 2].

The impingement occurs between complex proximal femur deformities as high-riding greater trochanter, short femoral neck, and reduced vertical distance between the head and the lesser trochanter against ilium, ischium, anteroinferior iliac spine (AIIS), and acetabular rim [3–6].

In most cases, there is a combination of extra-articular and intra-articular impingement resulting mainly from Legg–Calvé–Perthes Disease (LCPD), slipped capital femoral epiphysis (SCFE), post septic arthritis, or trauma [7, 8].

The clinical condition of most of these hips may be characterized by weakness of the gluteus medius and varying degrees of pain attributable to direct compression of soft-tissue structures or indirectly through the creation of abnormal stresses across the femoroacetabular articulation or impingement-induced instability [9].

A limited abduction in extension with an improvement of abduction in flexion because the high-riding trochanter slip posteriorly in flexion was described by MacNicol [10].

Classically, extra-articular impingement with associated abductor insufficiency are treated by trochanteric advancement [11]. Distalization of the greater trochanter was first described in 1969 by Jani [12], the purpose of this procedure was to eliminate bony impingement of the greater trochanter against the lateral ilium increasing the range of motion and the moment arm of the abductors as a result of the distal or lateral trochanteric advancement [13]. Free and Delp [14] in a computer model of total hip replacement showed a maximum increase of 11% for anterolateral transfer in a patient with normal anatomy but when the hip was shortened by the superior displacement of the hip center as in coxa brevis the moment arm of the abductor was not significantly improved with distal advancement. Based on a lab setting, Beck [15] concluded that in hips with high-riding trochanter the optimal position is at the level of the center of hip rotation and excessive distalization should be avoided. However, classic trochanteric advancement may increase the abductor force but cannot treat the impingement completely, this may leave intra-articular impingement and instability unaddressed [16]. The technique of surgical hip dislocation [17] in combination with a retinacular flap [1] allows the relative lengthening of the femoral neck associated with head–neck osteochondroplasty and eventual femoral head reduction osteotomy [18].

L. Turchetto (✉) · S. Saggin
Orthopedics and Traumatology Unit, Portogruaro Hospital, Portogruaro, Italy
e-mail: lturchetto@tin.it

R. Ganz
Faculty of Medicine, University of Bern, Bern, Switzerland

R. Ganz (ed.), *Modern Hip Preservation*, https://doi.org/10.1007/978-3-030-91967-2_11

11.2 Surgical Technique

The technique is called relative lengthening of the femoral neck because only the superior circumference of the neck becomes longer by trimming away most of the trochanteric massif prominence in its posterosuperior circumference, such that it becomes continuous with the smaller contour of the neck. Leg length remains the same but regarding the clearance for hip motion, the neck has been lengthened (Fig. 11.1). With further trimming of the superior contour, the neck becomes effectively more valgus [1].

The base of this surgical procedure is the safe surgical hip dislocation [17] combined with an extended retinacular soft-tissue flap, allowing visual protection of the femoral head blood supply during execution of extra- and intra-articular osteotomy [1, 20].

After hip dislocation [17], for the execution of the subperiosteal flap, the femoral head is reduced into the acetabular socket and the cancellous bone of the stable trochanter is exposed. Using a straight osteotome of 1.5 cm the bone mass of the stable trochanter is reduced piece by piece strictly subperiosteally. During these steps, the osteotome should not penetrate posteriorly out of the bone but it should be used to weaken the fragment that is manually bent and turned outward with a rongeur. In this way the fragment can be subperiosteally dis-

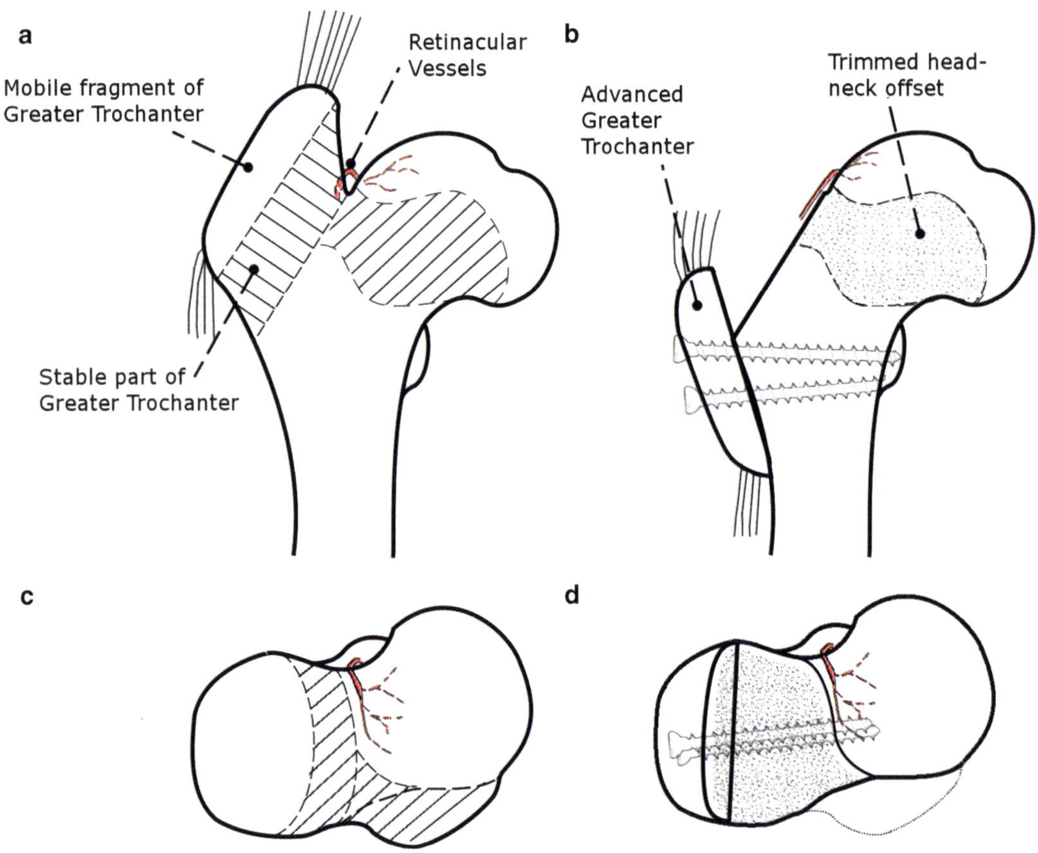

Fig. 11.1 (Modified from Tannast M et al. [19]). (**a**, **c**) Scheme of the relative femoral neck lengthening technique. (**b**, **d**) After osteotomy of the greater trochanter, the base of the greater trochanter is trimmed down and the trochanteric fragment is advanced distally. Care has to be taken to preserve the retinacular vessels of the medial femoral circumflex artery to the epiphysis (*colored in red*)

sected with a knife. This technique is repeated until the trochanteric surface is at the same levels of posterior and superior surface of the neck.

The periosteum over the femoral neck, anterior to the retinaculum, as well as the periosteum distal to the quadratus femoris muscle are incised longitudinally. The inferolateral border of the periosteum is now mobilized posteriorly and distally until the posterior surface of the lesser trochanter becomes visible. The periosteal flap includes the insertion of all the external rotators, the ramus profundus of the medial femoral circumflex artery (MFCA), its terminal branches and the retinacular vessels.

In case relative lengthening of the femoral neck is the only procedure, further dissection is not necessary.

If a neck osteotomy is planned, the flap is separated from the neck with a sharp periosteal elevator. It is important to achieve a long flap avoiding any tension on the vessels. Care must be taken proximally to avoid damages to the area where the retinacular vessels enter the femoral head. After this step the femoral head is dislocated and the periosteum is anteriorly incised at the femoral neck junction and the anterior subperiosteal flap is developed with a periosteal elevator. The flap includes the Weitbrecht ligament with the anteroinferior branch of the MFCA that supplies the inferomedial sector of the head.

After completion of this semi-tubular flap, two blunt Hohmann retractors can be placed from lateral and medial around the femoral neck, allowing sub-capital reorientation, neck osteotomy, or femoral head reduction osteotomy [1].

At the end of the procedure the borders of the periosteal tube are loosely approximated without any tension. The capsule is closed in the same way and the desired distal advancement of the trochanteric fragment is facilitated by a release of the long tendinous head of the gluteus minimus muscle along the anterior border of the mobile trochanteric fragment.

The definitive position of the trochanteric fragment is determined with a bone hook and a palpating finger near the undersurface of the trochanter to assess the position. The bone fixation is obtained with two 3.5 cortical screws.

11.3 Early Results

Relative neck lengthening in hips with complex deformities has shown promising results [5, 7]. The mid-term follow-up study by Albers et al. [3] resulted in reduced pain, improved function, and improved radiographic parameters of the proximal femur.

References

1. Ganz R, Huff TW, Leunig M. Extended retinacular soft-tissue flap for intra-articular hip surgery: surgical technique, indications, and results of application. Instr Course Lect. 2009;58:241–55.
2. Tannast M, Hanke M, Ecker TM, et al. LCPD: reduced range of motion resulting from extra- and intraarticular impingement. Clin Orthop. 2012;470:2431–40. https://doi.org/10.1007/s11999-012-2344-1.
3. Albers CE, Steppacher SD, Ganz R, et al. Joint-preserving surgery improves pain, range of motion, and abductor strength after Legg-Calvé-Perthes disease. Clin Orthop. 2012;470:2450–61. https://doi.org/10.1007/s11999-012-2345-0.
4. Albers CE, Steppacher SD, Schwab JM, et al. Relative femoral neck lengthening improves pain and hip function in proximal femoral deformities with a high-riding trochanter. Clin Orthop. 2015;473:1378–87. https://doi.org/10.1007/s11999-014-4032-9.
5. Anderson LA, Erickson JA, Severson EP, Peters CL. Sequelae of Perthes disease: treatment with surgical hip dislocation and relative femoral neck lengthening. J Pediatr Orthop. 2010;30:758–66. https://doi.org/10.1097/BPO.0b013e3181fcbaaf.
6. Ganz R, Slongo T, Turchetto L, et al. The lesser trochanter as a cause of hip impingement: pathophysiology and treatment options. Hip Int. 2013;23:S35. https://doi.org/10.5301/hipint.5000063.
7. Shore BJ, Novais EN, Millis MB, Kim Y-J. Low early failure rates using a surgical dislocation approach in healed Legg-Calvé-Perthes disease. Clin Orthop. 2012;470:2441–9. https://doi.org/10.1007/s11999-011-2187-1.
8. Mamisch TC, Kim Y-J, Richolt JA, et al. Femoral morphology due to impingement influences the range of motion in slipped capital femoral epiphysis. Clin Orthop. 2009;467:692–8. https://doi.org/10.1007/s11999-008-0477-z.

9. Ricciardi BF, Fabricant PD, Fields KG, et al. What are the demographic and radiographic characteristics of patients with symptomatic extraarticular femoroacetabular impingement? Clin Orthop. 2015;473:1299–308. https://doi.org/10.1007/s11999-014-4001-3.
10. Macnicol MF, Makris D. Distal transfer of the greater trochanter. J Bone Joint Surg Br. 1991;73:838–41.
11. Kelikian AS, Tachdjian MO, Askew MJ, Jasty M. Greater trochanteric advancement of the proximal femur: a clinical and biomechanical study. Hip. 1983;77–105.
12. Jani L. Die Entwicklung des Schenkelhalses nach der Trochanterversetzung. Arch Für Orthop Unf-Chir Mit Bes Berücksicht Frakturenlehre Orthop-Chir Tech. 1969;66:127–32.
13. Gore DR, Murray MP, Gardner GM, Sepic SB. Roentgenographic measurements after Müller total hip replacement. Correlations among roentgenographic measurements and hip strength and mobility. J Bone Joint Surg Am. 1977;59:948–53.
14. Free SA, Delp SL. Trochanteric transfer in total hip replacement: effects on the moment arms and force-generating capacities of the hip abductors. J Orthop Res. 1996;14:245–50.
15. Beck M, Krüger A, Katthagen C, Kohl S. Osteotomy of the greater trochanter: effect on gluteus medius function. Surg Radiol Anat. 2015;37:599–607. https://doi.org/10.1007/s00276-015-1466-z.
16. Ganz R, Campacci A, Grappiolo G, et al. Open intracapsular hip surgery. Minerva Ortop E Traumatol. 2014;65:53–7.
17. Ganz R, Gill TJ, Gautier E, et al. Surgical dislocation of the adult hip. A technique with full access to the femoral head and acetabulum without the risk of avascular necrosis. J Bone Joint Surg Br. 2001;83:1119–24. https://doi.org/10.1302/0301-620x.83b8.11964.
18. Ganz R, Horowitz K, Leunig M. Algorithm for femoral and periacetabular osteotomies in complex hip deformities. Clin Orthop. 2010;468:3168–80. https://doi.org/10.1007/s11999-010-1489-z.
19. Tannast M, Macintyre N, Steppacher SD, et al. A systematic approach to analyse the sequelae of LCPD. Hip Int. 2013;23(Suppl 9):S61–70. https://doi.org/10.5301/hipint.5000071.
20. Gautier E, Ganz K, Krugel N, et al. Anatomy of the medial femoral circumflex artery and its surgical implications. J Bone Joint Surg Br. 2018;83-B:149. https://doi.org/10.1302/0301-620x.83b1.0830149.

Indications and Results of Femoral Neck Osteotomy in Adults

12

Paulo Rego

12.1 Introduction

Proximal femoral intertrochanteric osteotomy (ITO) is a well-established realignment procedure for proximal femoral deformities [1, 2] or to prevent collapse in avascular necrosis (AVN) [3–5].

The use of ITO appears to be declining in current clinical practice [6]. Among the reasons there are a number of technical limitations: There is no direct access to intra-articular pathology. The correction being performed distant to the main anatomic distortion, creates a secondary deformity and eventually long-time loss of abductor strength [7]. The femoral shaft is either medialized or lateralized altering the mechanical axis of the lower extremity. The possible influence on limb length is a constant matter of concern [8, 9] (Fig. 12.1). Some studies also revealed that total hip replacement (THR) following ITO is technically more demanding, usually associated with increased operative time, increased blood loss, and higher infection rates [10, 11]. In caput valgum, with a short femoral neck and high riding trochanter, the varus ITO also has the potential to create an extra-articular impingement.

The possibility to perform safely a more proximal osteotomy, at the neck level, and a distal advancement of the trochanter [8] would have advantages over ITO: more efficiency with less angular correction, less residual deformity, especially less shortening of the limb, possibility to access the joint to check for femoroacetabular impingement, treat chondro-labral disorders and perform an osteochondroplasty.

In the last decade, a better comprehension of the vascular supply to the femoral head [12, 13], allowed the establishment of the technique of safe surgical dislocation of the hip [14] and generation of a soft tissue flap containing the hip short external rotators, the deep branch of the MFCA and the retinacular vessels [15]. Based on this flap, new approaches to the femoral neck have been developed and techniques, such as relative neck lengthening (RNL), sub capital and true femoral neck osteotomy (FNO) and femoral head reduction osteotomy (FHRO) have become real options [15, 16].

If the surgery is precisely executed, the risk of AVN is very low as it allows direct control of the vascular supply to the femoral head. The low complication rate, in particular AVN, in published series on sub capital realignment of SCFE demonstrates that it is a safe procedure [17–19].

Considering the more caudad level of ITO, the medial femoral circumflex artery (MFCA) seems to be protected against iatrogenic insult during surgery. However, several anatomic studies have shown that the deep branch propagates posteriorly about 5 to 10 mm proximal to the lesser trochanter [12, 13, 20, 21] (Fig. 12.2), precisely the area where the ITO cut exits the medial cortex.

P. Rego (✉)
Orthopedic Department, Hospital da Luz, Lisbon, Portugal

R. Ganz (ed.), *Modern Hip Preservation*, https://doi.org/10.1007/978-3-030-91967-2_12

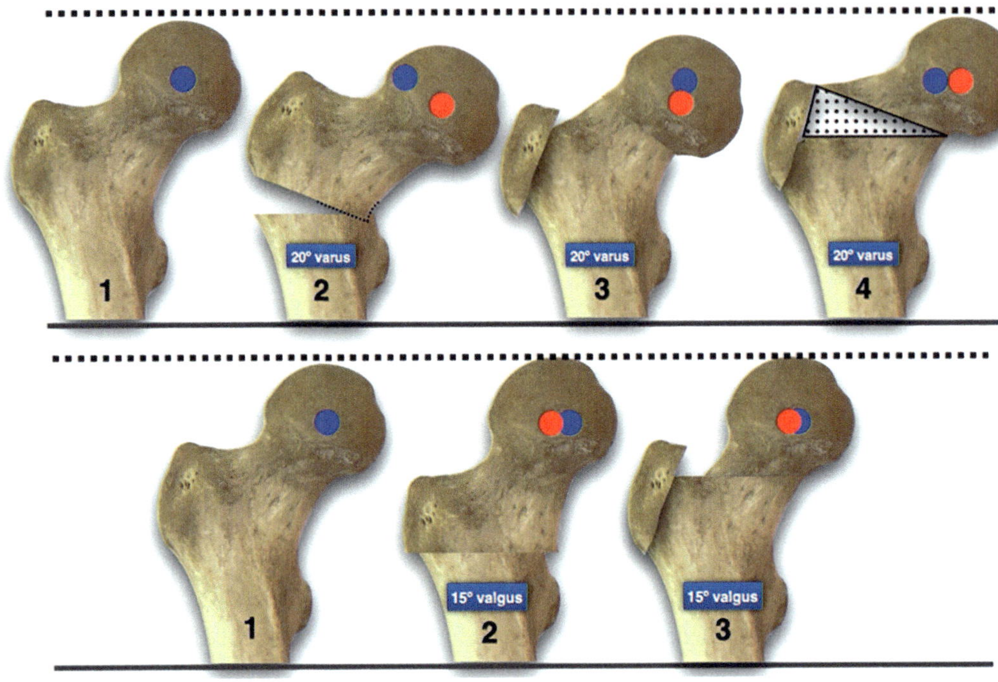

Fig. 12.1 *Above*: The effect of different types of 20° varus osteotomy: Normal proximal femur (*1*). Intertrochanteric varus osteotomy, even without wedge removal (*2*), shortens the leg more than varus close wedge neck osteotomy (*3*). Smallest shortening with open wedge neck osteotomy (*4*). Intertrochanteric varus osteotomy creates the largest lateral shift (*red circle* versus *blue circle*) of the femur when not compensated by active medialization. *Below*: The effect of different types of 15° valgus osteotomy: Normal proximal femur (*1*). The lengthening effect of intertrochanteric valgus can be controlled by removing a wedge (*2*). The femoral shaft again has the biggest shift with the intertrochanteric osteotomy when compared to close wedge valgus neck osteotomy (*3*)

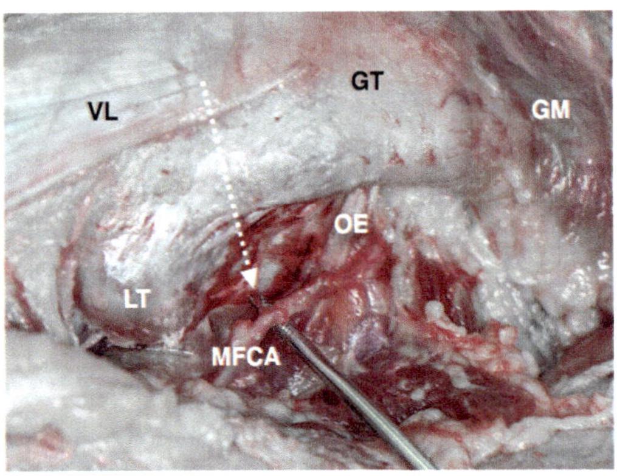

Fig. 12.2 Close relation of the *MFCA* to the lesser trochanter. The *dotted line* represents the ITO (Inter Trochanteric Osteotomy) cut direction. *LT* lesser trochanter, *MFCA* deep branch of medial femoral circumflex artery, *OE* obturator externus tendon, *VL* vastus lateralis, *GT* greater trochanter, *GM* gluteus medius

Another advantage of FNO over ITO is the possibility of using screws for fixation. Compared to the prominent knee of the angled blade plate, there is much less trochanteric irritation and pain resulting from hardware [8, 9].

The aim of our study was to demonstrate that the technique of FNO to realign the femoral head is feasible and reproducible also in adults with primary or post traumatic deformity.

12.2 Materials and Methods

Since 2009, we have performed 13 cases of femoral neck osteotomy. We include in this series the 11 cases with a minimum follow-up of 3 years (maximum 8 years; average time 4 years).

All patients (ten females and one male) were adults with an average of 26 years old (range 26–37 years).

The main radiographic abnormality in six cases was a Coxa valga with high fovea, articulating with the roof cartilage. Three cases had a varus neck and high riding trochanter. Two cases resulted from femoral neck fracture sequelae. Of those, one case sustained a valgus malunion after impacted sub capital fracture and the other a varus non-union with hardware failure. In four cases there was concomitant acetabular dysplasia with a congruent joint. One hip suffered from acetabular dysplasia secondary to Morbus Perthes. One patient had a shorter ipsilateral limb (20 mm) and another a longer ipsilateral limb before surgery (15 mm). All patients suffered from trochanteric and inguinal pain, worse under axial loading. Internal rotation was frequently limited and the problem influenced their daily activities. The patient with valgus malunion was unable to walk without crutches.

As preoperative routines, all patients had standard AP pelvis and hip cross-table view x-rays. Abduction or adduction views (depending on the primary deformity) were also obtained to simulate the position of the femoral head after correction. The neck shaft angle (NSA), acetabular index (AI), lateral center edge (CE), and delta (δ) angles [22–24] were measured before and after surgery. Magnetic resonance imaging (MRI) with arthrography including radial sequences was performed before surgery in all except one case (broken screws in place) to study the head-neck junction contour and to evaluate labrum and cartilage damage.

The patients were evaluated using the non-arthritic hip score (NAHS) [25] before surgery, at 12, 24 months and then once in every year. For practical reasons we have used only the outcome score from the last visit.

All patients where operated using the surgical hip dislocation approach [14, 26, 27]. The circumference of the neck was developed with the extended retinacular flap in order to perform a safe femoral neck osteotomy [15, 16]. In lateral decubitus, the operative side was freely draped and placed on a bag with a tunnel for the opposite leg. Skin incision was straight longitudinally over the anterior third of the greater trochanter (GT). The proximal fascia lata was incised anterior to the gluteus maximus muscle.

The trochanteric osteotomy was performed using an oscillating saw. The osteotomy line was oriented in such a way that, proximally, 3–4 mm of the posterior portion of the gluteus medius muscle remained attached to the stable tip of the trochanter. Distally, the entire origin of the vastus lateralis muscle remained on the mobile trochanter. Releasing carefully the remaining gluteus medius fibers from the stable trochanter, the mobile part could be freely mobilized and flipped anteriorly. The maximum thickness of the trochanteric fragment never exceeded 13–15 mm. With this technique, most of the piriformis tendon remained attached to the stable trochanter protecting the capsular penetration area of the deep branch of the MFCA (Fig. 12.3). The exposure of the capsule started by developing the interval between the piriformis and gluteus minimus muscles. This was facilitated by hip flexion, external rotation and abduction. The use of a leg holder allowed for a much more stable positioning of the hip. The capsule was exposed and the surface of the external rotators remained untouched to preserve the anastomoses to the

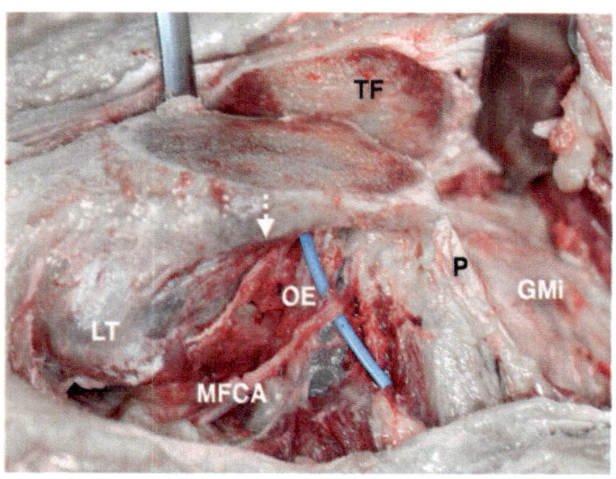

Fig. 12.3 The deep branch of *MFCA* (Medial Femoral Circumflex Artery) is crossing the obturator externus (*OE*). The greater trochanter fragment is flipped medially (*TF*) The piriformis muscle (*P*) remains attached to the stable trochanter. With the posterior intertrochanteric line (*arrow*) as reference there is a safety distance between osteotomy and deep branch. *LT* lesser trochanter; *GMi* gluteus minimus

deep branch of MFCA, coming from the inferior and superior gluteal arteries [13, 14]. The next step was Z shaped capsulotomy (for the right hip) allowing to inspect the joint for areas of abnormal contact during motion.

The hip was then dislocated after section of the ligamentum teres using specially curved scissors. With various positions and rotations of the leg, visualization of the entire acetabulum and the majority of the femoral head was possible. Morphologic abnormalities along with labral and articular cartilage lesions could be evaluated and treated. Osteochondroplasty of the head-neck junction was performed at this time in five patients.

After reducing the hip again, the extended retinacular flap was developed. Using a straight 15 mm osteotome, the posterior portion of the stable trochanter was carefully piecemealed. While performing this, the osteotome should not penetrate posteriorly out of the bone but should be used to weaken the fragment in a way that it could be manually bent and broken. The mobilized fragment was turned outwards, so that a strict subperiosteal dissection could be completed under direct vision (Fig. 12.4). At the superior circumference of the femoral neck, the periosteum

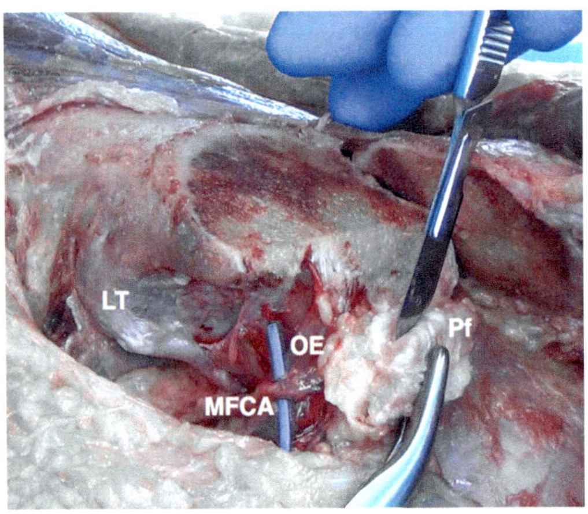

Fig. 12.4 Piece meal technique to remove the stable trochanteric bone. Safe distance to the deep branch (*MFCA*) (*blue rubber band*) and the eversion of the piecemeal fragment (*Pf*) being released from the short tendon's attachment. *OE* obturator externus, *LT* lesser trochanter

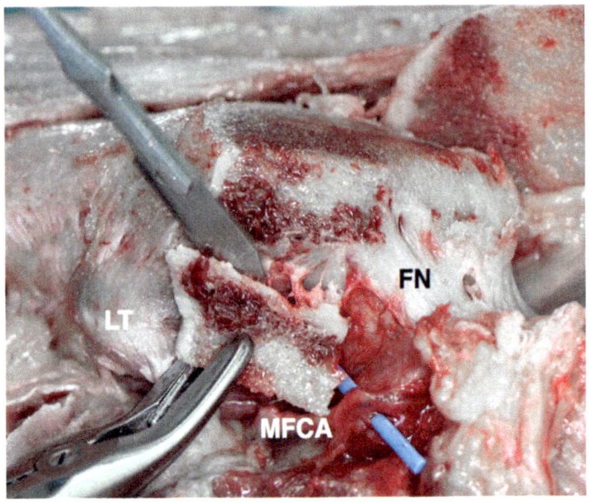

Fig. 12.5 Trimming of the posterior trochanteric bone to the level of the lesser trochanter and periosteal release. *LT* lesser trochanter, *FN* femoral neck, *OE* obturator externus, *MFCA* deep branch of the medial circumflex artery

anterior to the retinaculum was incised longitudinally and carefully dissected from the cortex.

This process was repeated until the osteotomy surface leveled the posterior and superior surface of the neck. The periosteum distal to the quadratus femoris muscle was also incised and mobilized posteriorly and distally (Fig. 12.5). The sub periosteal flap continued to be developed in this manner until the posterior surface of the base of the lesser trochanter became visible. The posterior part of the neck was exposed carefully using a small periosteal elevator until the tip of a curved retractor could pass around the neck and join the retractor placed around the neck from the anteromedial side for protection of the flap during osteotomy. For the medial retractor the respective subperiosteal dissection was executed with the head again dislocated. Care was taken to protect Weitbrecht's ligament, situated posteromedially; on top of this ligament runs the first branch of the MFCA, providing blood supply to a medial portion of the head [13, 21].

After completion of both dissections the flap represents an anteriorly open soft tissue tube containing all important vessels to the epiphysis. Due to its length, there is access to the entire neck area with low risk of overstretching the vessels during manipulations. The osteotomies are performed using a low vibration oscillating saw. Depending on the preoperative plan the cuts were done with the reduced hip (varus open wedge or valgus close wedge) or with the hip dislocated (varus close wedge). We used K-wires and a goniometer to control the precision of wedge and angular correction. In varus open wedge osteotomy with the hip reduced, the medial cortex was not completely separated, allowing gradual opening with a small bone spreader until the desired angle of correction is achieved. The gap was filled with bone from the piece meal resection of the trochanter. Correction was provisionally stabilized with two K-wires and after fluoroscopic control definitive fixation was achieved with two cortical 4.5 mm fully threaded screws to avoid compression and loss of correction. In varus close wedge osteotomy, the cuts were easier performed from anterior whit the hip dislocated (Fig. 12.6). In valgus close wedge osteotomy, the head remained again reduced and like in open wedge varus the medial cortex was not completely separated. In this condition, the gap was closed and secured with a reduction clamp while K-wires where placed. When closing a lateral gap, the retinacular flap became redundant and had to be carefully adapted to avoid kinking with potential stop of perfusion. Definitive fixation was carried out using two to three 4.5 mm cortical screws inserted parallel in femoral neck and head. The capsular flaps were adapted, but not tightly sutured. The trochanteric fragment was re-fixed using two 3.5 mm screws; care was taken that the capsular tissue was not compressed by the proximal screw. When needed, particularly in valgus close wedge osteotomies, the trochanter was advanced distally.

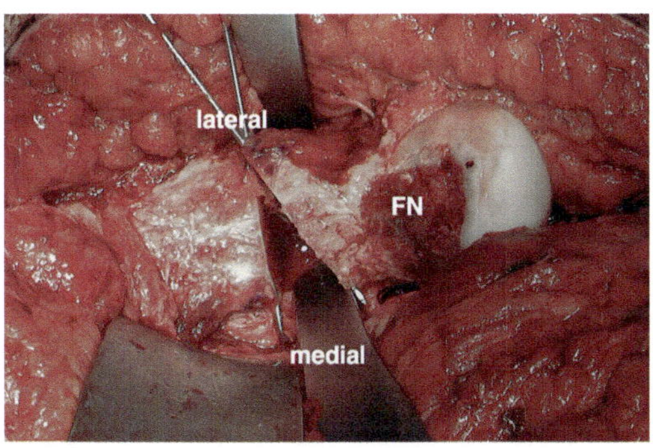

Fig. 12.6 Intraoperative picture of a 25° close wedge varus osteotomy with medial wedge removed to compensate for a longer ipsilateral limb. This osteotomy type was better performed with the hip dislocated. Osteochondroplasty at the head-neck junction for cam impingement before osteotomy (*FN*)

In five cases with acetabular dysplasia, we did an additional PAO. To profit from the lateral approach, the first and incomplete ischial osteotomy could be executed through the interval between the inferior gemellus and quadratus femoris muscles, allowing direct visualization and protection of the sciatic nerve with a soft tissue retractor. For the remaining PAO cuts the patient was turned into the supine decubitus [8]. In one of these patients the intraoperative radiography after the PAO did not show the expected congruency, although head and head-neck junction was treated with osteochondroplasty and relative neck lengthening was added. Therefore, the femoral approach was repeated and congruency was re-established with a valgus neck osteotomy (Fig. 12.7).

In the patient sustaining valgus malunion the procedure was the same as we used for a varus open wedge osteotomy. In the patient with neck non-union, broken screws and a distal shift of the proximal fragment, the base of the neck had to be developed for removal of the screw parts from the proximal fragment. A 10° laterally based wedge removal facilitated the approach to the screw ends and improved the plane of the non-union relative to the application of forces. Valgus ITO using a blade plate was disregarded for the interference to be expected with a femoral nail in situ (Fig. 12.8).

The postoperative regime included for all operated hips a 12-week period of toe touch walking. Full weight bearing was allowed when the femoral neck osteotomy and PAO were healed. All patients had abductor rehabilitation during at least 2 months after consolidation of the osteotomies.

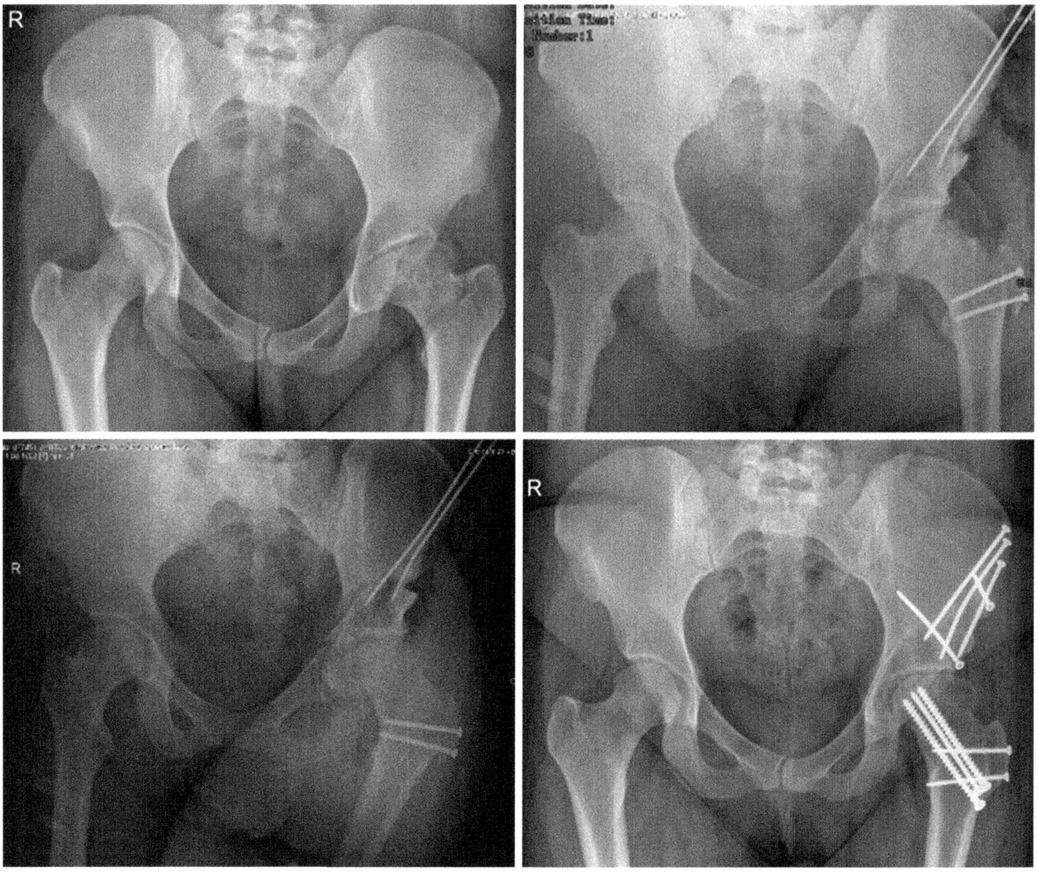

Fig. 12.7 Complex hip deformity after Perthes disease. With surgical hip dislocation shaping of the femoral head, relative neck lengthening and the ischial cut for PAO were performed. After completion of the PAO the intraoperative radiographies showed a degree of incongruence which was not anticipated. Therefore, the femoral approach was reopened and congruency re-established with a valgus neck osteotomy. The intertrochanteric level was discarded because a blade plate would not find good purchase in the neck after relative neck lengthening. The final picture shows good joint congruency

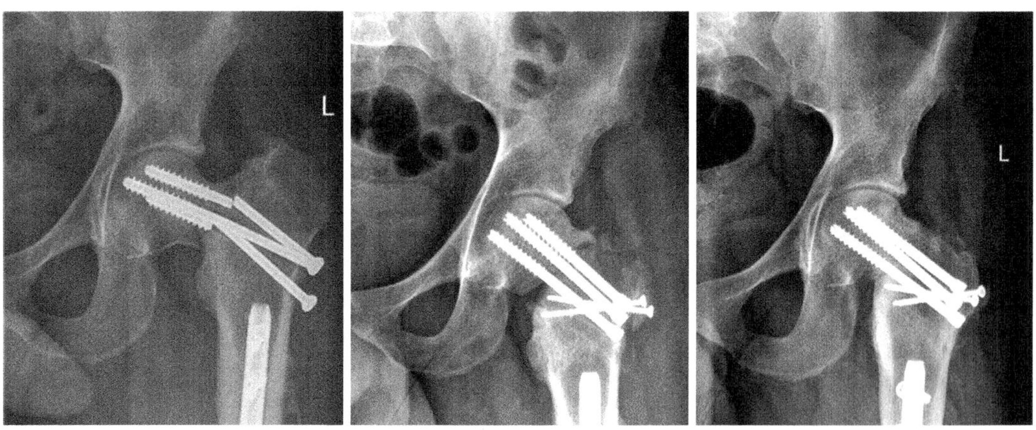

Fig. 12.8 Nonunion of the femoral neck with broken screws in a 26y old male. Safe mobilization of the nonunion for removal of the screw parts in the head was possible with the extended retinacular flap. Correction of the varus position with a laterally based wedge of the neck area. Intertrochanteric valgus osteotomy not possible due to the ipsilateral nail in place. 3 years result with slight residual varus, healed nonunion and without signs of AVN

12.3 Results

The neck shaft angle (range 150° to 120°) improved in all cases to a normal average value of 130°. The δ angle between the upper border of the fovea capitis and the medial border of the weight bearing area improved in valgus hips from −22° (range: −50 to −7) to 12.4° (range: −14 to 21). In the six cases with additional PAO, the CE-angle improved from 17.5° (range 11° to 22°) to 29° (range 22° to 40°) and the acetabular roof index from 20° (range 15° to 28°) to 3.8° (range −1° to 10°) (Fig. 12.9). The NAHS score improved from 37 points preoperatively (range 22 to 65) to 84 points postoperatively (range 76 to 98). All osteotomies healed in time without complications or hardware failure. No cases of AVN were observed at 3 years minimum follow-

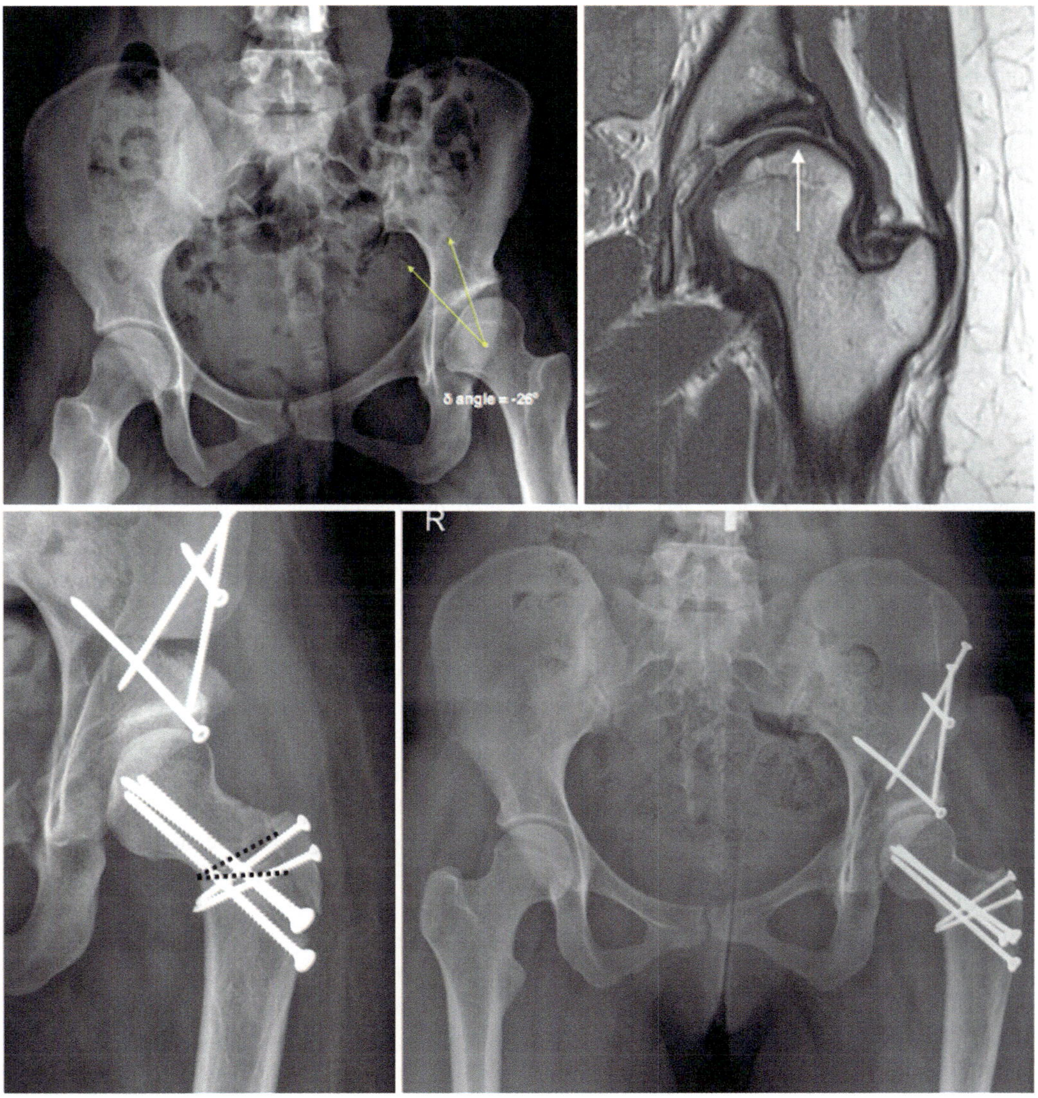

Fig. 12.9 Proximal focal femoral deficiency with residual acetabular dysplasia combined with caput valgum and high fovea capitis partly articulating with the acetabular cartilage. MRI with *white arrow* showing how far the fovea reaches into the weight bearing zone. To avoid overcorrection of the PAO with a resulting negative roof angle a femoral neck varus osteotomy was added. To avoid further shortening an open wedge osteotomy was performed (*dotted black lines*) 3.5 years result with good articular alignment and healed osteotomies

up, none of the patients needed reoperation for hardware removal and there were no cases of trochanteric pain caused by hardware.

We found no significant influence in leg length after surgery. The case with hardware breakage and non-union after a femoral neck fracture (Fig. 12.7) presented with shortening of 20 mm before surgery which remained nearly unchanged after the valgus osteotomy; using a shoe compensation, he is well adapted to activities of daily life with no major limitation. At follow-up, all patients had normal or near normal abductor function and a normal gait. Time of 3 months to osteotomy consolidation did not differ significant between patients who had just FNO and patients who had FNO plus PAO. We did also not find a significant discrepancy in healing time in varus open wedge osteotomies and close wedge osteotomies.

12.4 Discussion

In recent years, osteotomies of the adult proximal femur executed at the level of the inter- and subtrochanteric area became less indicated. When performed for established osteoarthritis, the results were frequently unpredictable and THR was preferred by doctors and patients [16]. Substantial leg length difference was another concomitant problem and many patients suffered from local pain produced by the prominent implants [7, 10, 11].

The possibility of safe surgical hip dislocation has not only led to a more detailed knowledge of hip impingement as important cause of osteoarthritis [14, 28], but allowed the development of a soft tissue flap [15] containing most of the vascular supply to the femoral head [12, 21, 29] and is the key for safe intracapsular osteotomy. The procedure is demanding but considered to be safe as long as the vascular structures are preserved and no tension is developed on the vessels during the surgical procedure.

The technique has been applied in children and adolescents to correct major deformities, resulting from slipped capital femoral epiphysis or Perthes disease, with good mid-term results [17–19, 30]. However, the literature is scarce when considering the extended retinacular flap in young adults to correct primary or acquired deformities of the proximal femur [15].

One may argue that the surgical technique of femoral neck osteotomy in the adult is even more demanding than in children and youngsters. In fact, the periosteum of the neck in adults is somewhat thinner and therefore the risk of laceration may be higher, however, meticulous dissection allows to avoid such complications. When compared with the modified Dunn procedure for sub capital realignment in SCFE it appears to be equally safe and efficacious in restoring hip anatomy and function. In our series, patients' satisfaction and improvement of the clinical outcome score were similar to other published younger patients series [17–19, 31–33]. Furthermore, we have successfully treated two posttraumatic deformities, conditions where retinacular scaring from the earlier injury is unforeseeable and may increase the risk of femoral head necrosis. Our small series confirms the consideration that patients like the reduced influence of the neck osteotomy on leg length and they are less bothered by the implant, an aspect that has a positive influence on the time for rehabilitation of the abductor muscle force. There are other advantages of FNO over ITO, mainly the possibility to access the intra-articular compartment to dynamically control the femoral head perfusion [34] and to treat impingement and labrum lesions.

Finally, reposition of the greater trochanter in the desired relation to the center of rotation is facilitated; it optimizes the muscle lever arm and can make easier a later conversion to THR. In the debate about the sequence in combined femoral and acetabular corrections the "femoral side first" attitude is favored; the additional direct protection of the sciatic nerve during the first ischial osteotomy is the strongest argument. Furthermore, femoral corrections are normally well defined and can be executed in this way; while acetabular osteotomies have a higher corrective potential and fine-tuning is easier. Exceptions are rare as in one of the demonstrated cases, where incongruency after acetabular correction made re-opening of the femoral approach and corrective osteotomy necessary. Varus neck osteotomies were not only performed to reduce a high CCD-angle, but even more important was the reduction of load sharing of the fovea capitis with the cartilage horseshoe of the acetabulum, an area which is already reduced in dysplastic hips [23].

On the other side, patients with a neck osteotomy had to accept a longer time on crutches by 1 month compared with an intertrochanteric osteotomy [9, 30, 35]. In contrast to the literature [15], our few cases with open wedge varus osteotomy did not have a longer consolidation time compared with the close wedge osteotomies. Major limitation to this study is the small number of our patient series, which together with the inhomogeneous pathomorphologies compromises general conclusions and made statistical analysis inappropriate. Nevertheless, we think femoral neck osteotomies can be used in selected adult patients with similar safety as capital realignment in children and adolescents and it has substantial advantages over inter- or sub trochanteric osteotomies.

References

1. Bartoníček J, Vávra J. Valgus intertrochanteric osteotomy for coxa vara of Bucholz–Ogden Types II and III in patients older than 30 years. Arch Orthop Trauma Surg. 2011;131:1211–7. https://doi.org/10.1007/s00402-011-1278-5.
2. Haverkamp D, Eijer H, Patt TW, Marti RK. Multi directional intertrochanteric osteotomy for primary and secondary osteoarthritis—results after 15 to 29 years. Int Orthop. 2005;30:15–20. https://doi.org/10.1007/s00264-005-0024-4.
3. Schneider W, Aigner N, Pinggera O, Knahr K. Intertrochanteric osteotomy for avascular necrosis of the head of the femur. J Bone Joint Surg Br. 2002;84-B:817–24. https://doi.org/10.1302/0301-620x.84b6.0840817.
4. Scher MA, Jakim I. Intertrochanteric osteotomy and autogenous bone-grafting for avascular necrosis of the femoral head. J Bone Jt Surg. 1993;75:1119–33. https://doi.org/10.2106/00004623-199308000-00001.
5. Jacobs MA, Hungerford DS, Krackow KA. Intertrochanteric osteotomy for avascular necrosis of the femoral head. J Bone Joint Surg Br. 1989;71-B:200–4. https://doi.org/10.1302/0301-620x.71b2.2925735.
6. Haverkamp D, Eijer H, Besselaar PP, Marti RK. Awareness and use of intertrochanteric osteotomies in current clinical practice. An international survey. Int Orthop. 2007;32:19–25. https://doi.org/10.1007/s00264-006-0270-0.
7. Leunig M, Puloski S, Beck M, et al. Proximal femoral osteotomy: current indications and techniques. Semin Arthroplast. 2005;16:53–62. https://doi.org/10.1053/j.sart.2004.12.006.
8. Ganz R, Horowitz K, Leunig M. Algorithm for femoral and periacetabular osteotomies in complex hip deformities. Clin Orthop. 2010;468:3168–80. https://doi.org/10.1007/s11999-010-1489-z.
9. Siebenrock K, Ekkernkamp A, Ganz R. The corrective intertrochanteric adduction osteotomy without removal of a wedge. Oper Orthopadie Traumatol. 2012;8:1–13. https://doi.org/10.1007/BF03181115.
10. Suominen S, Antti-Poika I, Santavirta S, et al. Total hip replacement after intertrochanteric osteotomy. Orthopedics. 1991;14:253–7.
11. Ferguson GM, Cabanela ME, Ilstrup DM. Total hip arthroplasty after failed intertrochanteric osteotomy. J Bone Joint Surg Br. 1994;76-B:252–7. https://doi.org/10.1302/0301-620x.76b2.8113286.
12. Gautier E, Ganz K, Krugel N, et al. Anatomy of the medial femoral circumflex artery and its surgical implications. J Bone Joint Surg Br. 2018;83-B:149. https://doi.org/10.1302/0301-620x.83b1.0830149.
13. Kalhor M, Beck M, Huff TW, Ganz R. Capsular and pericapsular contributions to acetabular and femoral head perfusion. J Bone Joint Surg Am. 2009;91:409–18. https://doi.org/10.2106/JBJS.G.01679.
14. Ganz R, Gill TJ, Gautier E, et al. Surgical dislocation of the adult hip. A technique with full access to the femoral head and acetabulum without the risk of avascular necrosis. J Bone Joint Surg Br. 2001;83:1119–24. https://doi.org/10.1302/0301-620x.83b8.11964.
15. Ganz R, Huff TW, Leunig M. Extended retinacular soft-tissue flap for intra-articular hip surgery: surgical technique, indications, and results of application. Instr Course Lect. 2009;58:241–55.
16. Leunig M, Ganz R. Relative neck lengthening and intracapital osteotomy for severe Perthes and Perthes-like deformities. Bull NYU Hosp Jt Dis. 2011;69:S62.
17. Leunig M, Casillas MM, Hamlet M, et al. Slipped capital femoral epiphysis: early mechanical damage to the acetabular cartilage by a prominent femoral metaphysis. Acta Orthop Scand. 2000;71:370–5. https://doi.org/10.1080/000164700317393367.
18. Ziebarth K, Zilkens C, Spencer S, et al. Capital realignment for moderate and severe SCFE using a modified Dunn procedure. Clin Orthop. 2009;467:704–16. https://doi.org/10.1007/s11999-008-0687-4.
19. Ziebarth K, Leunig M, Slongo T, et al. Slipped capital femoral epiphysis: relevant pathophysiological findings with open surgery. Clin Orthop Relat Res. 2013;471:2156–62. https://doi.org/10.1007/s11999-013-2818-9.
20. Al-Talalwah W. The medial circumflex femoral artery origin variability and its radiological and surgical intervention significance. Springerplus. 2015;4 https://doi.org/10.1186/s40064-015-0881-2.

21. Kalhor M, Horowitz K, Gharehdaghi J, et al. Anatomic variations in femoral head circulation. Hip Int J Clin Exp Res Hip Pathol Ther. 2012;22:307–12. https://doi.org/10.5301/HIP.2012.9242.
22. Tannast M, Siebenrock KA, Anderson SE. Femoroacetabular impingement: radiographic diagnosis--what the radiologist should know. AJR Am J Roentgenol. 2007;188:1540–52. https://doi.org/10.2214/AJR.06.0921.
23. Nötzli H, Müller S, Ganz R. Die radiologische Beziehung der Fovea capitis femoris zur azetabulären Belastungszone bei der normalen und dysplastischen Hüfte des Erwachsenen. Z Für Orthop Ihre Grenzgeb. 2001;319:502–6. https://doi.org/10.1055/s--2001-19231.
24. Beltran LS, Mayo JD, Rosenberg ZS, et al. Fovea Alta on MR images: is it a marker of hip dysplasia in young adults? Am J Roentgenol. 2012;199:879–83. https://doi.org/10.2214/ajr.11.8193.
25. Christensen CP, Althausen PL, Mittleman MA, et al. The nonarthritic hip score: reliable and validated. Clin Orthop. 2003;406:75–83. https://doi.org/10.1097/00003086-200301000-00013.
26. Lavigne M, Parvizi J, Beck M, et al. Anterior femoroacetabular impingement: part I. techniques of joint preserving surgery. Clin Orthop. 2004:61–6.
27. Beck M, Leunig M, Parvizi J, et al. Anterior femoroacetabular impingement: part II. Midterm results of surgical treatment. Clin Orthop. 2004:67–73.
28. Ganz R, Parvizi J, Beck M, et al. Femoroacetabular impingement: a cause for osteoarthritis of the hip. Clin Orthop. 2003:112–20. https://doi.org/10.1097/01.blo.0000096804.78689.c2.
29. Grose AW, Gardner MJ, Sussmann PS, et al. The surgical anatomy of the blood supply to the femoral head: description of the anastomosis between the medial femoral circumflex and inferior gluteal arteries at the hip. J Bone Joint Surg Br. 2008;90:1298–303. https://doi.org/10.1302/0301-620X.90B10.20983.
30. Leunig M, Slongo T, Ganz R. Subcapital realignment in slipped capital femoral epiphysis: surgical hip dislocation and trimming of the stable trochanter to protect the perfusion of the epiphysis. Instr Course Lect. 2008;57:499–507.
31. Huber H, Dora C, Ramseier LE, et al. Adolescent slipped capital femoral epiphysis treated by a modified Dunn osteotomy with surgical hip dislocation. J Bone Joint Surg Br. 2011;93-B:833–8. https://doi.org/10.1302/0301-620x.93b6.25849.
32. Ziebarth K, Domayer S, Slongo T, et al. Clinical stability of slipped capital femoral epiphysis does not correlate with intraoperative stability. Clin Orthop Relat Res. 2012;470:2274–9. https://doi.org/10.1007/s11999-012-2339-y.
33. Massè A, Aprato A, Grappiolo G, et al. Surgical hip dislocation for anatomic reorientation of slipped capital femoral epiphysis: preliminary results. Hip Int J Clin Exp Res Hip Pathol Ther. 2012;22:137–44. https://doi.org/10.5301/HIP.2012.9208.
34. Aprato A, Bonani A, Giachino M, et al. Can we predict femoral head vitality during surgical hip dislocation? J Hip Preserv Surg. 2014;1:77–81. https://doi.org/10.1093/jhps/hnu010.
35. Marti RK, Schuller HM, Raaymakers EL. Intertrochanteric osteotomy for non-union of the femoral neck. J Bone Joint Surg Br. 1989;71-B:782–7. https://doi.org/10.1302/0301-620x.71b5.2584247.

13 Subtrochanteric Osteotomy for the Management of Femoral Mal-Torsion

Mattia Loppini, Reinhold Ganz, Luigino Turchetto, Giuseppe Mazziotta, and Guido Grappiolo

13.1 Level of Evidence: IV, Case Series

13.1.1 Introduction

Torsional deformity of the femur is a common finding in patients affected by hip and groin pain [1]. It is rarely an isolated deformity. Associated deformities are primary and secondary acetabular dysplasia, coxa vara, Legg-Calvé-Perthes disease, and slipped capital femoral epiphysis [2, 3]. If untreated, pain and restricted function may continue after both open or arthroscopic preservation surgery [4, 5]. While in the past the exact pathomechanical impact on osteoarthritis (OA) was unclear [1, 6, 7], we know today that femoral mal-torsion can produce intra- and extra-articular impingement [8] and instability, both known as important initiators of OA [9, 10]. Low antetorsion of the femoral neck is an essential factor in traumatic posterior dislocation [11].

Rotational correction of the femur can be performed at several levels, such as intertrochanteric, subtrochanteric, diaphyseal, and supracondylar [2, 3, 6, 12–16], using more or less specially tailored fixation devices [2, 3, 6, 12–14, 16–21]. All procedures can be associated with complications including loss of fixation, errors in amount of correction, intraoperative fractures, or infection [18–20].

In complex hip deformities, the correction may be performed in association with other surgical procedures under the same anesthesia. When femoral derotation and other femoral procedures have to be combined with an acetabular correction it is advantageous to start with the femoral side; reasons for this sequence can be: the acetabular correction is only possible after the femoral correction; the femoral correction influences the amount of acetabular correction; under certain circumstances, one can even refrain from acetabular correction [22].

In the present report, we describe the surgical technique and report a two-center case series, which in part was already published earlier in the context of a bigger group [16]. The technique requires only a short extension of the proximal femoral incision and allows a mechanically stable alignment when the intertrochanteric region is involved by other procedures, such as greater trochanter advancement, relative lengthening of

M. Loppini (✉)
IRCCS Humanitas Research Hospital, Rozzano, Milan, Italy

Department of Biomedical Sciences, Humanitas University, Pieve Emanuele, Milan, Italy
e-mail: mattia.loppini@hunimed.eu

R. Ganz
Faculty of Medicine, University of Bern, Bern, Switzerland

L. Turchetto
Department of Orthopedics and Trauma Surgery, Ospedale di Portogruaro, Venice, Italy

G. Mazziotta · G. Grappiolo
IRCCS Humanitas Research Hospital, Rozzano, Milan, Italy

R. Ganz (ed.), *Modern Hip Preservation*, https://doi.org/10.1007/978-3-030-91967-2_13

the neck and head or neck osteotomy. Moreover, derotation can be associated with femoral shortening, as required in cases with high subluxation or dislocation. The necessary amount of rotational correction for optimal adjustment of the hip joint can be visually checked and fine-tuned on the open joint.

13.2 Patients and Methods

13.2.1 Demographics

We retrospectively reviewed nine hips in eight patients. The indication for rotational osteotomy was based on physical examination, the measured degree of abnormal torsion and on functional radiographies with compensated rotation of the femur.

Patients included one male and seven females, with an average age of 19.5 ± 4.2 years (range, 13–26) at the time of surgery. Preoperative diagnoses included: residual acetabular dysplasia after DDH (6), with arthrogryposis (1), with Larsen's syndrome (1), and with cerebral palsy (1). Four out of 8 patients had previous ipsilateral hip surgery, such as proximal femoral osteotomy (1), Chiari osteotomy (1), and unknown surgery (2).

In all patients, surgical hip dislocation was the first step. The subtrochanteric correction was in all cases a derotation to decrease a high femoral antetorsion. The additional procedures are listed in Table 13.1.

Outcome measures included serial plain radiographs and clinical evaluation performed in the follow-up consultations. All patients had a minimum follow-up of 1 year.

13.2.2 Preoperative Assessment

All patients had preoperative physical examination and plain radiographs of pelvis and affected hip. Preoperative standardized torsional imaging was not routinely performed.

Correction was performed using a sequential approach [22] in all patients. Therefore, preoperative planning could be adjusted intraoperatively based on the individual patient scenario including the intermediate result of an osteotomy step, e.g., in a Perthes deformity the true neck antetorsion became only visible after relative neck lengthening.

13.2.3 Surgical Technique

In all patients, surgery was performed with the patient placed in the lateral decubitus position on a standard operating table. The limb was prepared and draped allowing its free mobilization. Draping was extended when additional periacetabular osteotomy was planned. A U-shaped foam pillow was placed to protect the contralateral limb, and to stabilize the mobile leg with the hip in neutral abduction/adduction.

The derotation osteotomy was based on distal extension of the surgical dislocation approach, and executed as previously described [12]. General indication for a femoral derotation consisted in values of antetorsion over 20° or less than 0° (retrotorsion) in the setting of femoroacetabular conflict and/or joint instability. The latter was evaluated intraoperatively by observation of the head migration during range-of-motion with the open joint.

When an additional periacetabular osteotomy was indicated, the first step, the incomplete ischial osteotomy, was performed, according to the described technique [23], immediately after surgical dislocation of the joint. The intracapsular procedures, such as head-neck osteochondroplasty, relative lengthening of the neck, osteotomy of the neck, and/or osteotomy of the head, were also executed before the subtrochanteric procedure. Periacetabular osteotomy and capsular arthroplasty according to Codivilla-Colonna [24] were executed after the derotation ± shortening.

A provisional seven-hole, narrow, 4.5 mm dynamic compression plate was held against the lateral cortex in a way to allow proper placement and fixation of the proximal fragment. The osteotomy level was marked with an osteotome and a hole was drilled for the most proximal screw in the distal femur fragment (Fig. 13.1).

Table 13.1 Concomitant procedures performed with subtrochanteric derotation. Simultaneous surgical dislocation of the hip was performed in all hips before the other procedures

Patients	Age (year)	Gender	Side	Concomitant procedures	Type of fixation	Complications
1	21	Female	Left	RNL, head reduction osteotomy, capsular arthroplasty, SFO	Narrow 4.5 mm DCP, 6-hole, 4 screws	No
2	13	Female	Left	RNL, femoral osteochondroplasty	Narrow 4.5 mm DCP, 6-hole, 4 screws	No
3	26	Female	Left	RNL, PAO	Narrow 4.5 mm DCP, 7-hole, 4 screws	No
4	16	Female	Left	RNL, PAO, labral re-fixation	Narrow 4.5 mm DCP, 7-hole, 4 screws	No
5	22	Female	Left	RNL	Narrow 4.5 mm DCP, 7-hole, 4 screws	No
6	22	Female	Right	RNL, femoral osteochondroplasty, SFO, PAO	Narrow 4.5 mm DCP, 7-hole, 7 screws	No
7	20	Female	Left	RNL, femoral osteochondroplasty	Narrow 4.5 mm DCP, 6-hole, 4 screws	No
8	16	Male	Left	Femoral osteochondroplasty, PAO	Narrow 4.5 mm DCP, 6-hole, 4 screws	No

RNL relative neck lengthening, *PAO* periacetabular osteotomy, *SFO* shortening femoral osteotomy, *DCP* dynamic compression plate

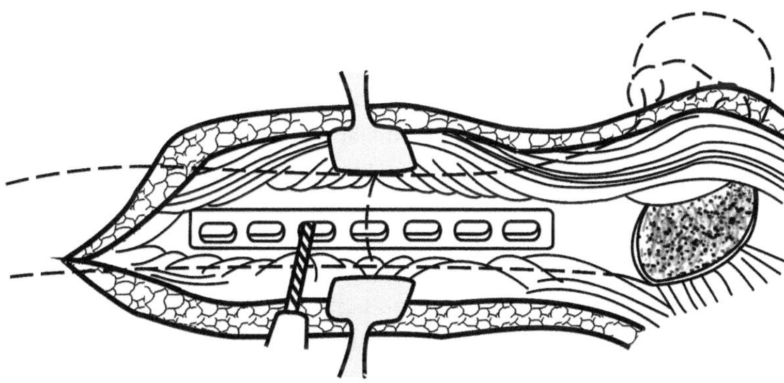

Fig. 13.1 Modified from Kamath et al. [16]. After surgical hip dislocation a plate is provisionally held in place to decide the level of the transverse osteotomy (*dashed line*). Prior to perform the femoral osteotomy, a hole is drilled distal to the planned osteotomy

After removal of the plate, an anterior and posterior decortication involving about two centimeters of bone proximal and distal to the osteotomy level was performed [25], using a sharp 10–15 mm straight osteotome (Fig. 13.2). The decortication should provide a continuous layer of bone chips with soft tissue attached. Anterior and posterior blunt retractors were placed between the decorticated flap and the diaphysis to prevent soft tissues injuries during the osteotomy.

The transverse osteotomy was performed using an oscillating saw with continuous irrigation (Fig. 13.3). Before doing so, the amount of rotatory correction can be indicated with two Kirschner wires introduced above and below the osteotomy level.

With the classic way to perform a subtrochanteric rotational osteotomy, the correcting move is performed on the distal fragment, a way that is accompanied by a rather laborious

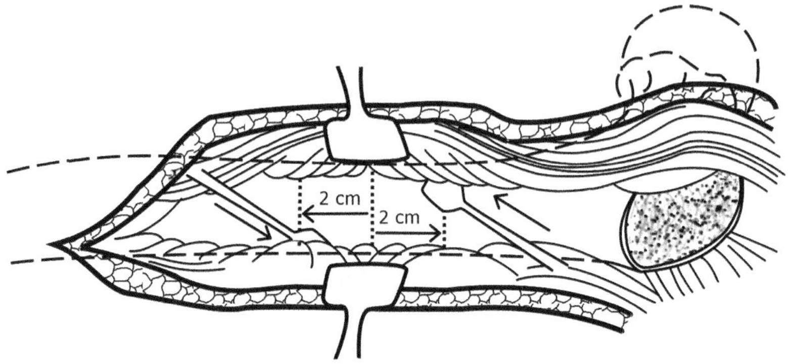

Fig. 13.2 Modified from Kamath et al. [16]. Decortication involving about two centimeters of bone proximal and distal to the osteotomy level is performed with a sharp osteotome developing a thin slice of bone with muscles attachment

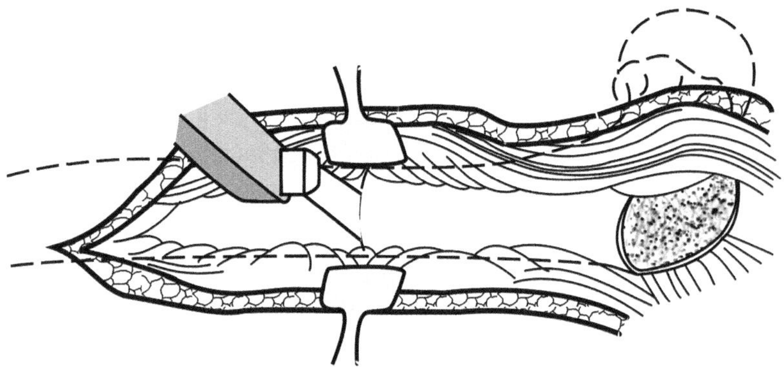

Fig. 13.3 Modified from Kamath et al. [16]. Transverse osteotomy is performed with an oscillating saw while blunt retractors prevent soft tissues damage

reduction and fixation maneuver. With the dislocated and relocated hip joint, the proximal fragment can be manipulated much easier while the distal fragment remains in a stable position. Optimal approximation of the distal fragment can be improved by fixation of the plate on the distal fragment in the already predrilled screw hole. The proximal fragment can now be rotated in place with the help of a bone clamp and the result can visually be controlled with the two Kirschner wires. The proximal segment is rotated anteriorly for correction of antetorsion or posteriorly for correction of retrotorsion. There is another, relatively easy way of control: the amount of antetorsion and the amount of correction can be shown with a wire held against the anterior neck. The other reference is the leg placed on the table in 90° knee flexion (Fig. 13.4). When the wire is perpendicular to the leg axis, neck torsion is zero. We normally aim for 10–15° of anteversion, however it may differ when an acetabular version is to be compensated on the femoral side. The final correction is than secured by introducing the first screw in the proximal fragment next to the osteotomy and using the compression mode for both screws (Fig. 13.5). Care must be taken to position the plate flush with the bone to avoid undesired fragment rotation during definitive driving home of the screws. Another way of compression is to use an articulating tensioning device, however this was not necessary in our cases.

Further aspects of intraoperative assessment in every case consisted of visual and/or fluoroscopic control of the overall rotational alignment, impingement-free motion, and the achieved joint congruency. For sufficient stability one more screw in each fragment was enough in all cases. Fluoroscopy may be used to document intraoperative osteotomy fixation and joint alignment. Subsequently, the capsule was sutured without tension and the trochanteric bone fragment was refixed with two 3.5 mm screws. This was followed by repair of the origin of the vastus lateralis muscle; the wound was closed in sequential layers.

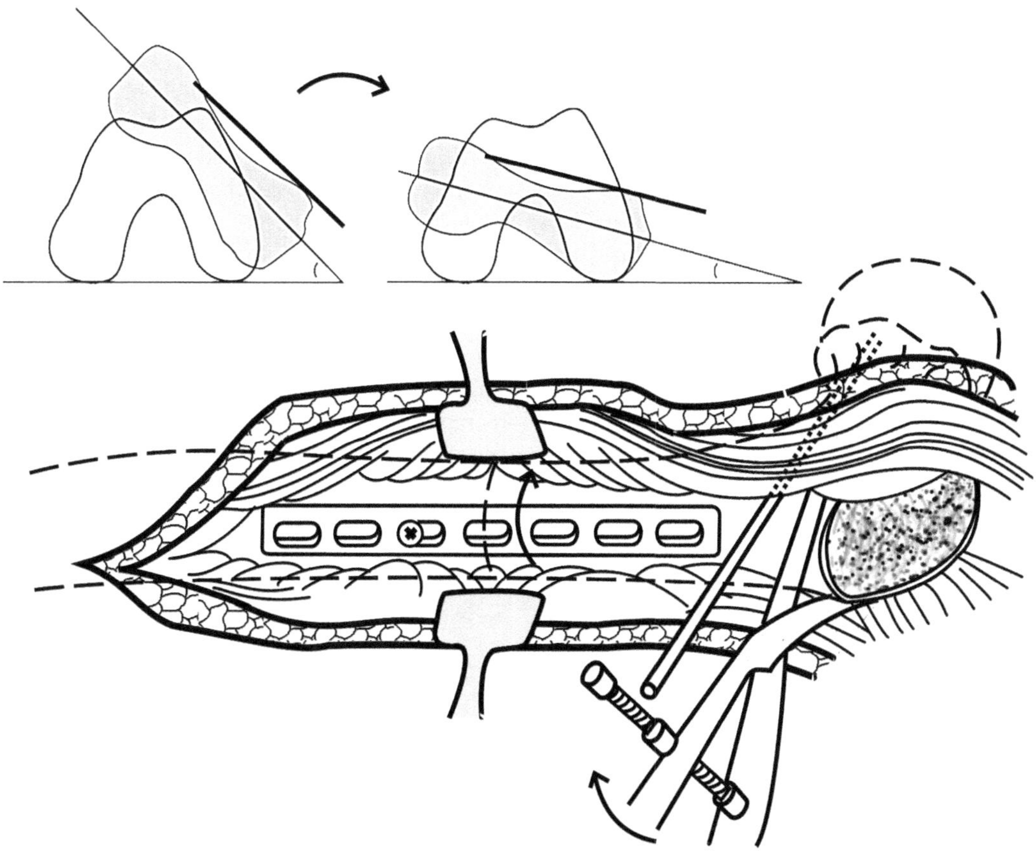

Fig. 13.4 Modified from Kamath et al. [16]. After fixation of the plate via the already drilled hole in distal fragment, the proximal fragment is rotated with a Verbrugge clamp. A Kirschner wire is placed along the anterior surface of the neck, and the amount of correction is evaluated measuring the angle between the Kirschner wire and the axis of the leg placed on the table in 90° knee flexion

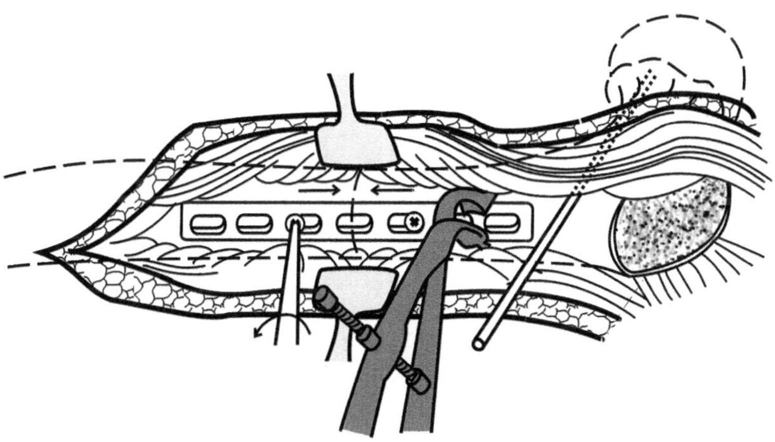

Fig. 13.5 Modified from Kamath et al. [16]. For definitive fixation, the plate is pushed proximally to bring the first screw in a compression mode position and the hole in the proximal fragment closest to the osteotomy is drilled again in the compression mode. By alternative driving home both screws and under constant control of the desired fragment position an ideal compression is achieved. After careful final check of joint stability and impingement free-motion, a second screw in each fragment is sufficient provided the bone quality is normal and the purchase of the screws is good

In patients who did not undergo additional osteotomies and concomitant procedures, walking was permitted with a 15-kg weight restriction. After 6 weeks, plain radiographs were performed to evaluate bone healing. Progressive weight bearing was allowed when callus bridging could be seen and the trochanter osteotomy showed consolidation. Abductor exercises were also initiated at this time.

13.3 Results

In all patients, the torsional deformity was an excessive antetorsion of the femoral neck. Therefore, an average derotation of 15–20° (maximum 40° of correction) was performed to achieve a final antetorsion of 10–15°.

All patients had concomitant procedures (Table 13.1). Of these, the most frequently performed were relative head-neck lengthening, anterior head-neck osteochondroplasty, and periacetabular osteotomy.

All patients showed union of all osteotomies at the latest follow-up (Fig. 13.6). Full weight bearing was allowed within 10–12 weeks after surgery in most patients, while radiographic findings of consolidation were seen at 6 weeks, and complete disappearance of the osteotomy line reached up to 16 weeks. No patients reported osteotomy-related problems, or major systemic complications.

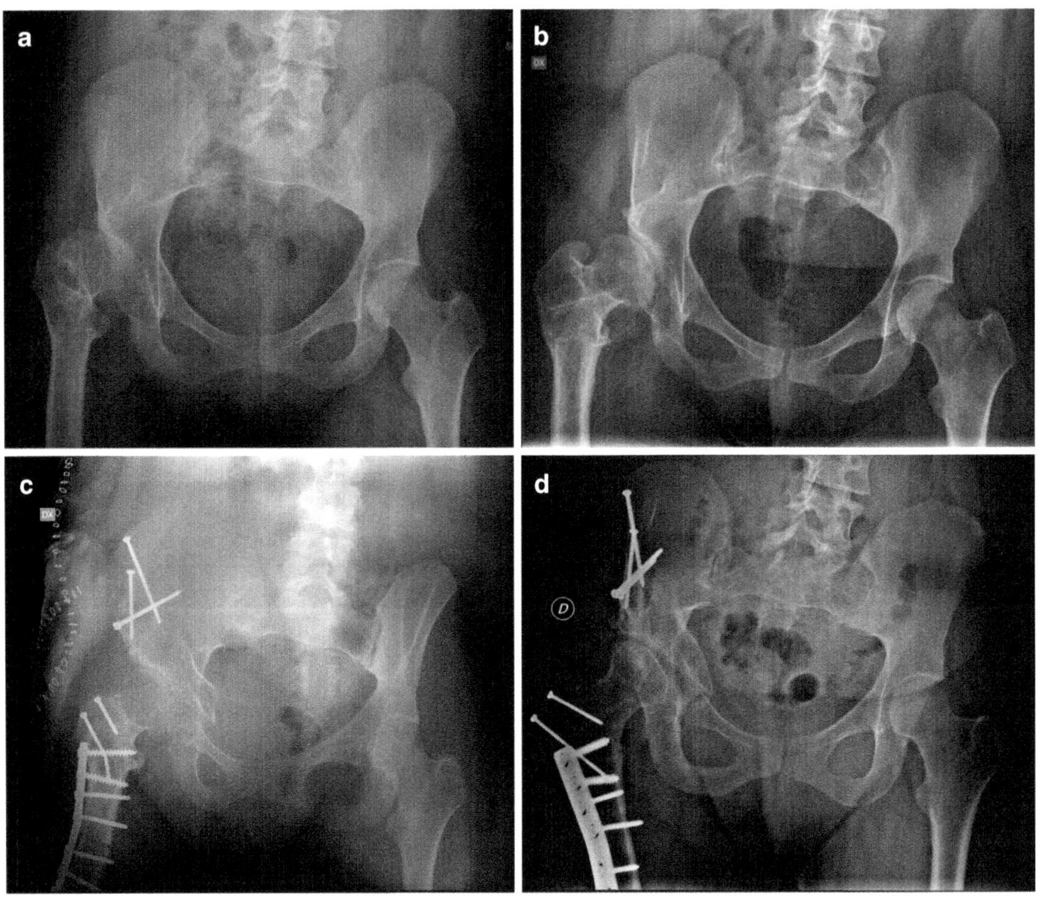

Fig. 13.6 21-year-old female affected by spina bifida with mixed neurological deficits. (**a**) Severe and painful subluxation based on complex acetabular and femoral deformities.(**b**) Radiography with abduction and internal rotation showing improved femoroacetabular relation and large joint space. (**c**) Postoperative radiography after relative neck lengthening, distal advancement of the trochanter, subtrochanteric derotation and periacetabular osteotomy. (**d**) 2 years follow-up radiography showing consolidation of all osteotomies. The patient is now pain free and has improved function of this leg

13.4 Discussion

Our series of subtrochanteric derotation osteotomy is small, the material comes from two centers of the GICCA group and was in part published earlier [16]. The technique differs from classic osteotomies at this level by taking advantage of the surgical dislocation approach [26]. Subtrochanteric derotation osteotomy may be indicated in patients with femoroacetabular impingement or joint instability due to pathologic femoral mal-torsion that is not sufficiently compensated with intra-articular procedures and/or additional acetabular correction.

In complex deformities, surgical hip dislocation offers a circumferential view of proximal femur and acetabulum and allows precise evaluation of functional problems as well as final indication of the necessary intra-capsular procedures, such as head-neck osteochondroplasty, relative lengthening of the neck, osteotomy of the neck, and/or osteotomy of the head. It permits final visual control of the femoral version and gives an idea about the eventual need of shortening together with a rotational correction. Especially in Perthes or Perthes-like hips, the true amount of pathological version of the femoral neck becomes visible only after relative lengthening of the neck.

When correction of both femoral and acetabular deformities is indicated, we advocate to address the femoral side first [22]. Some deformities do not allow acetabular reorientation or capsular arthroplasty before the femoral side has been corrected. Acetabular correction can be adapted easier than femoral corrections and occasionally, femoral derotation and trimming of the acetabular rim may be sufficient to achieve proper improvement in range of motion and stability, making acetabular reorientation not necessary. However, if periacetabular osteotomy is required, the first ischial cut can be performed via the femoral approach under direct visualization and optimal protection of the sciatic nerve [27].

The subtrochanteric osteotomy level has advantages over the intertrochanteric level with regard to implant application and construct stability. Beside the spatial interference with trochanteric, neck or head osteotomies, screw-plate or blade plate fixation is technically more demanding and does not allow optimal purchase in a proximal fragment with partial loss of the cortical mantel. In addition, re-fixation of the greater trochanter and even more so re-fixation with advancement would become technically difficult and less stable. In our experience, subtrochanteric plating is associated with a lower risk of lateral trochanteric pain and bursitis when compared with a more prominent blade plate. On the other side, the intertrochanteric level would allow the combination with varus- or valgus correction, which is hardly feasible at the subtrochanteric level.

Consolidation time of the subtrochanteric cortical bone is slightly longer compared with the cancellous intertrochanteric bone [28]. This may in part be compensated by the application of decortication to accelerate bridging callus leading to earlier stability of the montage [16]. However, the time to complete consolidation is less affected.

Appropriate stability is generally achieved with a 4.5 mm narrow dynamic compression plate, while the off-center arrangement of the screw holes in a large plate may determine undesired fragment rotation while inserting the screws. This problem becomes evident with the inevitable mismatch of surface curvature after rotation.

In literature several definitions of femoral mal-torsion have been provided [8, 29–32]. Fabricant et al. considered >25° as threshold for high anteversion [30]. Jackson et al. defined retroversion as −2° or less and excessive anteversion as 18° or greater [31]. However, we were less looking to achieve numeric corrections and followed more the intraoperative impression of achieved joint congruency, and stability as well as impingement-free motion. With the presented technique the risk of over- or under-corrections of femoral rotation deformity [20, 33] may be reduced.

The present study has some major limitations. The sample size is small. The study is performed in a retrospective fashion without any comparison with other fixation techniques. Therefore, we are not able to document the superiority over other techniques previously described. The sample is characterized by heterogeneity of underlying diagnoses and concomitant procedures; on the other side this supports the versatility of the presented technique across varying hip pathologies. Finally, a limitation is the lack of preoperative and postoperative standardized torsional imaging.

In conclusion, the management of femoral mal-torsion requires a dynamic intraoperative method of assessment to identify properly any intra- and extra-articular sources of impingement and/or instability. The subtrochanteric osteotomy of the femur performed with a straight compression plate and decortication, via a surgical dislocation approach, is a reproducible and safe technique. In the setting of complex joint preservation surgery, this technique can be associated with other femoral and/or pelvic procedures. It is recommended to start with the femoral side for an optimal sequential correction of the different pathomorphologies.

References

1. Tönnis D, Heinecke A. Diminished femoral antetorsion syndrome: a cause of pain and osteoarthritis. J Pediatr Orthop. 1991;11:419–31. https://doi.org/10.1097/01241398-199107000-00001.
2. Hamdy RC, Ehrlich MG. Subtrochanteric derotation osteotomy of the femur using three or four wires. A technical note. Clin Orthop. 1994;302:111–4.
3. Tomak Y, Piskin A, Ozcan H, Tomak L. Subtrochanteric derotation osteotomy using a bent dynamic compression plate in children with medial femoral torsion. Orthopedics. 2008;31:453–8. https://doi.org/10.3928/01477447-20110414-09.
4. Bogunovic L, Gottlieb M, Pashos G, et al. Why do hip arthroscopy procedures fail? Clin Orthop. 2013;471:2523–9. https://doi.org/10.1007/s11999-013-3015-6.
5. Clohisy JC, Nepple JJ, Larson CM, et al. Academic Network of Conservation Hip Outcome Researc M: persistent structural disease is the most common cause of repeat hip preservation surgery. Clin Orthop. 2013;471:3788–94. https://doi.org/10.1007/s11999-013-3218-x.
6. Reikerås O, Bjerkreim I. Idiopathic increased anteversion of the femoral neck. Radiological and clinical study in non-operated and operated patients. Acta Orthop Scand. 1982;53:839–45. https://doi.org/10.3109/17453678208992836.
7. Cordier W, Katthagen BD. Femoral torsional deformities. Orthopade. 2000;29:795–801. https://doi.org/10.1007/s001320050528.
8. Siebenrock KA, Steppacher SD, Haefeli PC, et al. Valgus hip with high antetorsion causes pain through posterior extraarticular FAI. Clin Orthop. 2013;471:3774–80. https://doi.org/10.1007/s11999-013-2895-9.
9. Tibor LM, Ganz R, Leunig M. Case reports: anteroinferior acetabular rim damage due to femoroacetabular impingement. Clin Orthop Relat Res. 2013;471:3781–7. https://doi.org/10.1007/s11999-013-2921-y.
10. Ganz R, Parvizi J, Beck M, et al. Femoroacetabular impingement: a cause for osteoarthritis of the hip. Clin Orthop. 2003;417:112–20. https://doi.org/10.1097/01.blo.0000096804.78689.c2.
11. Steppacher SD, Albers CE, Siebenrock KA, et al. Femoroacetabular impingement predisposes to traumatic posterior hip dislocation. Clin Orthop. 2013;471:1937–43. https://doi.org/10.1007/s11999-013-2863-4.
12. Hoffer MM, Prietto C, Koffman M. Supracondylar derotational osteotomy of the femur for internal rotation of the thigh in the cerebral palsied child. J Bone Joint Surg Am. 1981;63:389–93.
13. Hau R, Dickens DR, Nattrass GR, et al. Which implant for proximal femoral osteotomy in children? A comparison of the AO (ASIF) 90 degree fixed-angle blade plate and the Richards intermediate hip screw. J Pediatr Orthop. 2000;20:336–43.
14. Gordon JE, Pappademos PC, Schoenecker PL, et al. Diaphyseal derotational osteotomy with intramedullary fixation for correction of excessive femoral anteversion in children. J Pediatr Orthop. 2005;25:548–53. https://doi.org/10.1097/01.bpo.0000158783.37602.cb.
15. Staheli LT. Torsion--treatment indications. Clin Orthop. 1989;247:61–6.
16. Kamath AF, Ganz R, Zhang H, et al. Subtrochanteric osteotomy for femoral mal-torsion through a surgical dislocation approach. J Hip Preserv Surg. 2015;2:65–79. https://doi.org/10.1093/jhps/hnv011.
17. Handelsman JE, Weinberg J, Friedman S. The role of the small AO external fixator in supracondylar rotational femoral osteotomies. J Pediatr Orthop Part B. 2005;14:194–7. https://doi.org/10.1097/01202412-200505000-00010.
18. Shim JS, Staheli LT, Holm BN. Surgical correction of idiopathic medical femoral torsion. Int Orthop. 1995;19:220–3. https://doi.org/10.1007/bf00185226.
19. Staheli LT, Clawson DK, Hubbard DD. Medial femoral torsion: experience with operative treatment. Clin Orthop. 1980;146:222–5.
20. Svenningsen S, Apalset K, Terjesen T, Anda S. Osteotomy for femoral anteversion. Complications in 95 children. Acta Orthop Scand. 1989;60:401–5. https://doi.org/10.3109/17453678909149306.
21. Winquist RA. Closed intramedullary osteotomies of the femur. Clin Orthop. 1986;212:155–64.
22. Ganz R, Horowitz K, Leunig M. Algorithm for femoral and periacetabular osteotomies in complex hip deformities. Clin Orthop. 2010;468:3168–80. https://doi.org/10.1007/s11999-010-1489-z.

23. Tomczak RJ, Guenther KP, Rieber A, et al. MR imaging measurement of the femoral antetorsional angle as a new technique: comparison with CT in children and adults. AJR Am J Roentgenol. 1997;168:791–4. https://doi.org/10.2214/ajr.168.3.9057536.
24. Ganz R, Slongo T, Siebenrock KA, et al. Surgical technique: the capsular arthroplasty: a useful but abandoned procedure for young patients with developmental dysplasia of the hip. Clin Orthop. 2012;470:2957–67. https://doi.org/10.1007/s11999-012-2444-y.
25. Souza RB, Powers CM. Concurrent criterion-related validity and reliability of a clinical test to measure femoral anteversion. J Orthop Sports Phys Ther. 2009;39:586–92. https://doi.org/10.2519/jospt.2009.2996.
26. Ganz R, Gill TJ, Gautier E, et al. Surgical dislocation of the adult hip. A technique with full access to the femoral head and acetabulum without the risk of avascular necrosis. J Bone Joint Surg Br. 2001;83:1119–24. https://doi.org/10.1302/0301-620x.83b8.11964.
27. Ganz R, Huff TW, Leunig M. Extended retinacular soft-tissue flap for intra-articular hip surgery: surgical technique, indications, and results of application. Instr Course Lect. 2009;58:241–55.
28. Schmidt J, Kumm D, Naughton S. Classification of bone healing after intertrochanteric osteotomies. Consequences for the surgical procedure and postoperative rehabilitation. Acta Orthop Belg. 1995;61:29–36.
29. Ejnisman L, Philippon MJ, Lertwanich P, et al. Relationship between femoral anteversion and findings in hips with femoroacetabular impingement. Orthopedics. 2013;36:e293–300. https://doi.org/10.3928/01477447-20130222-17.
30. Fabricant PD, Bedi A, De La Torre K, Kelly BT. Clinical outcomes after arthroscopic psoas lengthening: the effect of femoral version. Arthrosc J Arthrosc Relat Surg Off Publ Arthrosc Assoc N Am Int Arthrosc Assoc. 2012;28:965–71. https://doi.org/10.1016/j.arthro.2011.11.028.
31. Jackson TJ, Lindner D, El-Bitar YF, Domb BG. Effect of femoral anteversion on clinical outcomes after hip arthroscopy. Arthrosc J Arthrosc Relat Surg Off Publ Arthrosc Assoc N Am Int Arthrosc Assoc. 2015;31:35–41. https://doi.org/10.1016/j.arthro.2014.07.009.
32. Decker S, Suero EM, Hawi N, et al. The physiological range of femoral antetorsion. Skelet Radiol. 2013;42:1501–5. https://doi.org/10.1007/s00256-013-1687-3.
33. Kay RM, Rethlefsen SA, Hale JM, et al. Comparison of proximal and distal rotational femoral osteotomy in children with cerebral palsy. J Pediatr Orthop. 2003;23:150–4.

Surgical Hip Dislocation in Traumatology

14

Alessandro Aprato, Ettore Sabetta,
Matteo Giachino, and Alessandro Massè

14.1 Introduction

Fractures involving articular surfaces of the hip have been a major challenge for orthopedic surgeons because of joint exposure difficulty, along with the great importance of anatomical reduction. Rapid evolution toward osteoarthritis has been reported to happen in post-traumatic hips left with even small articular incongruences. This peculiarity makes the pursuit of anatomical reduction mandatory in most of the cases, basically through open reduction and internal fixation. Furthermore, it's demonstrated that surgical accuracy in joint reconstruction, especially regarding the weight-bearing surfaces, influences long-term outcomes [1–6].

Single incision approaches are the most commonly used to reduce and fix the fracture. However, each standard approach allows a partial exposition of the acetabulum and the reduction of complex fractures may be not easy because it's demanding to obtain a clear view over patterns involving both anterior and posterior columns or walls of the acetabulum. Solutions involving extensile or combined approaches are sometimes performed, but criticized because some authors found a higher rate of complications such as infections, heterotopic ossification, and muscle weakness [7–11].

A second significant handicap in common hip exposures is the opportunity of direct intra-articular control of fracture reduction, as only small portions of the acetabular cavity and femoral head are visible during standard procedures [12]. A precise assessment of articular surfaces during reduction and fixation maneuvers would allow the surgeon to better restore normal anatomy, in a district where even a 1 mm articular step can lead to secondary joint degeneration [4].

Safe surgical dislocation of the hip showed excellent results for treatment of nontraumatic hip pathologies, taking advantage of its intrinsic capability to give a complete view of the acetabulum and femoral head [12]. Subsequently it comes clear how it can be a valuable technique even in the field of traumatology, to support the treatment of complex fractures, while avoiding combined or extensile approaches.

14.2 Indications

A variety of hip injuries can be favorably treated with safe surgical dislocation of the hip. Considering the acetabular side of the joint, major advantages are obtained for reduction and fixation of transverse or T-type fractures, with or without involvement of posterior wall too. Our experience suggests that transtectal and juxtatectal more than infratectal patterns of fracture

A. Aprato (✉) · M. Giachino · A. Massè
School of Medicine, University of Turin, Turin, Italy

E. Sabetta
Arcispedale Santa Maria Nuova Hospital,
Reggio Emilia, Italy

R. Ganz (ed.), *Modern Hip Preservation*, https://doi.org/10.1007/978-3-030-91967-2_14

benefit from this technique Other indications are intra-articular assessment of reduction in extensive comminutions, removal of intra-articular fragments and evidence of extra-articular placement of screws [13].

Surgical indications for femoral head fractures are less delineated. The decision for operative treatment has to be made considering not only fracture pattern but also patient's clinical status, age, level of activity and bone quality. Young and active patients are generally managed with open reduction and internal fixation for Pipkin type II, III, and IV; Pipkin type I lesions are operatively treated if head fragments are displaced. Beyond surgical indication there is still some debate regarding the choice of surgical approach and the operative procedure, especially regarding the selection of fragments to be fixed and the consequences they have on the final outcome [14–18].

14.3 Surgical Techniques

Either Gibson or the Kocher–Langenbeck approach could be used; the latter offers more space for the positioning of posterior clamps, while the first one preserves the gluteus maximus. Trochanteric flip osteotomy is executed to obtain a fragment containing the insertion of the gluteus medius, vastus lateralis, and long tendon of the gluteus minimus muscles. To ensure that the major part of the piriformis tendon remains on the stable part of the greater trochanter, a small part of the most posterior portion of the gluteus medius tendon should be initially kept attached to the trochanter and sharply cut after osteotomy. Only then, is the superior border of the piriformis tendon dissected near the trochanteric insertion and the interval between the gluteus minimus and the piriformis muscles is isolated. This interval is safe regarding the risk of damage to the deep branch of the medial circumflex artery. The osteotomized trochanteric fragment is then flipped and slid anteriorly after releasing the origin of the gluteus minimus; debridement of the gluteus minimus could be performed at this stage if necessary (gluteus minimus injuries are very common in acetabular fractures). An anterosuperior capsulotomy (Z-shaped) is performed when the capsule is intact or completed if there is a partial capsular rupture. The femoral head is dislocated anteriorly through adduction and external rotation of the leg.

14.3.1 Acetabular Fractures

With manipulation of the leg, a 360° inspection of the acetabulum is performed, debris are removed from articular surfaces. Femoral head is then relocated and further debridement of injured tissues is carried on, visualizing external fracture lines. At this stage it must be decided whether fracture manipulation and fixation can be executed without myotenotomy of the external rotators. If the tendons have to be cut, this should be done at a minimal distance of 2 cm from the posterior trochanteric crest. The obturator externus tendon should be preserved in all events so as not to damage the deep branch of the medial femoral circumflex artery. The posterior wall and column are exposed, and posterior fracture lines should be clearly visible. At this stage a direct reduction maneuver has to be performed, based on the specific fracture pattern.

For transverse fractures, associated or not with posterior wall rupture (Figs. 14.1 and 14.2), there are different possibilities to achieve reduction. The most practical technique makes use of two 3.5 mm Jungbluth clamps (Matta Pelvic System, Stryker Trauma AG, Selzach, Switzerland), one placed in the anterior column and one in the

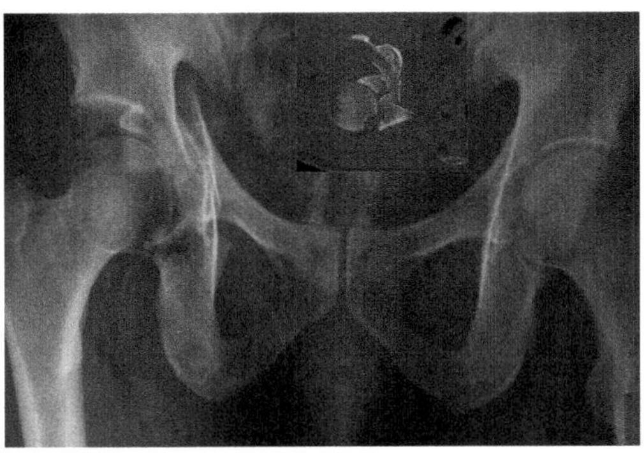

Fig. 14.1 Case 1: X-rays and CT scan showing a transverse plus posterior wall fracture

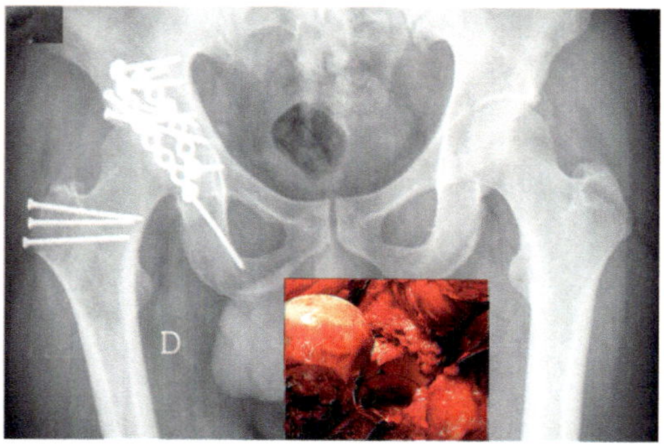

Fig. 14.2 Case 1: Intraoperative and postoperative views of the reduction and fixation

posterior one. The anterior clamp can be easily placed in juxtatectal and transtectal fractures, while for infratectal fractures often there is not enough space for the clamp to be put. In this case it's possible to combine the posterior 3.5 mm posterior clamp with a 3 mm Schantz screw placed in the anterior column. The posterior clamp is usually placed across the fracture rim between the area above the roof and the posterior border of the greater ischiatic notch. In case of using Gibson approach the posterior clamp should be positioned closer to the posterior wall in order to avoid excessive soft tissues tension.

Once the two clamps are placed, the reduction maneuver is usually a downward and external directed push of the inferior pelvic brim. If more derotation is needed, a supplementary Schantz screw drilled into the ischiatic tuberosity can be used.

When a satisfying reduction is achieved, fixation of the fracture can be realized with one or two 3.5 mm cortical screws inserted along the axis of the anterior column. The entry point for the screws is an approximately 2 cm wide circle situated 3–4 cm above the acetabular roof. The correct direction for screw placement can be felt by manually touching the medial aspect of the iliopectineal eminence from behind the posterior column and by direct inspection of the articular surface. In patients with a thick, soft tissues layer as in obese or muscular people it could be hard to find the correct direction of the screw, which tends to go medially and anteriorly.

At this stage the head is relocated and the posterior column is fixated with a reconstruction plate as described by Letournel and Judet. If the posterior wall is involved, its reduction can be performed before posterior column fixation; then, a second more lateral plate is placed after posterior column fixation.

Once both columns are fixed, femoral head is again dislocated to check intra-articular congruence of the fragments and the correct extra-articular placement of the screws.

T-type fractures could be reduced by transforming the T into a transverse fracture. This can be achieved by reducing the two columns distally to the transverse rim of the fracture with Schantz screws placed in the ischial tuberosity and in the anterior column; once the inferior parts of the columns are reduced, they can be temporarily fixed with one or two Kirschner wires drilled from posterior to anterior. Definitive reduction and fixation is then performed as previously described. The separate reduction of the columns is often more challenging, but it can be performed by placing a Schantz screw used as a joystick into the anterior column through articular cartilage or by using a collinear clamp (Synthes, Paoli, PA, USA). The collinear clamp can be inserted through the vertical branch of the T and allows a good reduction with minimal working space limitation. Final fixation of the anterior column is realized with one or two 3.5 mm screws. Reduction and fixation of the posterior column are obtained as described previously. Final intra-articular inspection for reduction and screws correct placement is then performed by femoral head dislocation.

The head is relocated in the acetabulum, retinaculum and capsule are sutured without any tension; the flipped trochanter is fixed with two or three screws [13].

14.3.2 Femoral Head Fractures

Femoral head dislocation must be carefully performed in Pipkin type III fractures and femoral neck should be previously temporary fixed with Kirschner wires. In Pipkin type I fractures the inferior fragment may be still attached to the ligamentus teres and/or the inferior retinaculum (Figs. 14.3, 14.4, 14.5 and 14.6); caution should

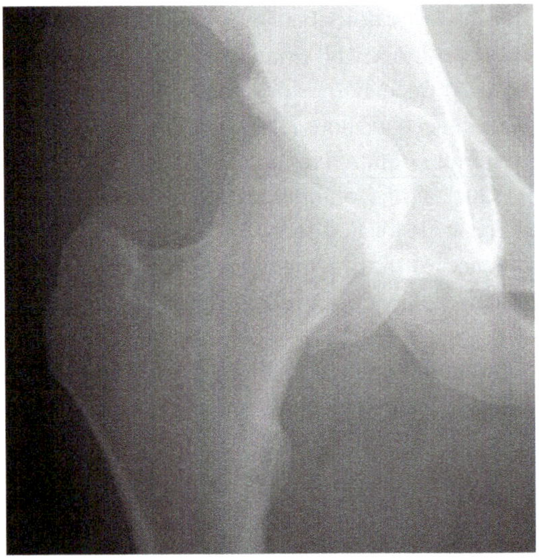

Fig. 14.3 Case 2: X-rays showing a Pipkin type I fracture

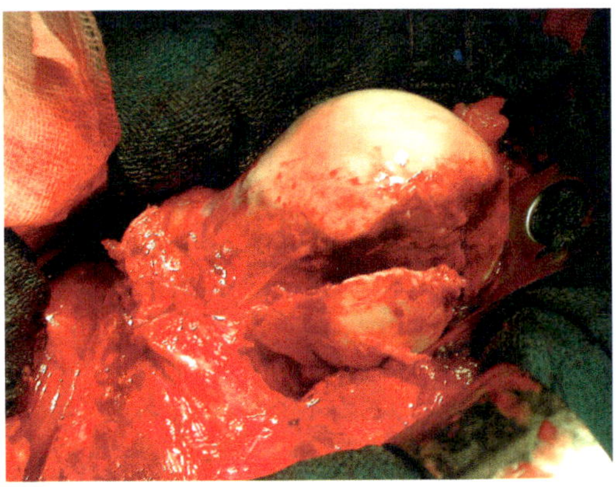

Fig. 14.4 Case 2: Intraoperative view of the Pipkin type I fracture

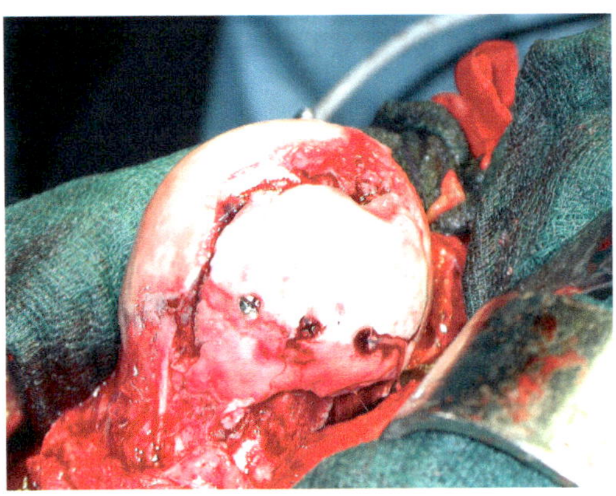

Fig. 14.5 Case 2: Intraoperative view of the reduction and fixation

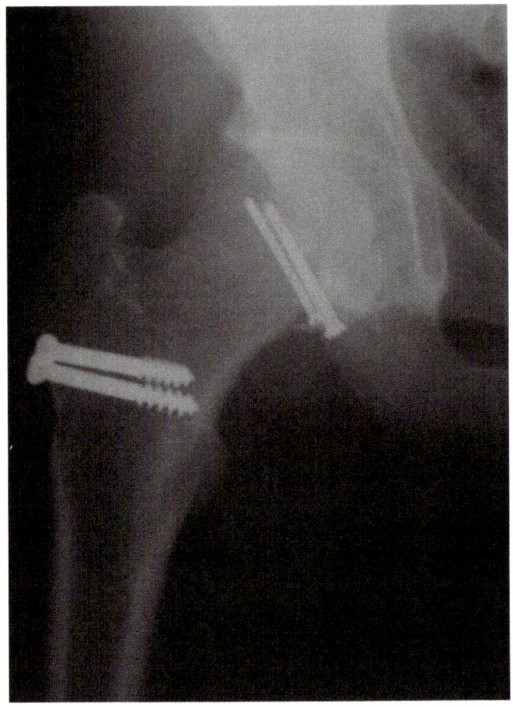

Fig. 14.6 Case 2: Postoperative view of the reduction and fixation

be made for meticulous section of the ligamentus with curved scissors, and preservation of the inferior retinaculum is mandatory to reduce the risk of AVN.

Femoral head fracture could be fixed through 2.7 mm nonabsorbable screws inserted from the articular side. The head of the screws should not protrude from articular surface and the weight-bearing area should be avoided, if possible. Eventually the head can be relocated in the acetabulum.

In Pipkin type III, after removal of previously placed K-wires, femoral neck is ultimately fixed with screws. In Pipkin type IV fractures the femoral head is relocated and posterior fractures lines are detected after debridement of destroyed tissues. Reduction maneuver is then performed based on fracture pattern; if a transverse fracture is associated, the previously described technique can be used [19].

14.4 Limitations

This technique has some limitations. Surgical exposure through safe dislocation of the hip is excellent, giving a complete view of the acetabulum, however the approach and the reduction maneuver of the anterior column is not always trouble-free. When the fracture rim goes medial to the iliopubic eminence the placement of the anterior reduction clamp could be challenging as the lower extra-articular portion of the anterior column is difficult to visualize. Another weakness of the technique could be the limited ability to achieve good compression and early stability of the anterior column during fixation, as only one or two cortical screws are placed.

From the femoral side, the first important risk during dislocation is the possibility of inferior vessels detachment from the inferior fragment. A higher rate of residual fracture displacement has also been found in femoral head fractures associated with transverse acetabular fractures treated in lateral position compared with those in prone, but there is no universal consensus on this topic [20].

14.5 Results

The overall rate of avascular necrosis reported in literature for patient with surgically treated acetabular fractures is 9.2% for patients with an associated posterior dislocation, while is 5% for not displaced injuries [7]. Data coming from fractures treated with surgical dislocation show a 6% rate of AVN, which is a comparable result, suggesting that the onset of necrosis depends on fracture pattern rather than surgical approach. A slightly higher incidence of AVN (7.7%) was observed in femoral head fractures, but it is again in line with literature large case series findings [21].

The rate of anatomical reduction obtained with surgical dislocation technique is calculated 65% following Matta's criteria, imperfect in 16% and poor in 19% [13]. This is in accordance with published data achieved with standard or extensive approaches, which report anatomical reduction attainment between 62% and 84% for the easiest patters of transverse and T-type fractures, while in more complex cases these percentages fall between 14.4% and 68% [7, 11, 17, 22–28]. Since there is no specific validated instrument to evaluate reduction quality for femoral head injuries, data are obtained using Matta's criteria as well. Anatomic reduction could be achieved in 61.5%, while suboptimal results in 38.5% [19].

Following the most recent studies excellent clinical results are reported in 21% of cases according to Merle d'Aubignè and Postel score, good in 48%, while fair or poor outcomes respectively in 17% and 14% [7]. Published data regarding acetabular fractures treated with standard approaches are essentially comparable with those obtained with surgical dislocation. Similar considerations can be made for femoral head fractures where, however, it seems to exist a slight benefit for dislocation compared to anterior and posterior approach.

Mean surgical time from incision to suture is estimated to be 150 min for surgical dislocation technique [19]. Extensive approaches use to have a longer operative duration, while conventional approaches tends to have a similar timing [11, 29].

Literature analysis suggests a significant rate of heterotopic ossification for trochanteric flip osteotomy in comparison to the posterior exposure, while the extended iliofemoral approach is reported to have the highest risk at all [7, 28, 30]. Findings from recent studies put safe surgical dislocation half the way between the two most common exposures in terms of heterotopic ossifications, suggesting that appropriated prophylaxis should be administered whenever possible.

14.6 Conclusion

Surgical dislocation of the hip is a safe technique for selected acetabular and femoral head fractures. Both surgical and clinical results seem to support the advantages of this approach for treatment of specific injuries of acetabulum and femoral head. After a period of appropriate training, surgeons working in centers with high volumes of acetabular or femoral head fractures should add this technique to their portfolio.

References

1. Heeg M, Klasen HJ, Visser JD. Operative treatment for acetabular fractures. J Bone Joint Surg Br. 1990;72:383–6.
2. Heeg M, Oostvogel HJ, Klasen HJ. Conservative treatment of acetabular fractures: the role of the weight-bearing dome and anatomic reduction in the ultimate results. J Trauma. 1987;27:555–9.
3. Letournel E, Judet R, Elson RA. Fractures of the acetabulum. 2nd ed. Berlin Heidelberg: Springer; 1993. p. 521–88.
4. Matta JM. Fractures of the acetabulum: accuracy of reduction and clinical results in patients managed operatively within three weeks after the injury. J Bone Joint Surg Am. 1996;78:1632–45.
5. Matta JM, Anderson LM, Epstein HC, Hendricks P. Fractures of the acetabulum. A retrospective analysis. Clin Orthop. 1986;205:230–40.
6. Mears DC, Velyvis JH, Chang C-P. Displaced acetabular fractures managed operatively: indicators of outcome. Clin Orthop. 2003;407:173–86. https://doi.org/10.1097/00003086-200302000-00026.
7. Giannoudis PV, Grotz MRW, Papakostidis C, Dinopoulos H. Operative treatment of displaced fractures of the acetabulum. A meta-analysis. J Bone Joint Surg Br. 2005;87:2–9.
8. Griffin DB, Beaulé PE, Matta JM. Safety and efficacy of the extended iliofemoral approach in the treatment of complex fractures of the acetabulum. J Bone Joint Surg Br. 2005;87:1391–6. https://doi.org/10.1302/0301-620X.87B10.16538.
9. Harris AM, Althausen P, Kellam JF, Bosse MJ. Simultaneous anterior and posterior approaches for complex acetabular fractures. J Orthop Trauma. 2008;22:494–7. https://doi.org/10.1097/BOT.0b013e3181830d2a.
10. Kaempffe FA, Bone LB, Border JR. Open reduction and internal fixation of acetabular fractures: heterotopic ossification and other complications of treatment. J Orthop Trauma. 1991;5:439–45. https://doi.org/10.1097/00005131-199112000-00009.
11. Kinik H, Armangil M. Extensile triradiate approach in the management of combined acetabular fractures. Arch Orthop Trauma Surg. 2004;124:476–82. https://doi.org/10.1007/s00402-004-0694-1.
12. Ganz R, Gill TJ, Gautier E, et al. Surgical dislocation of the adult hip. A technique with full access to the femoral head and acetabulum without the risk of avascular necrosis. J Bone Joint Surg Br. 2001;83:1119–24. https://doi.org/10.1302/0301-620x.83b8.11964.
13. Masse A, Aprato A, Rollero L, et al. Surgical dislocation technique for the treatment of acetabular fractures. Clin Orthop. 2013;471:4056–64. https://doi.org/10.1007/s11999-013-3228-8.
14. Gillespie P, Aprato A, Bircher M. Hip dislocation and femoral head fractures. In: European surgical orthopaedics and traumatology: the EFORT textbook. Berlin Heidelberg: Springer; 2014. p. 2179–202.
15. Alonso JE, Volgas DA, Giordano V, Stannard JP. A review of the treatment of hip dislocations associated with acetabular fractures. Clin Orthop. 2000;377:32–43. https://doi.org/10.1097/00003086-200008000-00007.
16. Solberg BD, Moon CN, Franco DP. Use of a trochanteric flip osteotomy improves outcomes in pipkin IV fractures. Clin Orthop. 2009;467:929–33. https://doi.org/10.1007/s11999-008-0505-z.
17. Stannard JP, Harris HW, Volgas DA, Alonso JE. Functional outcome of patients with femoral head fractures associated with hip dislocations. Clin Orthop. 2000;377:44–56. https://doi.org/10.1097/00003086-200008000-00008.
18. Swiontkowski MF, Thorpe M, Seiler JG, Hansen ST. Operative management of displaced femoral head fractures: case-matched comparison of anterior versus posterior approaches for Pipkin I and Pipkin II fractures. J Orthop Trauma. 1992;6:437–42.
19. Massè A, Aprato A, Alluto C, et al. Surgical hip dislocation is a reliable approach for treatment of femoral head fractures. Clin Orthop. 2015;473:3744–51. https://doi.org/10.1007/s11999-015-4352-4.
20. Collinge C, Archdeacon M, Sagi HC. Quality of radiographic reduction and perioperative complications for transverse acetabular fractures treated by the Kocher-Langenbeck approach: prone versus lateral position. J Orthop Trauma. 2011;25:538–42. https://doi.org/10.1097/BOT.0b013e31820b913d.
21. Giannoudis PV, Kontakis G, Christoforakis Z, et al. Management, complications and clinical results of femoral head fractures. Injury. 2009;40:1245–51. https://doi.org/10.1016/j.injury.2009.10.024.
22. Chiu FY, Chen CM, Lo WH. Surgical treatment of displaced acetabular fractures - 72 cases followed for 10 (6-14) years. Injury. 2000;31:181–5. https://doi.org/10.1016/s0020-1383(99)00277-6.
23. Li X, Tang T, Sun J. Results after surgical treatment of transtectal transverse acetabular fractures. Orthop Surg. 2010;2:7–13. https://doi.org/10.1111/j.1757--7861.2009.00056.x.
24. Liu Q, Wu D, Li P, Han S. Surgical treatment for complex acetabular fractures. Chin J Traumatol Zhonghua Chuang Shang Za Zhi. 2006;9:325–8.
25. Oh C-W, Kim P-T, Park B-C, et al. Results after operative treatment of transverse acetabular fractures. J Orthop Sci Off J Jpn Orthop Assoc. 2006;11:478–84. https://doi.org/10.1007/s00776-006-1045-6.
26. Onche II, Obiano SK, Udoh MK. A prospective evaluation of the management and outcome of

traumatic posterior dislocation of the hip--a preliminary report. Niger J Med J Natl Assoc Resid Dr Niger. 2008;17:163–7. https://doi.org/10.4314/njm.v17i2.37376.
27. Porter SE, Graves ML, Maples RA, et al. Acetabular fracture reductions in the obese patient. J Orthop Trauma. 2011;25:371–7. https://doi.org/10.1097/BOT.0b013e3181f974f4.
28. Triantaphillopoulos PG, Panagiotis T, Panagiotopoulos EC, et al. Long-term results in surgically treated acetabular fractures through the posterior approaches. J Trauma. 2007;62:378–82. https://doi.org/10.1097/01.ta.0000196540.81630.4e.
29. Iselin LD, Wahl P, Studer P, et al. Associated lesions in posterior wall acetabular fractures: not a valid predictor of failure. J Orthop Traumatol Off J Ital Soc Orthop Traumatol. 2013;14:179–84. https://doi.org/10.1007/s10195-013-0247-x.
30. Ghalambor N, Matta JM, Bernstein L. Heterotopic ossification following operative treatment of acetabular fracture. An analysis of risk factors. Clin Orthop. 1994;305:96–105.

15 Intra- and Juxta-Capsular Osteotomies for Childhood Deformities of the Hip. Surgical Technique and Follow-Up of Selected Cases

Luigino Turchetto and Reinhold Ganz

15.1 Introduction

Osteotomies of the growing hip are traditionally executed at a distance to the joint to avoid necrosis of the femoral head and injury to the growth plates. Such techniques can be successful with regard to joint reduction when the deformity is moderate and mainly extra-capsular. However, difficulties to successfully treat more complex problems increase when the deformity is located at the level of femoral head or acetabulum and even more so when the deformity is combined with joint subluxation. Intertrochanteric or subtrochanteric osteotomies can create substantial secondary deformities, especially varus as well as leg shortening, often without achieving sufficient centering and stabilization of the joint. Especially when correctly executed and tilted, the result of the frequently performed Salter osteotomy can be retroversion of the acetabulum, a deformity which may not be detected as damaging cause until early adulthood.

Intracapsular osteotomies of the femur and periacetabular osteotomies at or very close to the level of deformity are more effective, especially for joint stabilization and are accompanied with less secondary deformities. Although some may cross growth plates, we have learned over the past decades, that the dogmatic no-touch doctrine for growth plates around the hip can be replaced by a more differentiated attitude without risking substantial iatrogenic deformities during further growth.

In this chapter, we share our experience with the techniques of intra- and juxta-articular osteotomies for complex childhood hip deformities. We explain the indications and illustrate the results over time with typical examples.

15.2 Osteotomy Techniques

15.2.1 Bernese Periacetabular Osteotomy

The Bernese periacetabular osteotomy (PAO) is a reorientation procedure in which all osteotomy cuts are executed from the inner side of the pelvis [1] (Fig. 15.1). This approach allows to preserve the main blood supply coming from outside to the acetabular bone [2, 3]. The distance of the cuts to the joint is such that the periacetabular vascular circuit remains intact, allowing anastomotic compensation of localized vessel interruption [4]. The power of correction is high because the limiting sacro-spinal and sacro-tuberal ligaments remain on the spared posterior column. Moreover, the intact posterior column increases the stability of the hemi-pelvis and helps to protect the sciatic

L. Turchetto (✉)
Orthopedics and Traumatology Unit, Portogruaro Hospital, Portogruaro, Italy
e-mail: lturchetto@tin.it

R. Ganz
Faculty of Medicine, University of Bern, Bern, Switzerland

R. Ganz (ed.), *Modern Hip Preservation*, https://doi.org/10.1007/978-3-030-91967-2_15

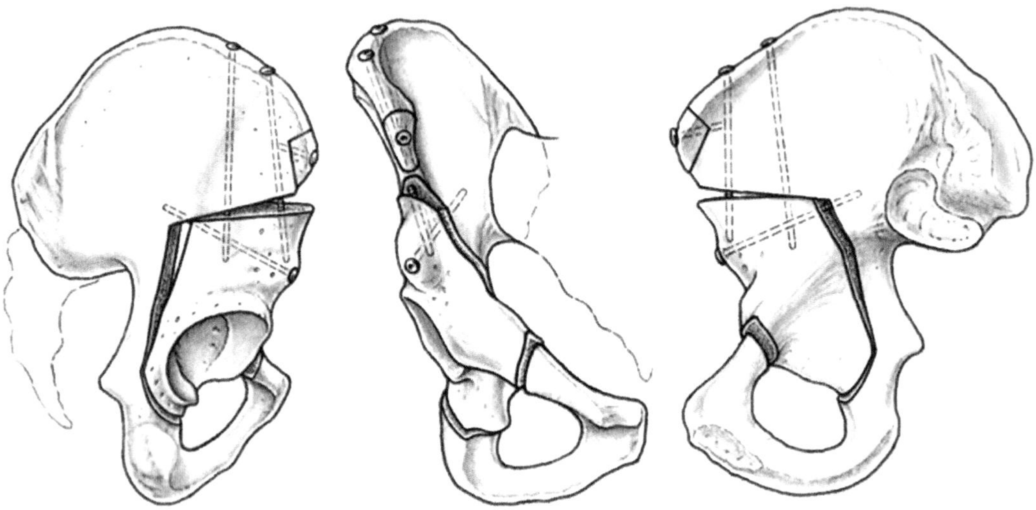

Fig. 15.1 Hemi-pelvis with the different PAO cuts, executed from anterior and medial, leaving the posterior column in continuity. The supra-acetabular cut starts next to the osteotomy of the ASIS in order to preserve the blood supply from superior and inferior gluteal artery to the supra-acetabular bone. When a femoral surgery is to be combined, the first ischial cut can be executed via the femoral approach with the advantage of a direct protection of the sciatic nerve. Fixation of the corrected acetabulum is sufficient with three screws in the demonstrated arrangement

nerve. A further advantage is the preservation of the birth canal, an important factor for natural childbirth. PAO was developed in 1984 and executed since with several modifications [5]. Based on ongoing publications, the procedure has reached a high level of acceptance [6].

The technical steps of the Bernese periacetabular osteotomy are explained in detail in several publications [7, 8] and visualized in video clips [9]. When combined with a femoral osteotomy, the first ischial cut can be executed safely via the femoral approach. One cut crosses the ischial part of the acetabular growth plate in its posterior aspect, reason why the procedure was excluded for many years from being used in children. However, perceptions from the study of the rare but distinct post-traumatic dysplasia made us reconsider such strict contraindication. So far, post-traumatic dysplasia was only seen when the injury to the ilio-ischial part of the acetabular growth plate took place before the age of five, although the overall incidence of pelvic fractures increased with older age [10, 11]. With this information in mind and motivated by the advantages of the procedure, we started to execute PAOs in older children with open acetabular physis. We felt reinvigorated all the more so as the ilio-ischial part of the growth plate is interrupted with a linear cut in its most posterior aspect, an injury being much less disturbing than a crush injury. With an experience over more than 20 years with a total of 25 hips in 21 children aged 5 1/2–12 years at the time of surgery, we can say that after the age of 9 years a disturbance of the overall acetabular growth is not to be expected [12].

An important difference to a PAO in adults is constituted by the periosteum. While it is thin and nearly negligible in the adult hip, it is thick in childhood and may resist the surgical moves for reorientation, if not incised carefully around the osteotomies of pubis and ischium.

15.2.2 Safe Surgical Dislocation of the Hip Joint

Not long ago, surgical dislocation of the hip joint was regarded as an intervention accompanied with a high risk of avascular necrosis of the femoral head regardless whether it was executed from anterior or posterior. Detailed studies of the vascular anatomy of the proximal femur revealed a

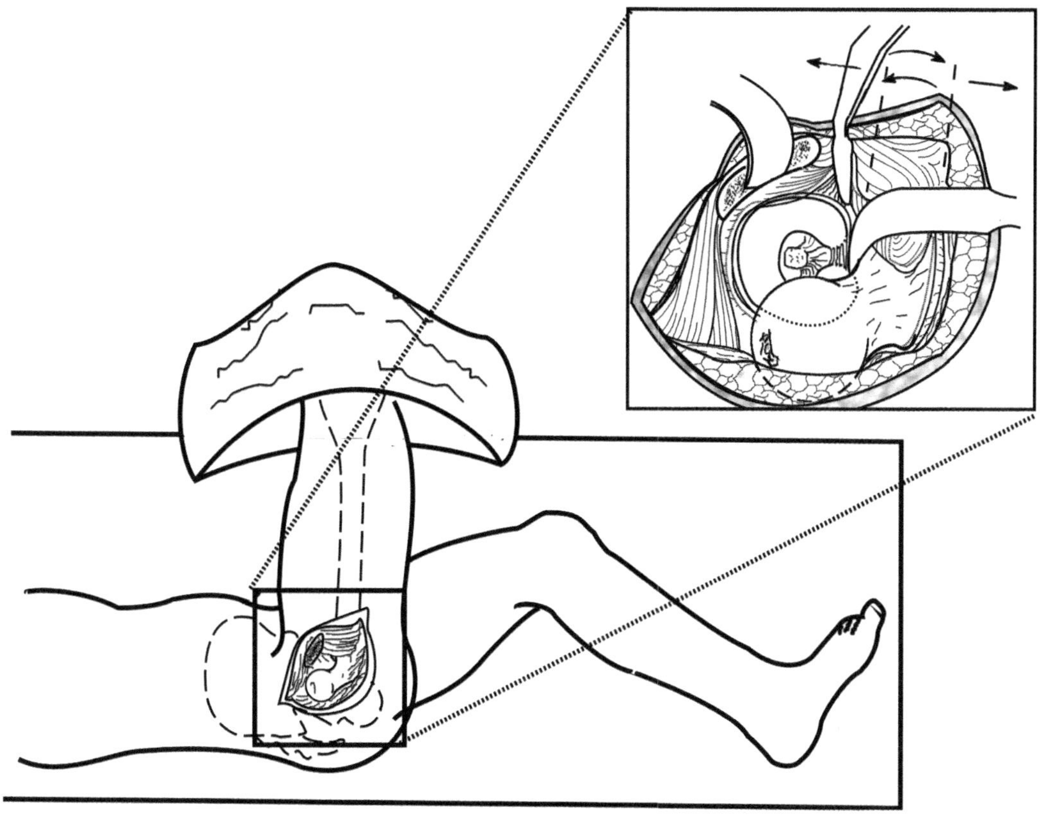

Fig. 15.2 Surgical dislocation of the hip is executed in lateral decubitus via a trochanteric flip osteotomy. With the leg placed in a sterile bag on the opposite side of the table, the joint is exposed with three retractors placed around the acetabulum. With different positions of the femur in flexion-extension and rotation, the entire acetabulum and the majority of the head surface can be visualized. (modified with permission from [15])

safe way to execute an anterior dislocation using a digastric trochanter flip osteotomy; it allows full access to acetabular cavity and femoral head for inspection and treatment [13, 14] (Fig. 15.2). After the first description of the technique [13], multiple articles have been published about the versatility including a multicenter study demonstrating the low morbidity of the procedure [16]. The technical details are also visualized in video clips [9]. Besides the possibility of intracapsular surgery [17], surgical hip dislocation allowed to observe and describe the different ways of hip impingement [18]. Together with an extended retinacular flap containing the vascular supply of the femoral head, it became the workhorse for a number of new intracapsular osteotomies [15].

15.2.3 Relative Lengthening of the Femoral Neck

In contrast to absolute neck lengthening [19], relative lengthening is the result of bone trimming of the intertrochanteric region at its superior and posterior circumference down to the level of the neck. By doing so, distal advancement of the greater trochanter is possible, extra- and intra-articular impingement can be eliminated resulting in increased joint clearance [15] (Fig. 15.3). Nearly always, posterolateral trimming of bone needs localized subperiosteal elevation of the retinacular fold containing the main vessels for femoral head perfusion [15]. Relative lengthening of the neck is rarely executed as an isolated

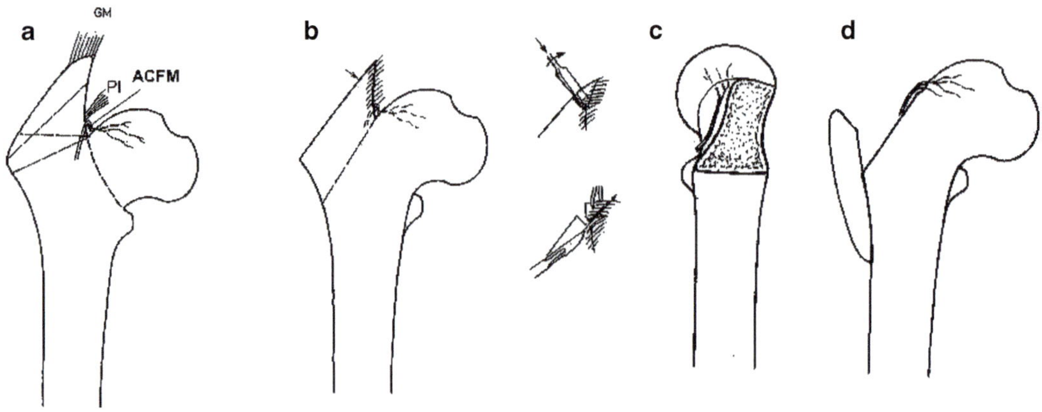

Fig. 15.3 (**a**) in the "no neck" configuration the retinacular vessels enter the head in the axilla between trochanter and head. The *proximal dotted line* in the trochanter marks the level of the digastric trochanter flip osteotomy, while the *distal dotted line* represents the final level of the new neck. (**b**) situation after trochanteric flip osteotomy. (**c**) preservation of retinacular vessels with strictly subperiosteal, piecemeal osteotomy down to the desired level of the new neck. (**d**) result with relative neck lengthening and preserved retinacular vessels

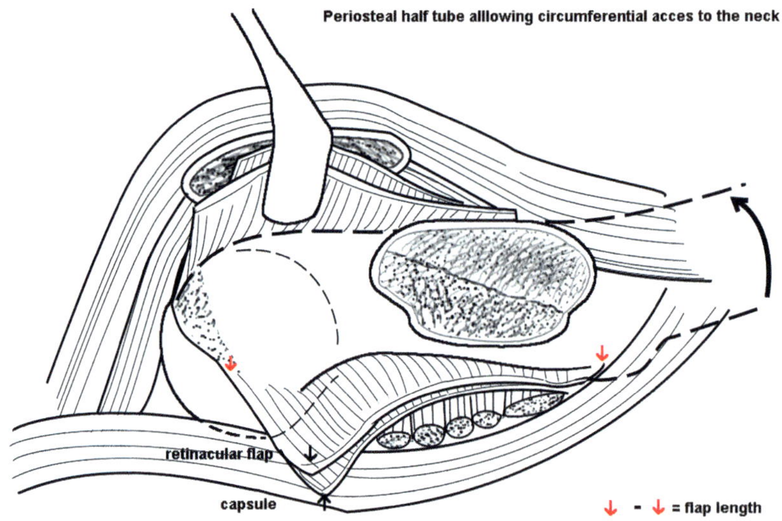

Fig. 15.4 Dislocated head with both retinacular flaps; the medial flap is held back with a retractor. The posterior facet of the trochanteric osteotomy results from piecemeal reduction of the stable trochanter down to the level of the neck

procedure [20], and more often part of other procedures of the femoral neck and head [15].

15.2.4 Extended Retinacular Flap

The first attempt to release the retinaculum from the neck for safer reduction of a slipped capital femoral epiphysis (SCFE) was published by Dunn [21]. Although combining it with a classic trochanteric osteotomy, the maneuvering space for reduction of the slipped epiphysis remained limited with some risk of overstretching or even rupturing the flap, the more so because it was executed without surgical dislocation of the joint. This problem was solved with safe surgical hip dislocation followed by trimming the bone of the stable part of the trochanter down to the level of the neck. By executing this strictly between periosteum and bone, the resulting soft tissue flap is extending distally as far as to the lesser trochanter, a fact, which increases the safety for the vessels. This extended surgical dislocation approach [15] offers the possibility to perform osteotomies of the neck and head with full attention of the epiphyseal perfusion (Fig. 15.4).

15.2.5 Sub-Capital Realignment

The understanding that SCFE is a prototype of impingement, as well as more recent publications reporting inferior results, have reduced the acceptance of pinning in situ. Sub-capital realignment based on surgical dislocation and extended retinacular flap has proven meanwhile to be safe, even in hips with complete disconnection; it allows anatomic correction of the deformity without undesired side deformities [22] (Fig. 15.5). In experienced hands the technique is not burdened with avascular necrosis of the head in stable slips, while in the series of disconnected hips the vascular insult could be related to other factors [23].

15.2.6 True Femoral Neck Osteotomy

Indications for osteotomies of the true neck are less frequent. Main indications are extreme coxa valga, deformities of SCFE after growth plate closure and post-traumatic deformities. It may be favored for unilateral deformities where an osteotomy at the intertrochanteric level would create substantial leg shortening. Most frequent type are varus and closed wedge osteotomy [24] (Fig. 15.6). The technical execution is somewhat easier compared with sub-capital reorientation, but fixation must meet higher requirements of stability and the time to consolidation is longer. This is especially the case, when an open wedge configuration is executed [15].

15.2.7 Head Size Reduction Osteotomy

Classic osteotomy techniques can hardly lead to satisfying results when a severe femoral head deformity after Perthes disease is leading to hinged abduction. Such deformity becomes even more complex due to the concurrent, reactive acetabular dysplasia. Quite often the deformity of the head is reminiscent to a saddle where the central deepening represents the necrotic area while the rounded margins correspond with the healthy parts of the epiphysis. The femoral head is simply too large in its horizontal diameter and often subluxated, to create a somewhat congruent containment with a classic femoral or acetabular osteotomy. In contrast, resection of the central deepening would allow to reduce the head size and create a more spherical contour by preserving and aligning the healthy margins. Detailed knowledge of the vascular supply to the femoral head [3, 13] as well as their intra-capital distribution and anastomoses [25] allowed to further evaluate such an osteotomy. According

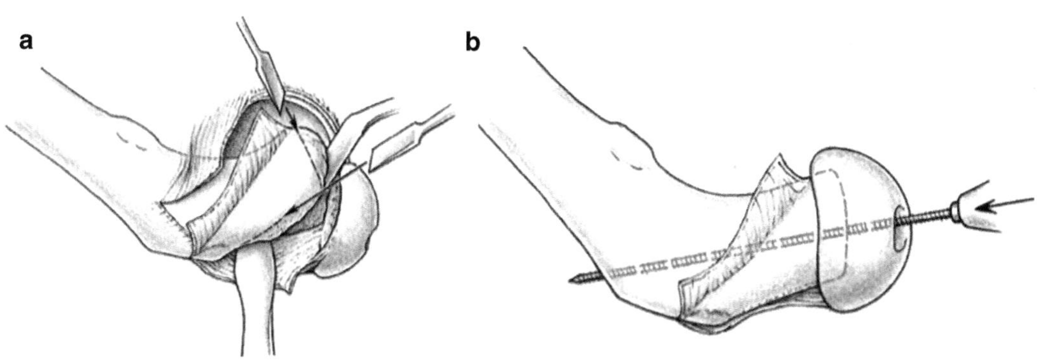

Fig. 15.5 (**a**) Reshaping of the metaphysis with dislocated joint. A cotton swab prevents the disconnected epiphysis from slipping back in the socket (not visible). Two retractors help to present the neck for resection of the posterior bone apposition. The top of the metaphysis is not shortened but only freed from debris of the growth plate (*arrows*). (**b**) with mobilization of the retinaculum down to the lesser trochanter, reposition of the epiphysis is possible without overstretching the retinacular vessels. A first transfixing K-wire is inserted in a retrograde manner, starting at the fovea

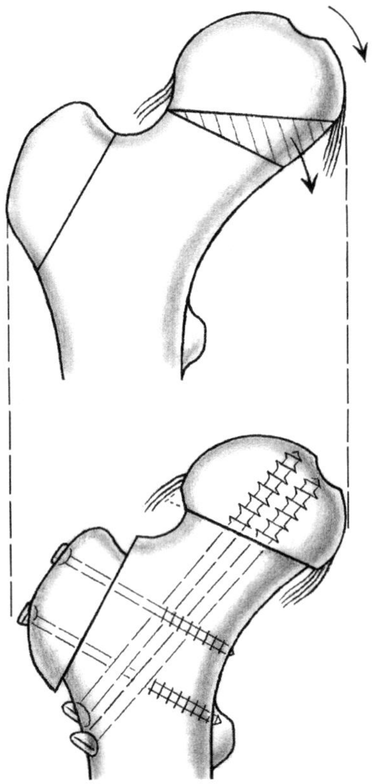

Fig. 15.6 Both, medial and lateral retinaculum are dissected. It results in an anteriorly open half tube of periosteum, allowing circumferential access to the neck bone. Varus osteotomy is the most frequent type; closed wedge is preferred over open wedge. The final osteotomy line should be oriented as horizontal as possible. Medially, both cortices should be aligned to allow cortical buttress. Two or three screws should be inserted as lag screws. The greater trochanter may be advanced to level the tip with the center of the head

to the vascular studies, the retinacular vessels of the MFCA perfuse the majority of the femoral epiphysis even when separated from the metaphysis, while the medial sector of the epiphysis gets the supply from the constant medial branch of the MFCA running on top of Weitbrecht's ligament. The medial segment remains united with the metaphysis, while the lateral segment is mobile, allowing three-dimensional shift, for alignment (Fig. 15.7a). To secure stable repositioning of the "new" head within the acetabular socket an additional PAO is nearly always necessary [15]. Good results of our first small series could be confirmed at 10 years [26] and are meanwhile repeated by others [27]. Pre-estimation of resection size and cut direction for optimal sphericity of the new head was largely facilitated by computer simulation and the use of cutting templates [28] (Fig. 15.7b, c).

15.3 Case Demonstration

15.3.1 Case 1

Nine-year-old male with Perthes disease, treated with an external splint to unload the hip for 1 year. In spite of that, ROM, especially abduction, decreased and pain increased. New radiography and MRI (Fig. 15.8) show slight increase of subluxation and incipient flattening of the acetabular roof. The apparent aggravation led to a change from conservative to operative treatment. Femoral varus osteotomy was discussed. It would be the easier procedure, but besides undesired leg shortening, the limitation of abduction may lead to postoperative adduction rather than improved containment. Acetabular reorientation (PAO), although technically more demanding, would allow more efficient coverage without major deformity, a result which was tested with fluoroscopy under anesthesia immediately before surgery.

The technical execution of the PAO followed the description above, knowing that the triradiate cartilage would be crossed by the retro-acetabular cut of the PAO. At the iliac crest, the apophysis was left intact and the exposure of the osseous wing was started posterior to the apophyseal growth plate. To facilitate correction of the freed

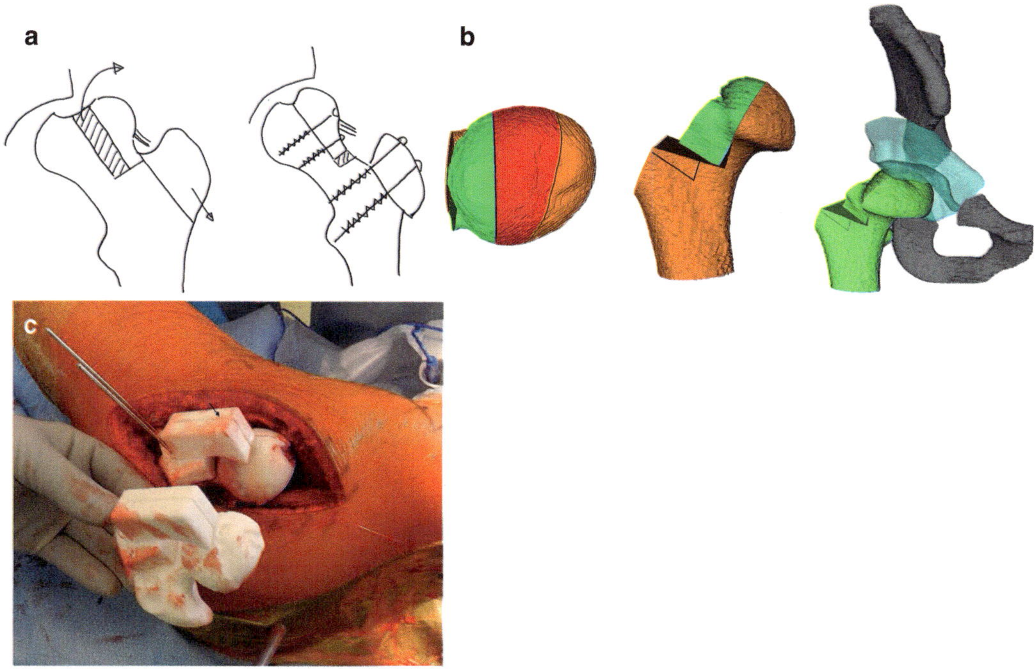

Fig. 15.7 (**a**) The osteotomy is performed on the dislocated femoral head. While the lateral retinaculum is dissected, the medial retinaculum remains in place. Size of the fragment to be resected (*hatched area*) and direction of cuts is best simulated on a computer model. Cutting devices guarantee the precision of the desired osteotomy directions. The mobile fragment, which is perfused from the retinacular vessels, can be shifted and rotated until the surface contours do match optimally. The new position is fixed with two 3.5 mm screws. Nearly always a substantial advancement of the greater trochanter is necessary. In the majority of the cases the acetabulum has also to be corrected; this part is done in the same anesthesia. (**b**) Individual Computer Simulation of head reduction osteotomy. *Left*: Red section to be resected. *Middle*: Best fit of green and orange section. *Right*: "New" head with optimal spatial correction of the acetabulum. (**c**) 3D Printed, personalized cutting blocks to be fixed on the anterior surface of the bone (*K-wires*). Slots for execution of precise cuts (*arrow*)

acetabulum, special care was taken to incise circumferentially the periosteum around the area of the pubic osteotomy. With regard to the impaired mechanical quality of the chronically diseased hip bone, correcting maneuvers were started only after the acetabular fragment was sufficiently mobile. Version was controlled with fluoroscopy placing a thin K-wire along the border of the anterior labrum.

The osteotomy healed sufficiently after 8 weeks. Unrestricted weight bearing was allowed at 3 months after surgery.

The patient rates his operated hip as normal. ROM is symmetrical, leg length is equal. He has no pain, works full time in an office job and is practicing jogging and bicycling on a regular basis.

15.3.2 Case 2

21-year-old female with a history of Perthes disease of the left hip, which started at the age of 9 years. She had no specific treatment but was monitored regularly over several years. A leg length difference of nearly 2.5 cm was only recently compensated for chronic lumbo-sciatic and gluteal pain, but resulted in only moderate relief. A herniated disc as well as a piriformis syndrome were discussed but not pursued further. Stretching exercises increased the pain.

With shoe elevation, limping did not completely disappear. Abductor strength, controlled in side position, was 4–5. ROM was substantially limited for external rotation and abduction and less for flexion, internal rotation and adduc-

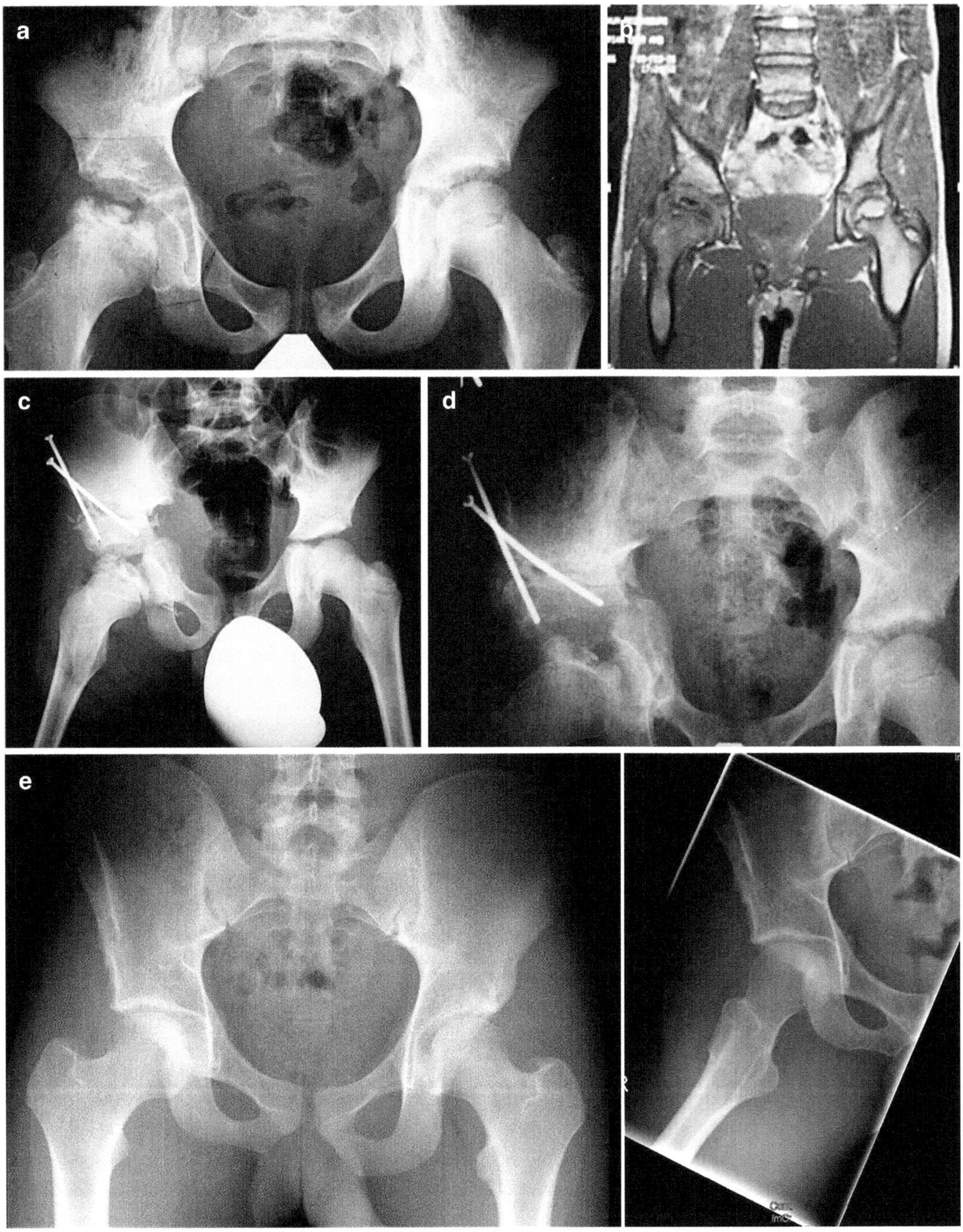

Fig. 15.8 (**a**, **b**) Perthes disease with incipient flattening of the roof and subluxation under treatment with an external splint. Coxa magna with slight extrusion. Lateral column of the epiphysis vital. Largely open acetabular growth plate. (**c**, **d**) Radiographies immediately and 3 months after PAO. Well recentered femoral head. (**e**) 22 years after surgery with a normally developed hip joint in both projections and only slightly deformed morphology of the iliac wing

tion. Terminal movements created moderate pain pointing to a complex intra- and extra-articular impingement. Lumbar spine and sciatic nerve were within normal limits.

Standard radiographies confirmed the clinical impression of a Perthes disease healed with a reasonably round and well covered head, a short neck and a high riding trochanter.

The surgical concept for this complex impingement was to perform relative lengthening of the neck with distal advancement of the greater trochanter to increase the pelvi-femoral clearance. It was thought to eventually perform an osteo-chondroplasty for a better anterior head neck waist. PAO seemed to be less necessary, but final decision should depend on intraoperative joint stability after neck lengthening. Eventual indication for femoral derotation to decrease the anteversion was also put up to intraoperative decision.

The procedure followed the steps as outlined in the schematic drawings of Figs. 15.2 and 15.3. Subperiosteal downsizing of the trochanteric massif to the level of the posterior neck was laborious. Osteo-chondroplasty was minimal to alleviate anterior impingement in flexion/internal rotation. Abduction and external rotation did not anymore lead to posterior impingement. Full extension and external rotation however produced subluxation, which could be related to an impingement of the lesser trochanter with ischium and posterior acetabular lip, a type of extraarticular impingement which has been observed occasionally [29]. The subluxation disappeared after osteotomy of the lesser trochanter; the fragment was finally refixed more distally using two screws. Thereafter, ROM was much improved in all directions without impingement or subluxation. Since the acetabulo-femoral relation seemed to be acceptable and the joint stability was high, femoral de-rotation and PAO were definitively renounced. The greater trochanter was advanced distally and was fixed with two screws about 2.5 cm distal of the original level. This position was controlled with fluoroscopy. Two crutches were administered for 6 weeks and one crutch for another 2 weeks. Active rehabilitation started at 4 weeks with special attention to abductor reinforcement. After 10 weeks and still on one crutch, the patient continued with her formation to become a hairdresser. At 1 year after surgery, ROM was nearly symmetrical, abductor force reached M5 and all symptoms were dissolved (Fig. 15.9b).

15 years after surgery, the patient remains pain free. ROM is nearly symmetrical. She gave birth to two children and works full time as hairdresser. The leg length discrepancy is not a problem for her; at work she wears shoes with length compensation. All in all, she is very happy with the result and denies the need for metal removal or a surgical procedure for leg lengthening.

15.3.3 Case 3

15-years-old male, slightly obese. When he was 5 years old, he was hit by a car when walking on a sidewalk together with his mother and younger brother. He was the only survivor, but his right leg had to be amputated at a sub-trochanteric level. When he was 13 years old, he started having pain in his left hip, but no medical investigation was induced, while ongoing problems with the amputation stump had priority. During the following 10 months, pain increased and hip motion decreased. Clinically, hip flexion was substantially limited and painful; spontaneously, the hip was held in fixed external rotation. There was normal active and passive mobility of the right hip.

Considering the severely reduced usability of the right lower extremity, there was a high demand on restoration of the left hip. Fixation in situ would prevent further slipping but would accept the deformation and therefore the mechanical limitation of the joint. Inter- or sub-trochanteric osteotomies may compensate for some parts of the deformity, but could not sufficiently eliminate the impingement problem at the head–neck junction. Only correction at the level of the deformity would be able to stop further

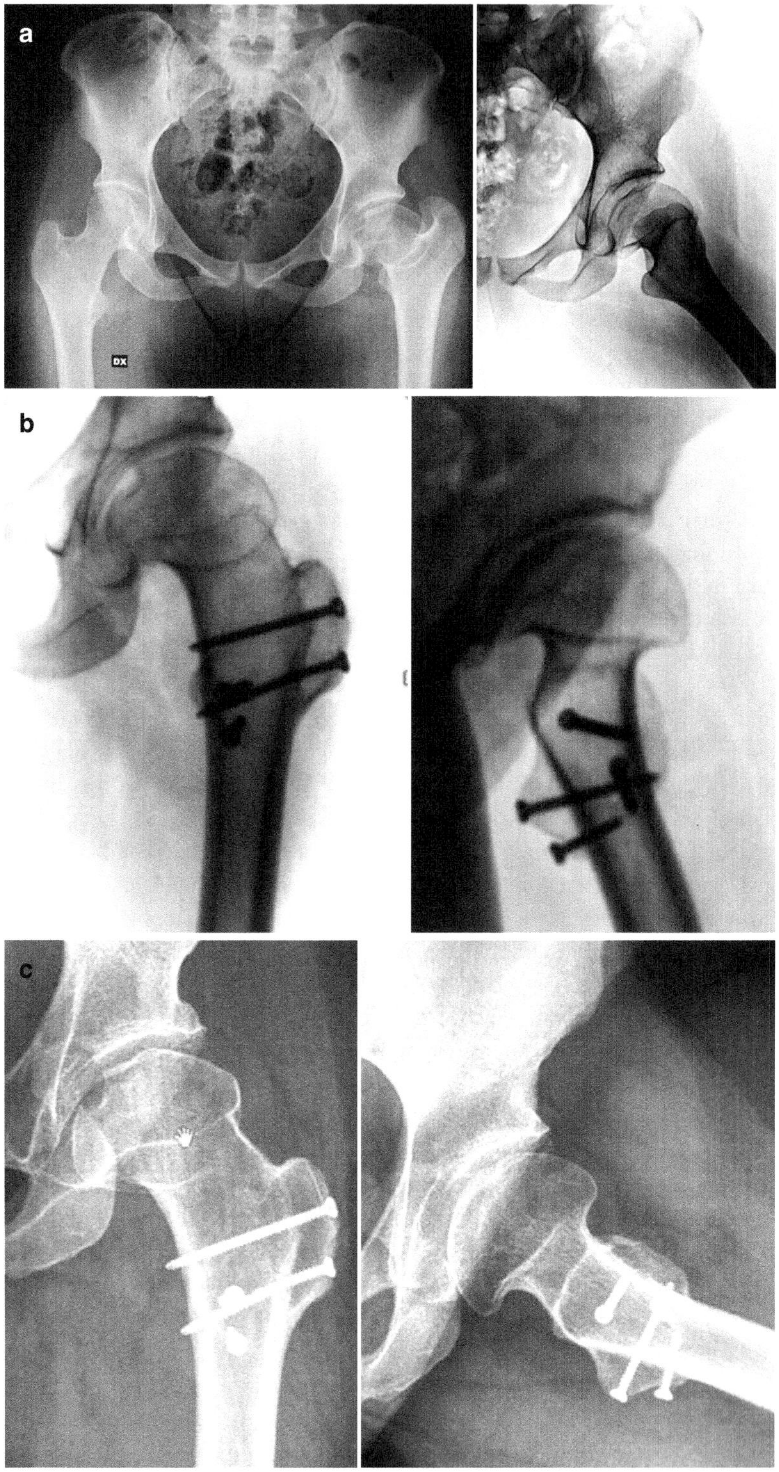

Fig. 15.9 (**a**) Radiographic appearance with a nearly spherical coxa magna, combined with markedly short neck and high riding greater trochanter. The head fits into a well-adapted acetabular cavity allowing high congruency in both planes. Due to the short neck the distance between lesser trochanter and postero-inferior acetabular lip was reduced. The anteversion of the neck seems to be rather high. (**b**) Radiographic result after 1 year. The relatively high anteversion of the neck as seen in the lateral view, is well tolerated. The patient had no complaints, gait was normal with a shoe lift; limitations in the daily life were denied. (**c**) Radiological result 15 years after surgery without morphological changes since postoperative appearance

slipping, correct the deformity and avoid further impingement. As such, it would ensure the best precondition against ongoing and rapid degeneration of the joint. Provided the surgeon has the necessary expertise with such a procedure, the risk of avascular necrosis would be calculable [22, 23]. The family agreed with this concept and was informed that an eventual joint instability after redirection of the epiphysis may necessitate a stabilizing PAO [30].

For the surgical dislocation approach the patient was placed in a lateral decubitus with a freely draped leg. Capsulotomy revealed some excessive and reddish tinged synovial fluid; the synovial fold was irritated and swollen. The epiphyseal cartilage in the periphery had a velvet like texture and the superior labrum was deformed and crashed as a result of chronic impingement with the antero-superior neck. As often in severe slips, external rotation of the hip for surgical dislocation was only possible after trimming of the stable part of the greater trochanter down to the level of the posterior neck surface. After sectioning the round ligament with scissors, immediate bleeding from its femoral stump could be observed. The final preparation of the posterolateral as well as of the posteromedial retinacular flap was less laborious than expected. After careful removal of some bone apposition on the posteromedial neck, a curved osteotome was advanced into the soft structure between epiphysis and underlying neck changing the direction several times. Special care was taken to avoid penetration of the instrument into the retinacular flap. Levering movements with the introduced osteotome finally allowed to break the epiphysis free. With external rotation of the femur the neck could be further exposed to allow removal of bone apposition at the posterior neck and to clean the inner side of the epiphyseal fragment from residual growth plate debris. Bleeding from this surface indicated preserved perfusion of the epiphysis. Manual anatomic reduction of the epiphysis was possible without creating adverse tension in the retinacular flap; shortening of the neck was not necessary. The achieved head position was fixed first with a fully threaded K-wire, inserted at the fovea capitis and penetrating the lateral cortex slightly distal to the prospected position of the greater trochanter (Fig. 15.10b). After fluoroscopic control of the optimal positioning of the epiphysis, two cortical screws were used for definitive fixation. The head was brought back into the socket and joint stability was tested carefully, before the joint capsule was readapted loosely and the trochanter was refixed, using small cortical screws.

The progress over the following 10 years was uneventful regarding the diseased hip, while the stump of the right leg created ongoing problems with breakdown of the scar and difficulties to adjust an external prosthesis. Since surgery he had never experienced pain in the left hip. ROM was free in all directions. Only the abductor force was with an M4 slightly reduced; this was probably related to the limited walking ability and practice. Radiologically, the left hip shows at 10 years peripheral edges, which however were already visible intraoperatively and on the 10 weeks picture. The width of the joint space over the years remained wide and regular. Considering the overall limited walking ability, the left hip may last long.

15.3.4 Case 4

23-year-old female, very active in mountaineering since childhood. For 3 years there was increasing left groin pain during running and less while climbing. Physiotherapy as well as several injections for trochanteric bursitis did not help. Finally, she was referred with the diagnosis of mild acetabular dysplasia.

Clinical examination did not reveal abnormalities of the hip except some reduced internal rotation in flexion which was painful in the end position. Standard anteroposterior radiography of

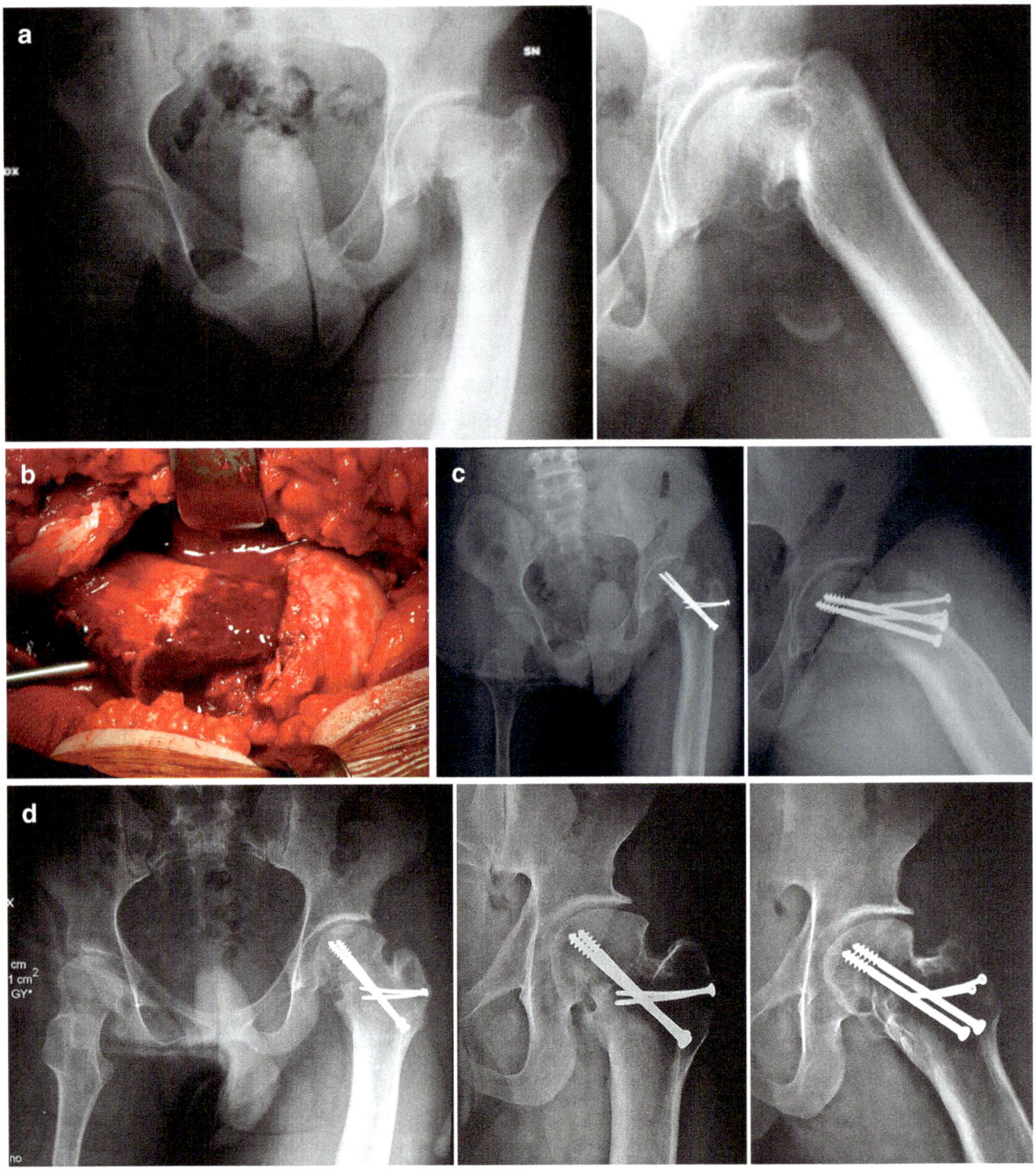

Fig. 15.10 (**a**) Radiographically, there was a chronic slip with severe medial and posterior tilt of the epiphysis. The sub-capital growth plate was still visible, but the width was reduced. The neck was additionally bent into some varus. The curvature of the acetabular roof was slightly flattened. Computer tomography or MRI were not available. (**b**) Intraoperative picture before reducing the head into the socket, showing the reduced epiphysis provisionally held in place with one Kirschner wire. (**c**) Anteroposterior and lateral view of the hip 10 weeks after surgery. The head is perfectly reduced into the acetabular socket. The neck osteotomy shows signs of healing and the trochanter is consolidated. (**d**) Follow-up series 3 and 10 years after surgery. There are no signs of necrosis of the femoral head. The joint space remains large and congruent over the years

the pelvis showed bilateral slight coxa valga with a large and high positioned fovea corresponding in part with the load bearing area of the acetabulum. The head coverage was borderline normal. Lateral radiography showed markedly reduced anterior head–neck waist.

Regarding treatment, PAO could improve coverage and would unload the fovea. However, in the presence of a horizontal roof, the correction would be achieved for the price of a negative roof angle. The abduction view helped to decide for surgery of the femur only, simply because the relation between acetabulum and head showed a normalized morphological appearance. Since the right hip was free of symptoms, surgery of this hip was unlikely to be necessary. Therefore, shortening of the left leg should be kept as small as possible. Consequently, the preferred level of correction was the femoral neck.

Surgery was executed in lateral decubitus. Dislocation of the hip followed the technique as described above in details [14]. For a femoral neck varus osteotomy, the greater trochanter was separated with a flat osteotomy. Dislocation of the joint was easy after cutting of the rather strong and flat ligamentum teres. The fovea capitis was larger than normal and localized higher on the head than normal. On the acetabular side the labrum was somewhat flattened along the anterior circumference. Th anterior head–neck junction had no waist, as it was expected from clinical and radiological findings (Fig. 15.11b). Dissection of the lateral and medial retinaculum was combined with molding of the anterior neck for a sufficient waist. No special treatment was necessary for the labrum. The neck osteotomy was conceived as a half diameter closed wedge osteotomy while the half wedge was inserted in the lateral gap. The achieved varus was about 15°. Fixation was with two 4.5 cortical screws. Ongoing perfusion of the heads fragment was controlled with bleeding from 2 mm drill holes in the head. After joint reduction impingement free hip motion was tested. After readaptation of the capsule, the greater trochanter was refixed with slight advancement.

Cornerstone of the aftertreatment was toe touch walking on two crutches. Active training of the abductor musculature started at 4 weeks and was increased after the 6 weeks radiography. Weight bearing was increased at 8 weeks. Full and unprotected weight bearing started at 3 months after surgery.

At latest telephone contact, 8 years after surgery, the patient is happy with the result. Leg length difference of 1 centimeter is neglected. Most important for her is that mountaineering is possible again without restrictions.

15.3.5 Case 5

A 12-year-old boy with slight overweight started having left hip pain when he was 6 years old. Soon after he was limping and refused to walk longer distances. First radiography was taken when he was seven (Fig. 15.12a). The a-p and lateral views showed already advanced flattening of the epiphysis, characteristic of Perthes disease. The boy was treated with a Thomas splint for 1 year and used crutches since, albeit inconsistently. The missing success finally forced the parents to look for surgical solutions.

Clinical examination revealed marked limping. When sparing himself, pain was minimal. The leg was spontaneously held in neutral position and was about 1.5 cm short. Marked muscle atrophy, especially around the thigh. ROM was limited, mainly for abduction and internal rotation; pain increased toward the end positions. The radiographic course over 5 years shows the process of epiphyseal flattening, extrusion and subluxation but also the amount of re-ossification in the area of the necrotic lateral pillar. It also

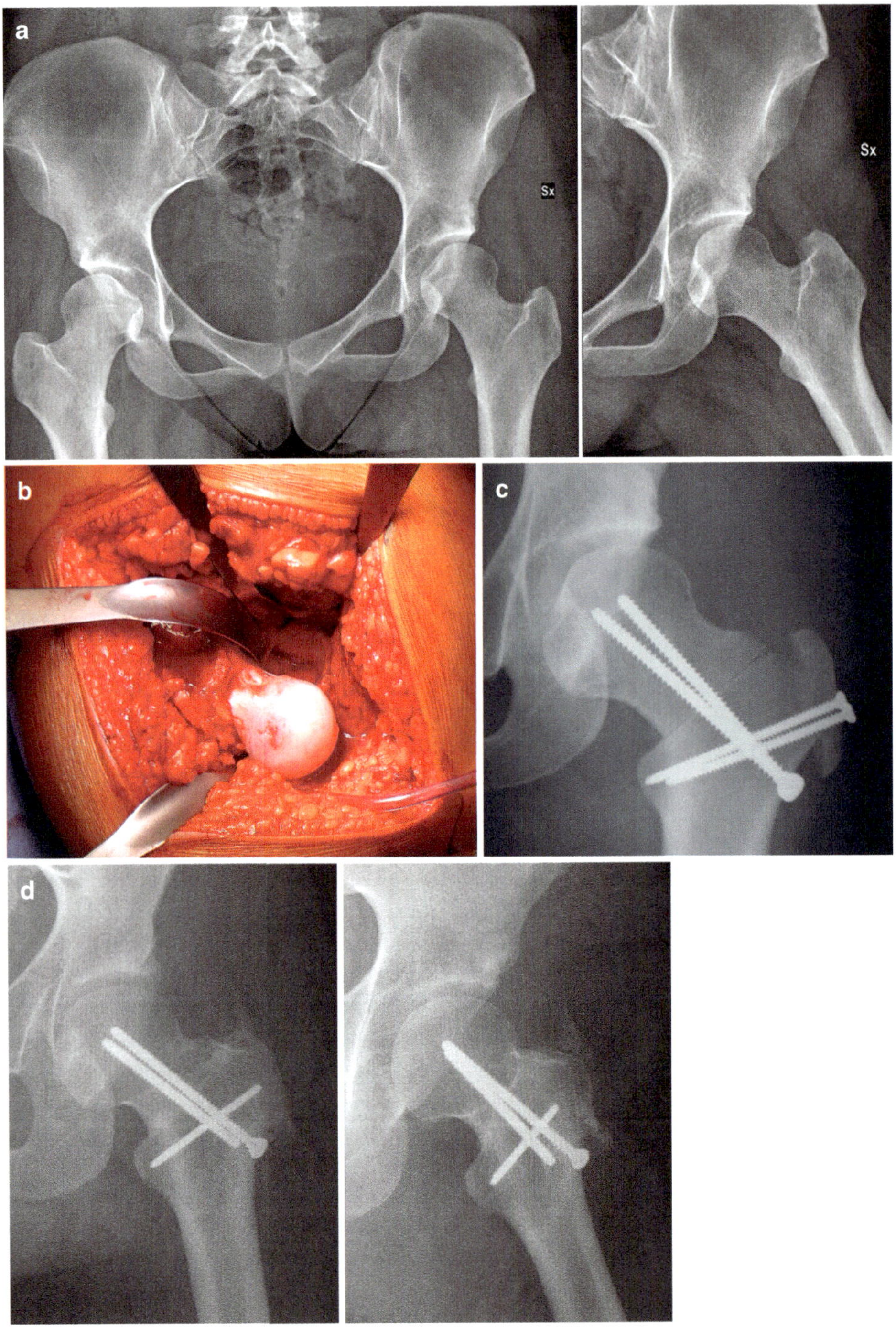

Fig. 15.11 (**a**) (Left) Radiography of the pelvis with moderate symmetrical coxa valga and high fovea capitis, corresponding with a substantial part of the acetabular weight bearing zone. Moderate acetabular dysplasia with horizontal roof and normal version. (Right). Abduction view of the left hip demonstrates improved femoroacetabular relation with a wide and congruent joint space. (**b**) Intraoperative picture with dislocated head, showing the flat anterior head–neck junction. Careful carving of a waist is necessary. (**c**) Radiography at 3 months showing advanced consolidation of the osteotomies. (**d**) Anteroposterior and lateral view 7 years after surgery. One year before, trochanteric pain disappeared completely after partial screw removal. The joint looks perfect. No signs of necrosis of the femoral head

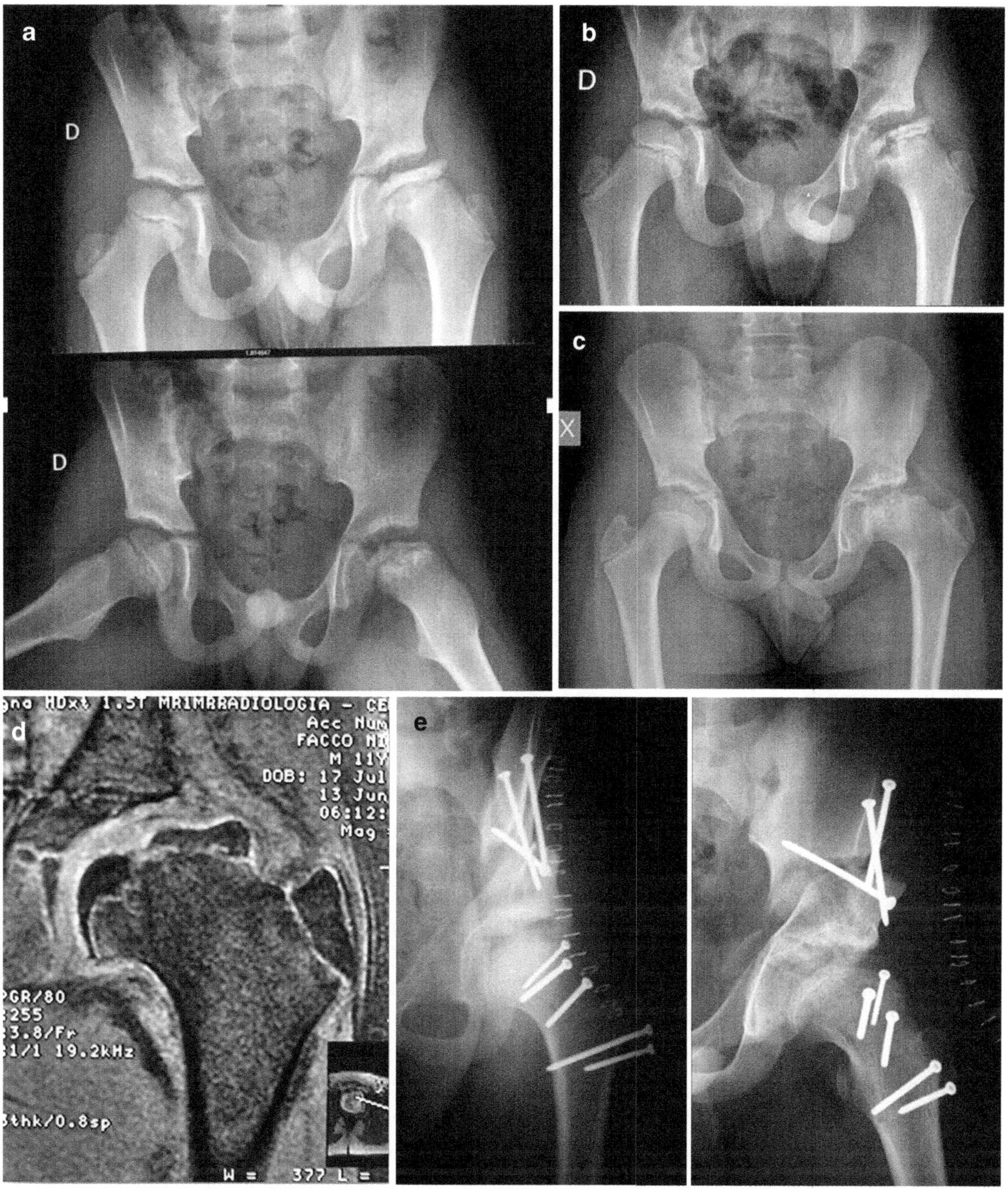

Fig. 15.12 (**a**) Perthes disease at the age of 7. Subtotal Involvement, slight subluxation. (**b**) At the age of 10 signs of re-ossification of the necrosis. (**c**) At age 12 visible acetabular adaptation to the deformed head. (**d**) MRI at 12 years showing re-ossification of the flattened and extruded lateral pillar. The osseous roof is losing its former concavity. (**e**) Postoperative X-rays after head reduction osteotomy and PAO. Good recentering of the head in the ap view. (**f**) 6 years result with large and congruent joint space, although the "new" head is not perfectly round. No signs of necrosis

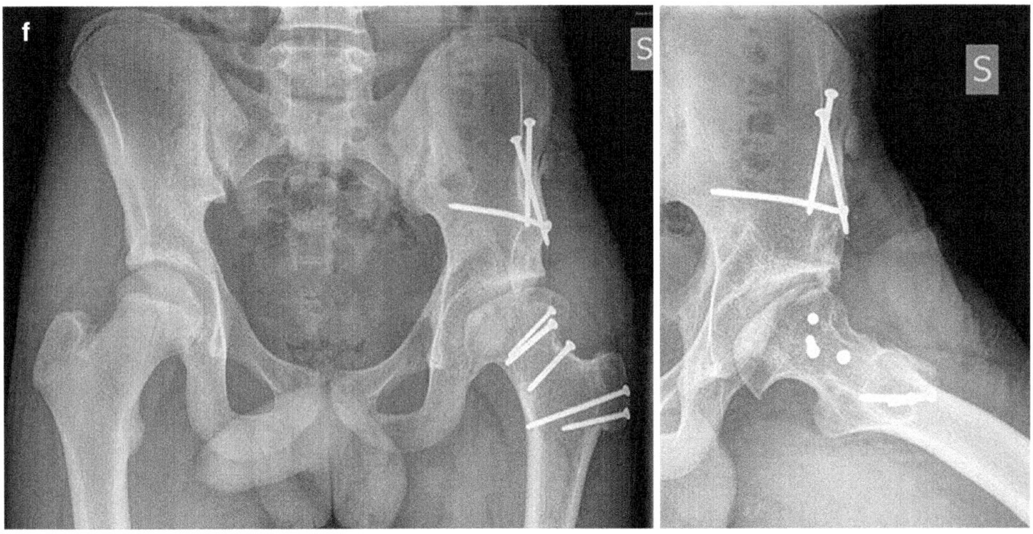

Fig. 15.12 (continued)

shows the adaptive flattening of the acetabular roof, indicative of chronic hinged abduction.

In the presence of markedly flattened and extruded head ruling out free abduction, an isolated varus-type femoral osteotomy would hardly lead to improved containment. An isolated acetabular reorientation would run a similar risk. Reduction of the head size by resecting a middle portion (see Fig. 15.7) is a more recent solution for such problems. However, the smaller "new" head may not find a stable position within the flattened acetabulum, reason why in the majority of such cases an additional PAO is recommended.

The surgical steps followed the description above. Simulation and cutting templates [28] were not yet available at the time of this surgery. The procedure started with the femoral part in lateral decubitus. Preparation of the skin and draping was done in a way to allow to change position for the acetabular surgery without re-draping.

The femoral approach was used to perform the first ischial cut of the PAO before dislocating the joint. In this early phase of the surgery blood impregnation of the tissues is minimal allowing easy preparation of the gap to the ischium between gemellus inferior and obturator externus muscles. This gap is not interfering with the deep branch of the MFCA and allows manual protection of the sciatic nerve. Furthermore, this approach to the ischium allows broad incision of the strong periosteum over the cut area.

Next step was dislocation of the joint followed by the dissection of the lateral retinaculum. The medial retinaculum and Weitbrecht's ligament were not dissected in this type of surgery. Most delicate decision making was about the size and shape of the part to be cutoff, a process which more recently became easier with computer simulation. The goal was to achieve a smaller head with optimal sphericity.

While the remaining mobile segment has its vascular pedicle via the lateral retinaculum, the stable medial segment is nourished by the medial branch of the MFCA running on top of Weitbrecht's ligament. For fixation 3 small screws were sufficient. After relocation of the "new" head and careful ROM testing, closure of the approach started with refixation of the greater trochanter, slightly distal to the original position.

After closure of the skin, the patient was turned into supine position for execution of the PAO. The approach was as described above, with the difference that the first ischial cut was already executed. Careful dissection of the strong periosteum was done for optimal displacement in the osteotomized pubis. Complete osteotomy of the retro-acetabular cut facilitated mobilization of the fragment. This step was controlled with fluoroscopy. Reorientation of the acetabular fragment was not attempted before complete mobilization, because the bone of the diseased hip was rather soft and Schanz' screws may break out of the bone easily. Version was controlled by fluoroscopy with a thin K-wire placed along the anterior labrum. Fixation was similar to fixation of the adult acetabulum.

Aftertreatment during the first 4 weeks comprised toe touch walking with two crutches. After 6 weeks range of motion was increased and abductor training was advised. All osteotomies were sufficiently consolidated after 8 weeks and unrestricted loading was allowed after 3 months.

At follow-up 6 years after surgery, the patient was pain free. His leg length was equal and walking was without limping. ROM was slightly reduced for internal rotation. Abductor force was symmetrical. He was playing soccer in a youth team. Metal removal was recommended. Thereafter the patient was lost to follow-up.

15.3.6 Case 6

9-year-old boy with unilateral congenital coxa vara combined with slight genu valgum. A first attempt to cure the deformity took place at the age of 4 but correction and fixation using Kirschner wires failed. At the age of 7, two cannulated screws were inserted to heal the nonunion, leaving the extreme deformity untouched for a later surgical intervention. The concomitant acetabular dysplasia was also not addressed. At presentation 2 years later, the nonunion was still present. Clinically there was much discomfort mainly due to leg shortening and abductor weakness. Beside a limited abduction, ROM was not reduced. Abductor strength in side position was M 3.

In lateral decubitus, the basically straight skin incision was including the former scar. Damage to abductor and vastus lateralis muscles as well as to the external rotators was minimal. As proposed earlier for combined corrections of acetabulum and femur, the first ischial cut of the PAO was performed via the femoral approach allowing active protection of the sciatic nerve during execution [32]. Preparation of the sciatic nerve would also allow visual and manual control of the nerve tension during the massive valgus correction resulting in an expected leg lengthening of about 2 cm.

After L-shaped anterior mobilization of the vastus, the screw heads and washers could easily be identified and removed. No attempt was made to find the hidden broken wire from the first surgery. Under fluoroscopic control, the hole for the second screw of the T-plate was drilled parallel to a Kirschner wire placed in the hole of the former proximal screw.

After definitive closure of the approach, the patient was turned back into supine position to complete the PAO using the modified Smith Petersen approach [7, 8]. Since the first ischial cut was already executed via the femoral approach, there was no need to open the gap between capsule and iliopsoas to reach the ischium from anterior. Special care was taken to separate the periosteum at the osteotomy levels, which finally allowed easy manipulation of the acetabulum without much force to be exerted on the Schanz' screw. The acetabular reorientation added up to a sufficient coverage of the femoral head.

Overall surgery time for both procedures was 4:05 h (2:15 and 1:15). Function of the sciatic nerve was regularly controlled during the first 3 days after surgery. Two units of blood had to be given on day two. Stay in hospital was 12 days and time on crutches reached 5 months.

At the age of 15.5 years, hip parameters are within normal ranges (Fig. 15.13h) Compared with the preoperative acetabular morphology, the shape of the inner contour did not change, the medial osseous bottom did not enlarge and there was also no acetabular retroversion, all morphological changes typical for an essential damage of the ischial part of the growth plate [9, 10].

The hip is pain free, ROM, and abductor force are nearly symmetrical. Leg length difference is 2 cm; with a shoe race of 1.5 cm the gait pattern is normal. Surgical equalization of leg length is not an option for the patient so far. He lives a normal life with moderate sportive aspirations.

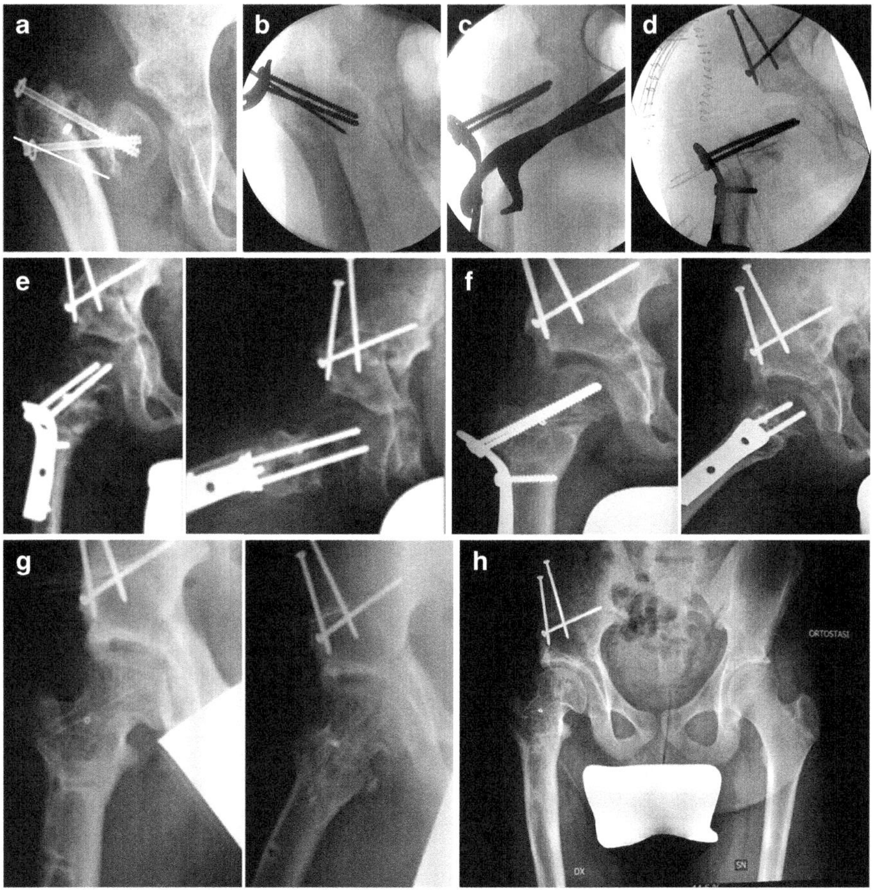

Fig. 15.13 (**a**) Radiologically, the nonunion is now located closer to the shaft and callus formation attached to the head is mimicking a neck. CCD angle is about 50°. The epiphysis is vital and congruent with the dysplastic acetabulum. Wiberg CE angle is slightly negative. It was planned to combine a valgus osteotomy and a correction of the acetabulum in one anesthesia. A screw/T-plate construct, allowing optimal adaptation to the individual possibility of correction [31], was thought to be the best solution for fixation. The proximal screw from last surgery was perfectly aligned with the middle axis through trochanter and head in both planes (see also Fig. 15.13d). Its channel could therefore be used as guide for the implant screws securing the plate in the head–neck fragment. The osteotomy level was planned to start at the distal screw head and should end medially just below the inferior head contour (*continuous white line*). Intraoperative fluoroscopy in adduction showed that the stretch ability of the abductors would allow a valgus correction of more than 60°. Fluoroscopy also showed no tendency for subluxation of the head in this position. Fluoroscopy in maximal abduction showed that it would be critical to achieve sufficient acetabular reorientation before femoral correction. Both information helped for the decision to start the surgery on the femoral side. (**b**) A T-plate for 3.5 mm screws with a 3-hole shaft was bended to allow 60° valgus, which was tested with a provisional application of plate and screws. Next step was to mark the direction of the osteotomy. While it would start on the lateral cortex at the level of the distal screw hole, the medial exit point was determined with a Kirschner wire placed under fluoroscopic control (see also *continuous white line in* Fig. 15.13a). (**c**) After completion of the osteotomy and careful separation of periosteal bridges the pre-bended T-plate was definitively fixed on the proximal fragment by firmly tightening the two screws. Instead of tilting up the proximal fragment, the safer way was to abduct the femur toward the shaft of the plate. The sciatic nerve was under constant visual and manual control. Shortening at the femoral shaft to allow the correction was not necessary. Since fluoroscopy showed suboptimal up-righting of the proximal fragment, the plate was removed again and re-bent to gain another 10–15° correction. Tension of the sciatic nerve was still not excessive as long as the hip was not flexed; it was completely relaxed when the knee was additionally flexed. Anteversion of the neck was controlled with the direction of the screws in the neck. Two screws in the plate shaft gained sufficient purchase in the proximal femur. (**d**) Final fluoroscopy showed sufficient correction with a CCD angle of about 120°. (**e**) The result after 6 weeks shows beginning consolidation of nonunion and osteotomies. (**f**) After 3 years, the triradiate growth plate is still open. At this time plate and screws were removed because the upper edge of the plate was somewhat prominent and painful. The development of the acetabular cavity is uneventful. (**g**) At 5 years, the growth plate is closed but the acetabular cavity remains unchanged showing good containment in both planes. (**h**) At age 15.5 (6.5 years after surgery) the final stage of joint molding is reached

15.4 Conclusion

The patho-morphological diversity of the presented hips shall demonstrate the capacity of modern intra- and juxta-articular surgery to channel further growth toward normal development or to save a young adult hip from discomfort and rapid deterioration. It is longstanding experience, that open growth plates around the hip in patients 10 years old or older is not a contraindication for crossing osteotomies. Key for such surgery is precise knowledge of the vascular supply to hip and pelvis. Careful evaluation before surgery increases the predictability of the result. For precise decision making, imaging includes more than standard radiographies; advanced resonance imaging and/or computer tomography are indispensable tools. Preoperative planning is a must, frequently on the basis of 3D models and with simulation of the individual procedure.

Nevertheless, the definitive decision can be difficult, especially when the anatomic conditions are extreme; other factors like age, expectations as well as the social environment may play an important role. Failure cannot be excluded and possibilities of complications have to be discussed beforehand. Surgical techniques are subject to ongoing improvement; a clear example is the periacetabular osteotomy, which emerged from a rather lengthy procedure to a less invasive and very predictable surgery with little blood loss. Routine is another key element to achieve satisfying results. Routine comes from ongoing training and a sufficient caseload. In other words, such surgery should be performed in specialized centers.

References

1. Ganz R, Klaue K, Vinh TS, Mast JW. A new periacetabular osteotomy for the treatment of hip dysplasias. Technique and preliminary results. Clin Orthop Relat Res. 1988;232:26–36.
2. Beck M, Leunig M, Ellis T, et al. The acetabular blood supply: implications for periacetabular osteotomies. Surg Radiol Anat SRA. 2003;25:361–7. https://doi.org/10.1007/s00276-003-0149-3.
3. Kalhor M, Beck M, Huff TW, Ganz R. Capsular and pericapsular contributions to acetabular and femoral head perfusion. J Bone Joint Surg Am. 2009;91:409–18. https://doi.org/10.2106/JBJS.G.01679.
4. Hempfing A, Leunig M, Nötzli HP, et al. Acetabular blood flow during Bernese periacetabular osteotomy: an intraoperative study using laser doppler flowmetry. J Orthop Res. 2003;21:1145–50. https://doi.org/10.1016/S0736-0266(03)00083-4.
5. Kalhor M, Gharehdaghi J, Leunig M, et al. Surgical anatomy of the rectus sparing approach for PAO. A cadaveric study. JBJS Essential Surgical Techniques; 2021.
6. Wells J, Schoenecker P, Duncan S, et al. Intermediate-term hip survivorship and patient-reported outcomes of periacetabular osteotomy: the Washington University experience. J Bone Joint Surg Am. 2018;100:218–25. https://doi.org/10.2106/JBJS.17.00337.
7. Leunig M, Siebenrock KA, Ganz R. Rationale of periacetabular osteotomy and background work. JBJS. 2001;83:438.
8. Kalhor M, Collado D, Leunig M, et al. Recommendations to reduce risk of nerve injury during bernese periacetabular osteotomy (PAO). JBJS Essent Surg Tech. 2017;7:e34. https://doi.org/10.2106/JBJS.ST.17.00017.
9. MEM MEDIA Foundation. Kursorganisation und Videoproduktion. https://www.memmedia.ch/de/home. Accessed 22 Jan 2021.
10. Trousdale RT, Ganz R. Posttraumatic acetabular dysplasia. Clin Orthop Relat Res. 1994:124–32.
11. Dora C, Zurbach J, Hersche O, Ganz R. Pathomorphologic characteristics of posttraumatic acetabular dysplasia. J Orthop Trauma. 2000;14:483–9. https://doi.org/10.1097/00005131-200009000-00004.
12. Blümel S, Leunig M, Turchetto L, Ganz R. Periacetabular osteotomy before closure of the triradiate acetabular growth plate. In preparation.
13. Gautier E, Ganz K, Krügel N, et al. Anatomy of the medial femoral circumflex artery and its surgical implications. J Bone Joint Surg Br. 2000;82:679–83. https://doi.org/10.1302/0301-620x.82b5.10426.
14. Ganz R, Gill TJ, Gautier E, et al. Surgical dislocation of the adult hip. A technique with full access to the femoral head and acetabulum without the risk of avascular necrosis. J Bone Joint Surg Br. 2001;83:1119–24. https://doi.org/10.1302/0301-620x.83b8.11964.
15. Ganz R, Huff TW, Leunig M. Extended retinacular soft-tissue flap for intra-articular hip surgery: surgical technique, indications, and results of application. Instr Course Lect. 2009;58:241–55.
16. Sink EL, Beaulé PE, Sucato D, et al. Multicenter study of complications following surgical dislocation of the hip. J Bone Joint Surg Am. 2011;93:1132–6. https://doi.org/10.2106/JBJS.J.00794.
17. Beck M, Leunig M, Parvizi J, et al. Anterior femoroacetabular impingement: part II. Midterm results of surgical treatment. Clin Orthop Relat Res. 2004;418:67–73.
18. Ganz R, Parvizi J, Beck M, et al. Femoroacetabular impingement: a cause for osteoarthritis of the hip.

Clin Orthop Relat Res. 2003;417:112–20. https://doi.org/10.1097/01.blo.0000096804.78689.c2.
19. Hasler CC, Morscher EW. Femoral neck lengthening osteotomy after growth disturbance of the proximal femur. J Pediatr Orthop B. 1999;8:271–5.
20. Albers CE, Steppacher SD, Schwab JM, et al. Relative femoral neck lengthening improves pain and hip function in proximal femoral deformities with a high-riding trochanter. Clin Orthop Relat Res. 2015;473:1378–87. https://doi.org/10.1007/s11999-014-4032-9.
21. Dunn DM. The treatment of adolescent slipping of the upper femoral epiphysis. J Bone Joint Surg Br. 1964;46:621–9.
22. Leunig M, Casillas MM, Hamlet M, et al. Slipped capital femoral epiphysis: early mechanical damage to the acetabular cartilage by a prominent femoral metaphysis. Acta Orthop Scand. 2000;71:370–5. https://doi.org/10.1080/000164700317393367.
23. Ziebarth K, Leunig M, Slongo T, et al. Slipped capital femoral epiphysis: relevant pathophysiological findings with open surgery. Clin Orthop Relat Res. 2013;471:2156–62. https://doi.org/10.1007/s11999-013-2818-9.
24. Rego P, Mascarenhas V, Mafra I, et al. Femoral neck osteotomy in skeletally mature patients: surgical technique and midterm results. Int Orthop. 2021;45:83–94. https://doi.org/10.1007/s00264-020-04822-4.
25. Sevitt S, Thompson RG. The distribution and anastomoses of arteries supplying the head and neck of the femur. J Bone Joint Surg Br. 1965;47:560–73.
26. Siebenrock KA, Anwander H, Zurmühle CA, et al. Head reduction osteotomy with additional containment surgery improves sphericity and containment and reduces pain in Legg-Calvé-Perthes disease. Clin Orthop Relat Res. 2015;473:1274–83. https://doi.org/10.1007/s11999-014-4048-1.
27. Clohisy JC, Pascual-Garrido C, Duncan S, et al. Concurrent femoral head reduction and periacetabular osteotomies for the treatment of severe femoral head deformities. Bone Joint J. 2018;100-B:1551–8. https://doi.org/10.1302/0301-620X.100B12.BJJ-2018-0030.R3.
28. Fürnstahl P, Lanfranco S, Leunig M, Ganz R. Computer simulation and jig cutting of femoral head reduction osteotomy in severe Perthes' deformities. Br Editor Soc Bone Joint Surg. 2018:81–1.
29. Ganz R, Slongo T, Turchetto L, et al. The lesser trochanter as a cause of hip impingement: pathophysiology and treatment options. Hip Int. 2013;23(Suppl 9):S35–41. https://doi.org/10.5301/hipint.5000063.
30. Aprato A, Leunig M, Massé A, et al. Instability of the hip after anatomical re-alignment in patients with a slipped capital femoral epiphysis. Bone Joint J. 2017;99-B:16–21. https://doi.org/10.1302/0301-620X.99B1.BJJ-2016-0575.
31. Elzohairy MM, Khairy HM. Fixation of intertrochanteric valgus osteotomy with T plate in treatment of developmental coxa vara. Clin Orthop Surg. 2016;8:310–5. https://doi.org/10.4055/cios.2016.8.3.310.
32. Ganz R, Horowitz K, Leunig M. Algorithm for femoral and periacetabular osteotomies in complex hip deformities. Clin Orthop Relat Res. 2010;468:3168–80. https://doi.org/10.1007/s11999-010-1489-z.

GPSR Compliance

The European Union's (EU) General Product Safety Regulation (GPSR) is a set of rules that requires consumer products to be safe and our obligations to ensure this.

If you have any concerns about our products, you can contact us on ProductSafety@springernature.com

In case Publisher is established outside the EU, the EU authorized representative is:

Springer Nature Customer Service Center GmbH
Europaplatz 3
69115 Heidelberg, Germany

Batch number: 09699300

Printed by Printforce, the Netherlands